AF382865

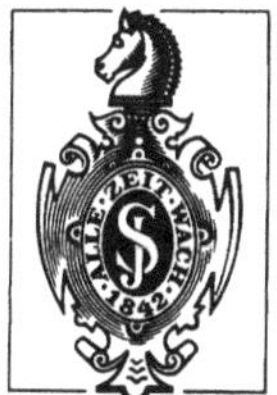
ALLE·ZEIT·WACH·
S
1842

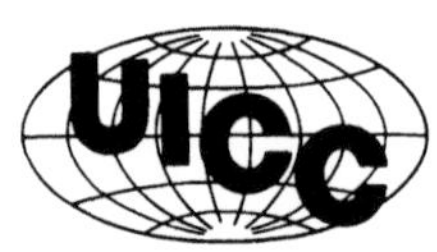 International Union Against Cancer

---

The series *Current Treatment of Cancer* consists of the following volumes:

Cancer in Children, 2nd edition (1986)

Hematologic Malignancies (1986)

Lung Tumors (1988)

Breast Cancer

Gynecological Tumours

Urogenital Tumours

Cancer of the Digestive Tract

Skin, Soft Tissue and Bone Tumours

Head and Neck Tumours

Tumours of the Nervous System

General Principles of Oncology

Lung Tumors

Lung, Mediastinum, Pleura, and Chest Wall

Edited by
B. Hoogstraten   B. J. Addis   H. H. Hansen
N. Martini   S. G. Spiro

With Contributions by

B. J. Addis   M. S. Bains   M. E. Burt   P. Goldstraw
H. H. Hansen   F. R. Hirsch   M. E. Hodson   L. R. Kaiser
N. Martini   P. M. McCormack   A. H. Pomerantz
M. Rørth   R. Souhami   S. G. Spiro   J. S. Tobias
T. Treasure   J. R. Yarnold

With 100 Figures

Springer-Verlag Berlin Heidelberg New York
London Paris Tokyo

UICC, Rue du Conseil-Général 3, CH-1205 Geneva

Editors:

Barth Hoogstraten
Medical Director Cancer Treatment Center
Bethesda Hospital, Inc.
629 Oak Street, Suite 409
Cincinnati, OH 45206, USA

Bruce J. Addis
Brompton Hospital
Cardiothoracic Institute, Fulham Road
London SW3 6HP, United Kingdom

Heine H. Hansen
Department of Oncology ONB
Finsen Institute, 49, Strandboulevarden
2100 Copenhagen, Denmark

Nael Martini
Thoracic Service
Department of Surgery
Memorial Sloan-Kettering
Cancer Center
1275 York Avenue
New York, NY 10021, USA

Stephen G. Spiro
Brompton Hospital
Fulham Road
London SW3 6HP
United Kingdom

ISBN-13: 978-3-540-16920-8   e-ISBN-13: 978-3-642-82873-7

DOI: 10.1007/978-3-642-82873-7

Library of Congress Cataloging-in-Publication Data
Lung tumors : lung, mediastinum, pleura, and chest wall / edited by B. Hoogstraten . . . [et al.] ;
with contributions by B.J.Addis . . . [et al.].
p. cm. – (Current treatment of cancer) "International Union against Cancer" – P. facing t.p.
Includes bibliographies and index.

1. Lungs - Tumors. 2. Respiratory organs - Tumors. I. Hoogstraten, Barth. II. Addis, B.J. (Bruce J.)
III. International Union against Cancer.
[DNLM: 1. Lung Neoplasms - therapy. 2. Mediastinal Neoplasms - therapy. 3. Pleural
Neoplasms - therapy. WF 658 L9644] RC280.L8L87 1988 616.99'224 - dc19 DNLM/DLC
for Library of Congress 87-37639 CIP

Typesetting and bookbinding: Appl, Wemding; printing: aprinta, Wemding
2121/3140-543210

Members of the UICC Current Treatment of Cancer Project Committee

Charles M. Balch
M. D. Anderson Hospital
and Tumor Institute
6723 Bertner Avenue
Houston, TX 77030, USA

H. Julian G. Bloom
23 Raymond Road
Wimbledon
London SW19 4AD
United Kingdom

Ian Burn
British Association
of Surgical Oncology
Charing Cross Hospital
Fulham Palace Road
London W6 8RF
United Kingdom

Jerzy Einhorn
Karolinska Sjukhuset
Radiumhemmet
10401 Stockholm, Sweden

Ismail Elsebai (Chairman)
National Cancer Institute Cairo
Kasr El-Aini Street
Cairo, Egypt

Barth Hoogstraten
Cancer Treatment Center
Bethesda Hospital, Inc.
629 Oak Street, Suite 409
Cincinnati, OH 45206, USA

Herbert M. Pinedo
Free University of Amsterdam
De Boelelaan 1117
Amsterdam, The Netherlands

Foreword

This series on the treatment of cancer is sponsored by the UICC. The editors and authors feel strongly that more standardization in cancer therapy is needed on a worldwide basis. This, of course, is only possible if experts from all countries subscribe to a joint policy of making their treatment designs available to practising oncologists all over the world.

Current Treatment of Cancer discusses all the equipment and methods now in use in cancer therapy. It covers all types of cancer, thus providing the reader with comprehensive information on cancer management.

In recent decades there has been a tremendous improvement in the treatment of cancer, and there is hope for even further success in this fight. We are convinced that this series will help us to make a concerted response to the challenge of cancer.

UICC
Treatment and Rehabilitation Programme
Ismail Elsebai
Chairman

Preface

Part I

Members of two institutions, the Brompton Hospital in London and the Finsen Institute in Copenhagen, were invited to write on lung cancer, and after reading the manuscripts it was decided that the contents of three pairs of chapters overlapped sufficiently for them to be combined. Spiro and Hansen are thus co-authors of a chapter on early detection and screening, as well as of one on diagnostic procedures. Spiro and Rørth also combine their efforts in the discussion of clinical features. The excellent chapters by Addis on the pathology of lung cancer and by Hirsch on the histopathology complement each other.

The authors are in agreement on the treatment on non-small-cell lung cancer (NSCLC). At present there is no evidence that adjuvant chemotherapy has any influence on survival and it should not be used except as part of a study. In patients with advanced disease, a comparison of supportive treatment only with supportive care plus chemotherapy has shown no difference in median survival times. Surgery continues to be the main mode of treatment. At the Brompton Hospital, Goldstraw stresses very detailed preoperative assessment of the patients and careful preparation prior to surgery. Haste is definitely not called for in patients with lung cancer, and pulmonary function studies are absolute necessities. Both British and American surgeons favor pneumonectomy or lobectomy, and reserve segmentectomy or wedge resections only for the physiologically compromised patient. The latter two procedures do not constitute adequate operative treatment. About half of the NSCLC patients present with N_2M_0 disease and when the contralateral lymph nodes are involved none of the institutions consider the patient a surgical candidate. Only when ipsilateral nodes appear to be involved will a complete resection with lobectomy or pneumonectomy plus dissection of mediastinal nodes be attempted. This is possible in approximately 20% of cases with N_2 disease and results in 30% 5-year survival. Postoperative radiation to the mediastinum and tumor bed may be of benefit.

The role of radiation therapy is limited, and in the opinion expressed by the members of the three institutions there is no place for radiation therapy if the resection is complete. A combination of surgery and curative radiotherapy is recommended for the following disease presentations:

1. Residual disease after resection
2. All N_2 disease undergoing complete resection
3. Superior sulcus tumor

For the latter tumor, the MSKCC recommends 4000 rad preoperative external radiation, followed by complete resection. This, however, is possible in only 20%-30% of the patients. When feasible, the MSKCC suggests including intraoperative implantation of radioisotopes in visible tumor that is not resected, and then adding further postoperative external radiotherapy.

Chemotherapy is at present the first treatment of choice for small-cell lung cancer (SCLC). Hansen and his colleagues at the Finsen Institute have long been in the forefront of the management of this disease, as has Spiro at the Brompton Hospital. At both institutions, the two drugs most frequently used in combinations of agents are cyclophosphamide (Cytoxan) and doxorubicin (Adriamycin), with vincristine and etoposide (VP-16) added as a third or alternative choice. Drs. Hansen and Spiro tend to be less aggressive than American investigators when it comes to drug doses and surprisingly, cisplatin is mentioned in neither chapter. The median survival times of 709 patients with SCLC seen in Copenhagen during 1973-1981 are disappointing, 11 months and 7 months respectively, for limited and extensive disease. At Brompton, these figures are 15 and 9 months.

In the United States, the doses of drugs for the most frequently used combination are usually as follows:

CAV - (Cyclophosphamide, 1000 mg/m^2; Adriamycin 50 mg/m^2; Vincristine 1.4 mg/m^2).
Etoposide (60 mg/m^2 for 5 days) can be added to this combination.

The role of cisplatin has been emphasized by Einhorn, who combined it with etoposide because it proved to be a highly synergistic combination in many animal models. A frequently used course consists of cisplatin (60 mg/m^2) on days 1 and 22 plus etoposide (120 mg/m^2) on days 4, 6, 8, 25, 27, and 29. Studies from the Finsen Institute have shown that another epidophyllotoxin, teniposide (VM-26), may be at least as active as etoposide and deserves further investigation. Using the Goldie-Coldman hypothesis, several oncologists are now alternating CAV with cisplatin plus etoposide. The reader may be recommended to read the proceedings of a 1986 symposium on the treatment of lung cancer (*Seminars in Oncology* 13, suppl. 3). On pages 83-86, Natale, McCracken, T. Evans, Greco, Bunn, Aisner, Murray, W. Evans, and Einhorn, representing nine different cooperative groups or institutions, each outlined how they would treat a new patient with limited SCLC and a new patient with extensive SCLC cancer, both off protocol. Seven of the nine said they would give cisplatin/etoposide and chest radiation for limited disease, and seven of the nine selected CAV alternating with platinum/etoposide in extensive disease.

X

Part II

In this part, Addis gives an impressive description of the numerous tumors to be found in the mediastinal structures and in the chest wall. In the thymus alone, he differentiates 10 malignancies on cytological and histological grounds. The excellent photographs should be of great assistance to the pathologist and the clinician. The signs and symptoms of these tumors vary greatly, and Treasure emphasizes the need for a careful diagnostic investigation and attempts at biopsy before an operation is planned.

Malignant mesothelioma presents very much as a separate entity with which Hodson, working with Law, has extensive experience. Unfortunately, we still have no effective treatment for this tumor, and oncologists are well advised to avoid extensive surgery or radiotherapy. A sporadic response to an anthracycline has been observed, but otherwise chemotherapy remains experimental.

Tobias puts emphasis on the "mantle" technique for patients with mediastinal Hodgkin's disease and gives detailed guidelines for the use of radiotherapy for chest-wall and pleural tumors. He stresses the need for interaction with the surgeon, and discusses tumor radiosensitivity, disadvantages of radiotherapy, and alternative treatment. Histology in large part dictates the chemotherapy which can be given, since the drug regimens do not change from those used for tumors with the same histology but located in other parts of the body.

A fourth revision of the TNM classification was published, while production of this volume was already in progress. (TNM Classification of Malignant Tumours, 4th edn, Springer-Verlag, Heidelberg 1987). In this latest revision, the surgical staging (sTNM) has been eliminated and combined into the clinical or cTNM. This cTNM (pretreatment clinical classification) is based on evidence acquired before treatment. Surgical exploration is not regarded as therapy. The pathological classification, designated pTNM, entails resection of the primary tumor or biopsy adequate to evaluate the highest pT category. The reader is encouraged to use the revised system where appropriate.

Barth Hoogstraten

Contents

Part I. Lung Tumors

12. Treatment at Brompton Hospital and Royal Marsden Hospital . . 133

P. Goldstraw, S. G. Spiro, and J. R. Yarnold

13. Prognosis and End Results 163

S. G. Spiro

Part II. Tumors of the Mediastinum, Pleura, and Chest Wall

14. Pathology of Mediastinal Tumors 169

B. J. Addis

Contributors

Bruce J. Addis
Brompton Hospital
Cardiothoracic Institute
Fulham Road
London SW3 6HP
United Kingdom

Manjit S. Bains
Thoracic Service
Department of Surgery
Memorial Sloan-Kettering Cancer
Center
1275 York Avenue
New York, NY 10021
USA

Michael E. Burt
Thoracic Service
Department of Surgery
Memorial Sloan-Kettering Cancer
Center
1275 York Avenue
New York, NY 10021
USA

Peter Goldstraw
Brompton Hospital
Fulham Road
London SW3 6HP
United Kingdom

Heine H. Hansen
Department of Oncology ONB
Finsen Institute
49, Strandboulevarden
2100 Copenhagen
Denmark

Fred R. Hirsch
Department of Oncology ONB
Finsen Institute
49, Strandboulevarden
2100 Copenhagen
Denmark

Margaret E. Hodson
Brompton Hospital
Cardiothoracic Institute
Fulham Road
London SW3 6HP
United Kingdom

Larry R. Kaiser
Thoracic Service
Department of Surgery
Memorial Sloan-Kettering Cancer
Center
1275 York Avenue
New York, NY 10021
USA

Nael Martini
Thoracic Service
Department of Surgery
Memorial Sloan-Kettering Cancer
Center
1275 York Avenue
New York, NY 10021
USA

Patricia M. McCormack
Thoracic Service
Department of Surgery
Memorial Sloan-Kettering Cancer
Center
1275 York Avenue
New York, NY 10021
USA

Arthur H. Pomerantz
Thoracic Service
Department of Surgery
Memorial Sloan-Kettering Cancer
Center
1275 York Avenue
New York, NY 10021
USA

Mikael Rørth
Department of Oncology ONB
Finsen Institute
49, Strandboulevarden
2100 Copenhagen
Denmark

Robert Souhami
University College Hospital
London WC1
United Kingdom

Stephen G. Spiro
Brompton Hospital
Fulham Road
London SW3 6HP
United Kingdom

Jeffrey S. Tobias
University College Hospital
London WC1
United Kingdom

Tom Treasure
The Middlesex Hospital
Mortimer Street
London WIN 8AA
United Kingdom

John R. Yarnold
The Royal Marsden Hospital
Downs Road
Sutton
Surrey SM2 5PT
United Kingdom

Part I

Lung Tumors

1. Epidemiology

S. G. Spiro

Introduction

Carcinoma of the bronchus is the commonest cancer in the Western world among men, while in women only cancers of the breast, large bowel, and skin have a higher incidence. Since lung cancer is predominantly caused by smoking, future trends in the disease will be largely determined by what happens to smoking habits over the next few decades. There are, however, a number of other factors involved in the pathogenesis of lung cancer and examination of the epidemiological data for the past 30 years suggests that some changes can be expected independently of changes in smoking habits.

In both the United Kingdom and the United States deaths from lung cancer have been increasing steadily since the 1930s in line with increases in cigarette smoking (Figs. 1, 2). Despite improvements in treatment the fatality rate remains high – with 35 000 deaths a year currently in England and Wales. Four-fifths of the

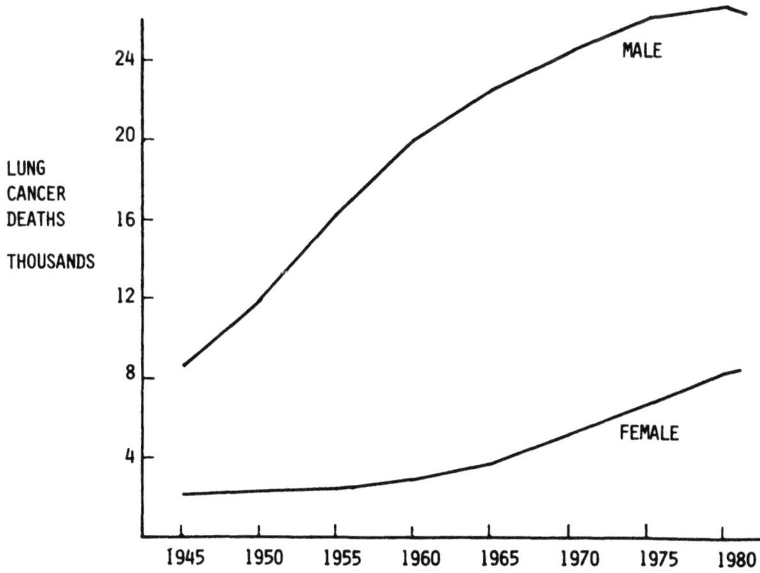

Fig. 1. Increase in lung cancer deaths since 1945 in men and women in England and Wales

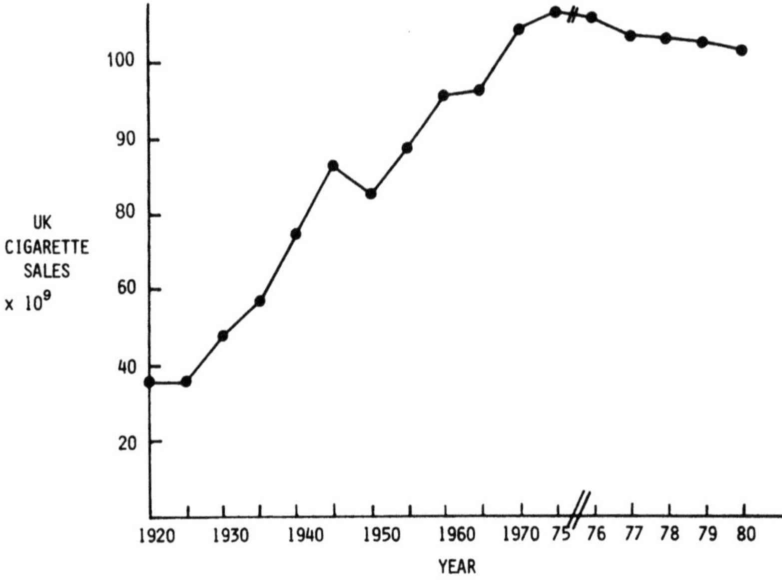

Fig. 2. Cigarette sales in millions in the United Kingdom since 1920

deaths occur in men. There has been an epidemic of lung cancer in the western world over the course of this century. Recently, however, deaths in men have stabilized and are now beginning to fall while deaths in women are continuing to increase. The increase in women is entirely consistent with the increase in popularity of smoking among women since the Second World War, but the changes in men are more difficult to explain. The decline in male mortality is earlier than might have been expected from changes in smoking habits and more detailed analysis shows that age-specific mortality rates are continuing to increase in older age groups and falling in men under 60 years. Again smoking habits alone are an insufficient explanation.

Etiologic Considerations

An analysis of the geographical distribution of lung cancer (Table 1) helps to provide clues about factors other than smoking which may be responsible. In the first place different countries have very widely different mortality rates even when smoking habits are taken into account. For example, the United Kingdom and Germany fare much worse than France and Italy. Although differences in tobacco and smoking techniques may play some part, it seems likely that heavy industry and coal burning have also been important. Secondly, analysis by county in the United States shows an association between lung cancer deaths and counties with chemical, petroleum, ship building, and paper industries. Furthermore, detailed

4

Table 1. Age-adjusted incidence of lung cancer per
100000 population for the ten countries with the greatest world incidence. (Silverberg and Luben 1983)

Country	Men	Women
1. Scotland	83.9	17.1
2. England and Wales	73.7	14.8
3. Netherlands	70.6	4.4
4. Belgium	69.5	5.6
5. Czecheslovakia	66.4	5.5
6. Finland	64.4	4.2
7. Luxembourg	54.1	3.8
8. Northern Ireland	53.0	11.0
9. Austria	51.8	7.0
10. United States	51.2	12.2

Table 2. Industrial products and processes known to cause or suspected of causing lung cancer

Known causes
Nickel refining

    Underground hematite mining (with exposure to radon)
    Arsenic and arsenic compounds
    Asbestos
    Bis(chloromethyl)ether and technical grade chloromethyl methyl ether
    Chromium and certain chromium compounds
    Mustard gas
    Soots, tars, and oils

Suspected causes
    Acrylonitrile
    Beryllium and beryllium compounds
    Dimethyl sulfate

studies of specific occupational pollutants also give a clear message. For example, asbestos exposure acts in synergy with cigarette smoking to contribute to an increased lung cancer risk: individuals with dual exposure have an 80- to 90-fold increased risk as compared with a 10- to 20-fold increase in those exposed to cigarettes alone. All the available data point to a conclusion that industrial and environmental pollution are important risk factors for the development of lung cancer. They probably contribute little to the risk in isolation but exert a powerful effect in determining which smoker will develop lung cancer and which will not. A list of industrial products and processes which are known or suspected to cause bronchial carcinoma is given in Table 2. In terms of the number of cases produced asbestos is the most important and may account for as many as 5% of deaths from lung cancer in the United States. Apart from hematite mining the hazards are all more prevalent in industrial towns and cities than in the rural areas and so contribute to the urban-rural gradient in existence.

The increasing awareness of the importance of environmental and industrial pollution has led to legislation to ensure cleaner air. As a result both environmental and occupational atmospheric pollution have fallen dramatically in the past 30 years and this fall has preceded any change in smoking habits. When differences in age and sex are taken into account the mortality from lung cancer in conurbations of England and Wales is 1.5 times that in rural districts. A similar excess of mortality in urban areas has been observed in the United States. Urban air contains several known lung carcinogens including asbestos and arsenic as well as polycyclic aromatic hydrocarbons from the incomplete combustion of fossil fuel; but the importance of these pollutants is difficult to establish because the exposure of individuals cannot be reliably estimated. It follows, however, that there is a cohort of people passing through the population who have both smoked and also breathed polluted air for many years. These people have a very greatly increased risk of lung cancer but with today's cleaner air the younger smoker will have a lower risk. This would account for the clustering of cases in the older population and the falling age-specific death rates in the under 60s.

There are two main conclusions from all this evidence. First, as the at risk cohort ages and dies the death rates from lung cancer may begin to fall sooner and faster than might be expected from smoking habits alone. Secondly, countries where smoking is now becoming widespread can expect a dramatic increase in lung cancer but this may be in part mitigated if attention is paid to pollution as well as to smoking.

Trends in Tobacco Consumption

Antismoking propaganda has built up during the past decades in the United Kingdom and United States. As a result, the general population and politicians in Western countries have become aware of the health risks of smoking, and measures have been taken to restrict advertising and to increase the cost of tobacco products. These measures, together with the direct impact of the antismoking propaganda, have led to changes in tobacco consumption in these two countries. While overall consumption increased steadily from 1900 to 1970 it has stabilized since then and is now falling. Many smokers have switched from cigarettes to other "safer" tobacco products and the trend is best seen in the decline in cigarette sales since 1975 (Fig.3). Furthermore the proportion of the population who are regular smokers has been falling steadily in men since 1972, and has become stable in women. Also, wide differences in smoking habits between social classes have developed, with 57% of male unskilled manual workers smoking as compared with only 21% of male professional workers (Table 3).

It is likely that these trends will continue and that the rate at which people give up smoking may very well increase. If this happens we can predict a steady reduction in deaths from lung cancer during the next few decades in the Western world and this will happen first in the higher socioeconomic groups. The risk of the disease, however, remains high for many years after stopping smoking. For example, the 16-fold risk in a current smoker falls to about 5-fold after 10 years, and only approaches the nonsmoker's risk after 15 years. Changes in lung cancer deaths will, therefore, lag behind changes in smoking by at least a decade.

6

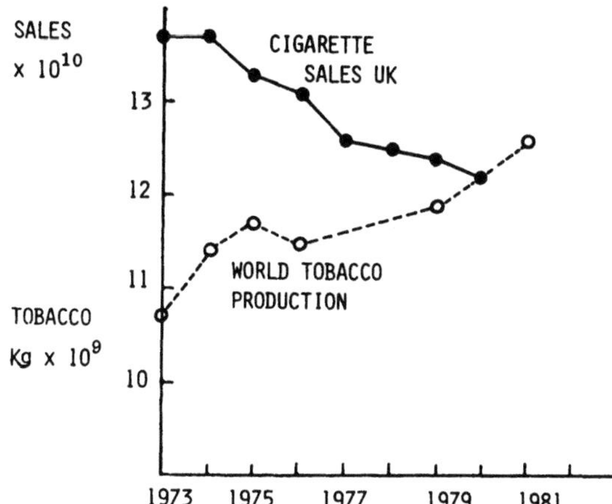

Fig. 3. Cigarette sales in the United Kingdom compared with world tobacco production in the past 10 years

Table 3. Cigarette smoking by social class in Britain

Class	Males (%)		Females (%)	
	1972	1980	1972	1980
A	33	21	33	21
B	44	35	38	33
C	45	35	38	34
D	57	49	42	39
E	64	57	42	41
ALL	52	42	42	37

As the death rates begin to fall the distribution of histological types may also change. This is because different tumors grow at different speeds and so the more rapidly growing small cell lung cancer grows to a size which causes symptoms more quickly than the slow-growing squamous or adenocarcinoma. If all smokers, therefore, were to stop today, one might predict that small cell cancer would diminish in frequency before the other histological types. Such predictions, however, depend upon major changes in smoking habits that will certainly not be realized during this century. In the developing world the picture is precisely the opposite. Reliable figures on smoking habits and tobacco consumption are not available, but estimates have been made and suggest a rapid increase in smoking in the Third World. Probably the simplest dependable way of predicting long-term trends in lung cancer throughout the world is to look at total tobacco production (Fig. 3). This has continued to increase steadily during the past decade in spite of the reduction in smoking in the developed countries. The increased consumption must therefore be taking place predominantly in the Third World and an impending epidemic of smoking-related diseases in Africa, Asia, and Latin America therefore seems inevitable. The delay between the onset of smoking and the development of a disease is so long that today's politicians need take little blame for tomorrow's catastrophe and, ironically, in the short term the Third World will benefit from an increase in smoking. This is because tobacco is a rich crop which yields money quickly and so gives an immediate advantage to the economies of many developing countries.

The tobacco companies are investing heavily to develop Third World markets and their advertising skills seem to be more than a match for those used by the antismoking lobby. In particular, they are aiming at the younger section of the population and most new smokers tend to be aged between 20 and 40. Thus, while Western countries begin to contain the epidemic and confine the disease to the elderly, it is probable that the new wave of Third World lung cancers will occur in the younger age groups. History is therefore all set to repeat itself.

Passive smoking is now known to be harmful. Both in Greece and in Japan passive smoking by wives has been reported to increase the risk of lung cancer, but these studies have been criticized on statistical grounds. Others have found very little if any increased risk among American nonsmoking women who were married to smokers.

Further Reading

Doll R, Peto R (1976) Mortality in relation to smoking: 20 years observations on male British doctors. Br Med J 2: 1525-1527

Mason TJ, McKay FW, Hoover R, Blot WJ, Fraumeni JF (1975) Atlas of cancer mortality for US counties 1950-1969. US Govt Printing Office, Washington DC

Selikoff IJ, Hammond EC, Churg J (1968) Asbestos exposure, smoking and neoplasia. JAMA 204: 106-112

Trichopoulos D, Kalandidi A, Sparros L, MacMahon B (1981) Lung cancer and passive smoking. Int J Cancer 27: 1-4

2. Early Detection: Screening

S. G. Spiro and H. H. Hansen

From many studies it is quite clear that the prognosis for lung cancer is best if it is detected in a presymptomatic stage. It is therefore natural to conceive that the overall mortality of lung cancer could be diminished through screening of high-risk groups with chest X-rays and/or sputum cytology and/or fiber optic bronchoscopy or by other innovative methods. Through early detection more and more patients could undergo resection and the overall survival-rate improve, and since the population at risk can be clearly defined (e.g. male smokers aged over 45 years), the possibility of screening for early diagnosis and more effective treatment is highly attractive.

In some, but not all studies focusing on this subject, there is a tendency that the cases detected by screening have an improved 5-year survival compared with the average patient. This can, however, easily be explained by a selection factor and it does not *per se* prove that the screening procedure is of any value. Different tumors have selected locations, which give symptoms that might lead the patients to the physicians within a short period. Screening has to be done with an interval of at least some months, and it favors thereby the detection of tumors with a long presymptomatic period, low aggressiveness, and thereby a better long-term prognosis.

Another pitfall in the interpretation of uncontrolled screening evaluation is the *lead time bias,* which causes that the time zero for observations of the course in cases detected by screening is placed earlier in the natural history of the disease. This phenomenon might itself automatically lead to an apparent improvement of the results on a short-term basis. If one considers a very slow growth rate in some lung tumors, 7–10 years observation time may be necessary if the latter pitfall is to be eliminated. In order to test whether or not the screening method is of value, prospective studies are necessary, where the mortality in a screening group and a non-screening group is compared. Certain conditions focusing on the accuracy of the diagnosis of the disease in the population are also important. They include an evaluation of the sensitivity and specificity of the methods, the cost in connection with the screening program, and also possibly negative influences on morbidity and mortality. Important conclusions can be drawn from two comprehensive and well-conducted studies.

The Philadelphia Pulmonary Neoplasm Project

All men aged 45 years or over who came to the Philadelphia Tuberculosis and Health Association for a free chest X-ray were invited to join; 6136 men were enrolled between 1951 and 1955 and were interviewed for occupation and respiratory symptoms and screened with 70-mm chest fluorograms every 6 months for 10 years. Of the participants, 86% were smokers or ex-smokers.

Eighty-four prevalence cases of lung cancer were discovered on the first visit, and 121 incidence cases were diagnosed subsequently. Clearly, only incidence cases can be used to evaluate the benefits of screening.

Compliance was only moderately good, with an average probability of two consecutive 6 monthly attendances of 57%. The interval between detection of a tumor and a prior negative film exceeded 7.5 months in 45% of the incidence cases. Survival in the incidence cases was disappointing; 8% were alive at 5 years and, if those who missed appointments are excluded and only the 6-monthly attenders considered, the 5-year survival was only 12%. These figures are similar to those reported in patients diagnosed in the normal way, and while part of the poor survival may be because treatment was sometimes delayed or refused, in general they provide little support for the value of screening. Only 19 of the 121 incidence cases were considered ideal candidates for surgery (young, localized disease, otherwise well).

The Mayo Lung Project

Men aged over 45 years who were chronic "excessive" smokers were enrolled and randomly allocated to two groups. The control group was asked to attend annually for chest X-ray and sputum cytology, while the "close surveillance group" underwent chest X-ray and sputum cytology every 4 months. Between 1971 and 1976, a total of 11 001 patients were entered and 91 prevalence cases of lung cancer were discovered on the first visit. From 1972 to 1982, 9211 men were followed. Final results are not yet available, but in a report published in 1981 there had been 78 incidence cases in the control group and 109 in the close surveillance group. In the close surveillance group, 81% of the patients were discovered because of a chest X-ray abnormality and so the impact of sputum cytology was small. Survival data are not yet available, but about half of the patients were suitable for "curative" surgery.

These two studies allow the following conclusions:

1. The detection rate of new cases of lung cancer is very low in comparison to the work and expense involved.
2. No benefit in terms of survival has yet been demonstrated.
3. Sputum cytological examination adds little to chest X-rays as a screening technique.

It is very unlikely that these results will lead to widespread screening programmes in the future. At present any prospective screening of at risk subjects cannot be recommended.

Further Reading

Weiss W, Boucot KR, Seidman H (1982) The Philadelphia pulmonary neoplasm research project. Clin Chest Med 3: 243–256
Woolner LB, Fontana RS, Sanderson DR, et al. (1981) Mayo lung project. May Clin Proc 56: 544–547

3. Biology of Lung Cancer

H. H. Hansen, F. R. Hirsch and M. Rørth

Within the past decade, considerable research activity has taken place focusing on the biology of malignant lung tumors. This has provided important knowledge of the patho- and histogenesis of lung cancer and the interrelationship between the various histologic types.

The present review presents a status of the most important aspects of the biological research which in the future might have some clinical implications for the management of lung cancer.

Growth Characteristics

In many ways, lung cancer offers a reasonably good opportunity for cytokinetic studies:

1. It is a common disease.
2. The tumor is often accessible by bronchoscopy, thoracotomy, or sampling of metastatic lesions.
3. The size of the primary tumor can usually be followed by X-ray.

The clinical tumor doubling times of primary lung tumors are listed in Table 1.

The doubling time of adenocarcinoma is significantly longer than that of the other types of lung cancer. Correspondingly, the [^{3}H]-thymidine labeling index appears to be especially low in adenocarcinoma in contrast to the high index for small cell carcinoma (Table 2).

Flow cytometric DNA-analyses of malignant tumors have demonstrated that 70%–90% of the tumors have aneuploid DNA content. Most of the tumors are hyperdiploid, with the majority being hypotetraploid. Although all lung cancers have

Table 1. Clinical tumor doubling time of lung cancer

Histology	No. of patients	Mean doubling time (days)
Squamous cell	102	100
Small cell	65	55
Adenocarcinoma	45	185
Large cell	5	95

Table 2. Labeling indices in lung cancer

Histology	[^{3}H]-thymidine labeling index
Small cell carcinoma	0.24
Large cell carcinoma	0.11
Squamous cell carcinoma	0.08
Adenocarcinoma	0.05

a wide range of aneuploidy and chromosome content, "non-small cell" tumors have a higher percentage of aneuploidy and higher DNA content than small cell tumors.

Chromosomal Studies

Chromosomal banding studies have demonstrated a deletion involving the short arm of chromosome 3 associated with many small cell lung tumors (3p(14-23)). However, the deletion, of 3p has also been demonstrated in some "non-small cell" tumors, and thus this chromosomal abnormality might not be as specific for small cell carcinoma of the lung (SCCL) as thought initially. Whether the defect represents an absolute deletion of 3p or a translocation of 3p material to another chromosome is still unclear. The chromosome defect has been demonstrated in human tumors, cell lines, and also heterotransplants. Future studies are needed to elucidate the role of this abnormality related to the development and biological behavior of the tumor.

In Vitro Clonogenic Assays

Clonogenic assays have been developed to study in vitro growth of tumor cells from lung cancer. The intention of developing this method has primarily been to produce an easily accessible drug-testing system before initiating therapy.

In general, the tumor cells are disaggregated into single cells and suspended in semisolid growth medium overlying a firmer base layer. The tumor "stem" cell then forms colonies, but the colony-forming efficiency varies considerably, depending on the material used. The plating efficiency is highest in specimens from bone marrow and effusions while the rates of tissues from solid tumors are much lower. The overall colony-forming efficiency is low ($p < 0.001\%-0.1\%$/plated cell and 0.1%-1.6%/plated tumor cell), which means that only a small fraction of the tumor cell population is being studied.

The usefulness of the clonogenic assay as a drug-testing system for malignant lung tumors is still under investigation. Preliminary studies have reported an accuracy of 100% for negative prediction, while the positive predictions vary from 50% to 75%, depending on the methods applied.

Monoclonal Antibodies

Since the somatic cell hybridization technique was developed, great emphasis has been put into the search for specific monoclonal antibodies for the various types of lung cancer. The studies have included tumor tissue as well as cell lines. The investigations have demonstrated that the percentage of antigen-positive cells may vary considerably (10%-90%) in the individual cell lines, and that the different types of lung cancer may share certain common antigens, as well as express more specific antigens. The exact specificity of these antibodies is at present uncertain. The monoclonal antibodies appear to have the following potential clinical applications:

1. Detection of circulating antigens in preclinical screening
2. Histopathologic diagnosis of morphologic subtypes with different clinical behavior
3. Detection of micrometastases with or without use of isotope-labeled antibodies for nuclear scanning
4. Therapeutic use of antiboidies provided that they can be conjugated with cytotoxic drugs
5. Elimination of tumor cells from bone marrow by monoclonal antibodies prior to subsequent reinfusion of marrow when using bone marrow transplantation in combination with intensive combination chemotherapy.

Heterotransplantation

About 45%-60% of the lung cancer will form tumors after subcutaneous injection into nude mice, provided an adequate number of cells is present ($10^5/mm^3$). The tumors usually have a local progressive growth, and only seldom do they grow invasively and/or metastasize. The tumor-inducing dose for *intracranial* growth is 10- to 1000-fold less than that for subcutaneous injection, and the nude mouse brain assay may be a useful method of growing tumor cells for drug testing. Heterotransplanted tumors have a higher success rate for establishing continuous cell lines than fresh tumor specimens. Currently, the heterotransplanted tumors are being tested as predictors of drug sensitivity.

Tumor Markers

The endocrine biochemistry of lung cancer has recently attracted great interest, especially the SCCL. Biochemical studies have, in general, demonstrated that some biochemical characteristics may separate SCCL from non-SCCL.

The enzyme *L-dopa-decarboxylase* has been found in high concentration intracellularly in SCCL, but very seldom in non-SCCL tumors. However, measurable blood levels have not been recorded and, therefore, the substance cannot be used as a clinical tumor marker. *Neuron-specific encolase* has also been found in high concentration in SCCL, in contrast to non-SCCL. Clinical studies with the latter substance have demonstrated a good correlation of serum concentration and tumor bulk/tumor response during chemotherapy, and it is conceivable that this marker might play an important role for monitoring in the future. Likewise, the *creatinine kinase* (especially the brain-type isoenzyme) occurs in exceedingly high concentrations in SCCL tumors in contrast to non-SCCL tumors. Also, the peptide *bombesine* has been demonstrated in high concentrations in SCCL.

Despite an extensive search for a potential clinical marker for lung cancer, no ideal marker has, until now, been detected, perhaps reflecting the considerable heterogeneity of the malignant lung tumors.

Tumor Heterogeneity

One of the main obstacles in the treatment of malignant lung cancer today is the considerable heterogeneity of these tumors. The biological knowledge accumulated recently has given clear evidence of the heterogeneity of the lung tumors demonstrated in the following areas: (a) clinical pathology, (b) flow cytometric DNA analyses, (c) in vitro clonogenic assays, (d) biochemical studies, and, (e) studies with monoclonal antibodies.

With respect to clinical pathology, consecutive studies of surgically removed lung tumors have demonstrated that about 15%–20% of the tumors contain more than one cell type based on conventional staining methods. Selective studies by electron microscopy have verified the high proportion of lung tumors with ultrastructural features of multiple cell types.

4. Pathology of Lung Cancer

B.J. Addis

Cancer of the lung arises by neoplastic transformation of the normal lining epithelium. Tumors probably begin as a single malignant clone but rapid division and mutation result in different subpopulations and this is reflected in a wide variety of histological patterns, often suggesting differentiation in more than one direction. Nevertheless the majority of lung carcinomas are readily classified into four main types:

Squamous cell (epidermoid) carcinoma	50%
Adenocarcinoma	20%
Large cell carcinoma	10%
Small cell carcinoma	20%
(Carcinoid	1%)

The relative frequency of each type of carcinoma varies considerably between different series. Surgical series are particularly misleading because patients are selected according to operability. The incidence given above is taken from the Mayo Clinic Lung Project.

A number of classifications of lung carcinoma have been proposed, but that produced in 1981 by the World Health Organization is most widely used. This is a modification of the original 1967 classification and, with minor changes, forms the basis of the description given below (Table 1). Premalignant change and benign squamous cell lesions are included as they are part of the spectrum of neoplastic change seen in the lower respiratory tract.

Premalignant Change and Early Carcinoma

In cigarette smokers and other high-risk groups invasive carcinoma may be preceded by a sequence of changes in bronchial epithelium in response to low-grade chronic irritation combined with inhaled carcinogens. These changes are focal, with an abrupt transition from normal to abnormal epithelium, and are most frequently seen in segmental bronchi. Squamous metaplasia and dysplasia, although usually seen together, probably occur independently.

Table 1. Classification of lung carcinoma

1. Premalignant change and early carcinoma
   a) Squamous metaplasia
   b) Dysplasia and carcinoma in situ
   c) Early carcinoma

2. Bronchial papillomas and papillary carcinoma
   a) Squamous cell papilloma
   b) "Transitional" papilloma
   c) Papillary carcinoma

3. Squamous cell (epidermoid) carcinoma

4. Adenocarcinoma
   a) Acinar
   b) Papillary   } Well or moderately differentiated
   c) Bronchioloalveolar
   d) Solid with mucin production   Poorly differentiated

5. Adenosquamous carcinoma

6. Large cell undifferentiated carcinoma
   Variants: giant cell carcinoma
             clear cell carcinoma

7. Spindle-cell carcinoma and carcinosarcoma

8. Small cell carcinoma
   a) Oat cell type
   b) Intermediate cell type   } Classic oat cell type
   c) Combined small cell type
   d) Small cell-large cell type

9. Lung tumors of low-grade malignancy
   a) Carcinoid tumors
   b) Tumors of bronchial gland origin

Squamous Metaplasia

Squamous metaplasia results from continued proliferation of basal cells in bronchial epithelium. Surface ciliated and mucous cells are retained at first but as the process continues specialized surface cells are lost and the epithelium becomes stratified, often with keratinization of surface layers.

Dysplasia and Carcinoma In Situ (Fig. 1)

The features of malignant change are hyperchromatic nuclei, increased mitotic rate, and a disorderly growth pattern. These may be superimposed at the stage of basal cell hyperplasia, involve the deeper layers in an area of squamous metaplasia, or extend through the full thickness of the metaplastic epithelium (carcinoma in situ). At this preinvasive stage the malignant cells remain confined by the epithelial basement membrane. This sequence of changes is detectable by sputum cy-

18

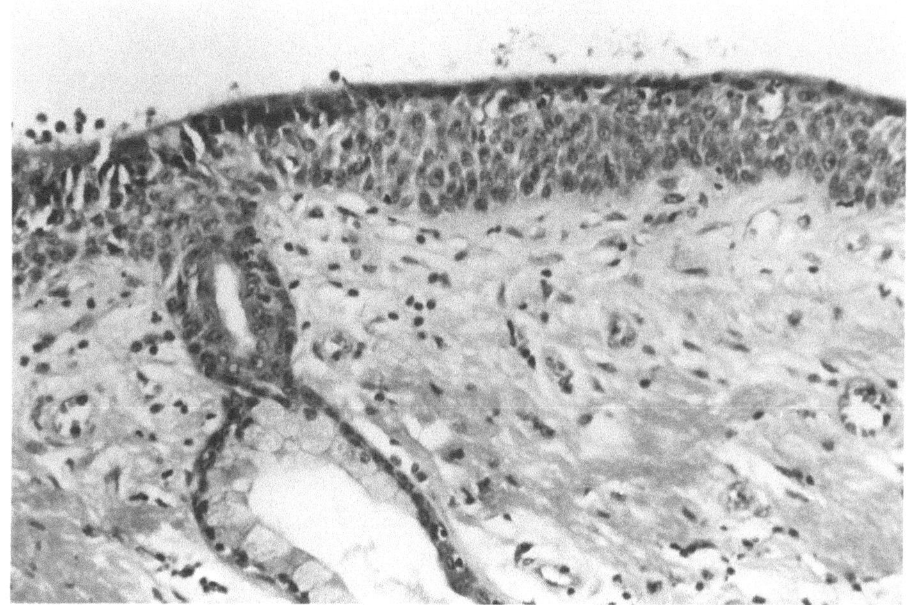

Fig. 1. Dysplasia of bronchial epithelium. Ciliated cells are preserved over several layers of atypical cells with a disorderly growth pattern. Abnormal epithelium extends into the neck of a bronchial gland duct

tology and the cytological appearances of carcinoma in situ may be difficult to distinguish from invasive squamous carcinoma.

Early Bronchial Carcinoma

This term is used for occult tumors that have breached the epithelial basement membrane to become invasive but remain confined to the bronchial wall. They are squamous cell tumors that arise centrally in subsegmental or larger bronchi. Although not apparent radiologically they are detectable by sputum cytology.

Bronchial Papillomas and Papillary Carcinoma

Squamous Cell Papillomas

These are benign tumors occurring in a younger age group in which the papillary processes are covered by stratified squamous epithelium with scattered mucous cells. They are often multiple and the association with laryngeal papillomatosis suggests a viral origin. Malignant change is rare.

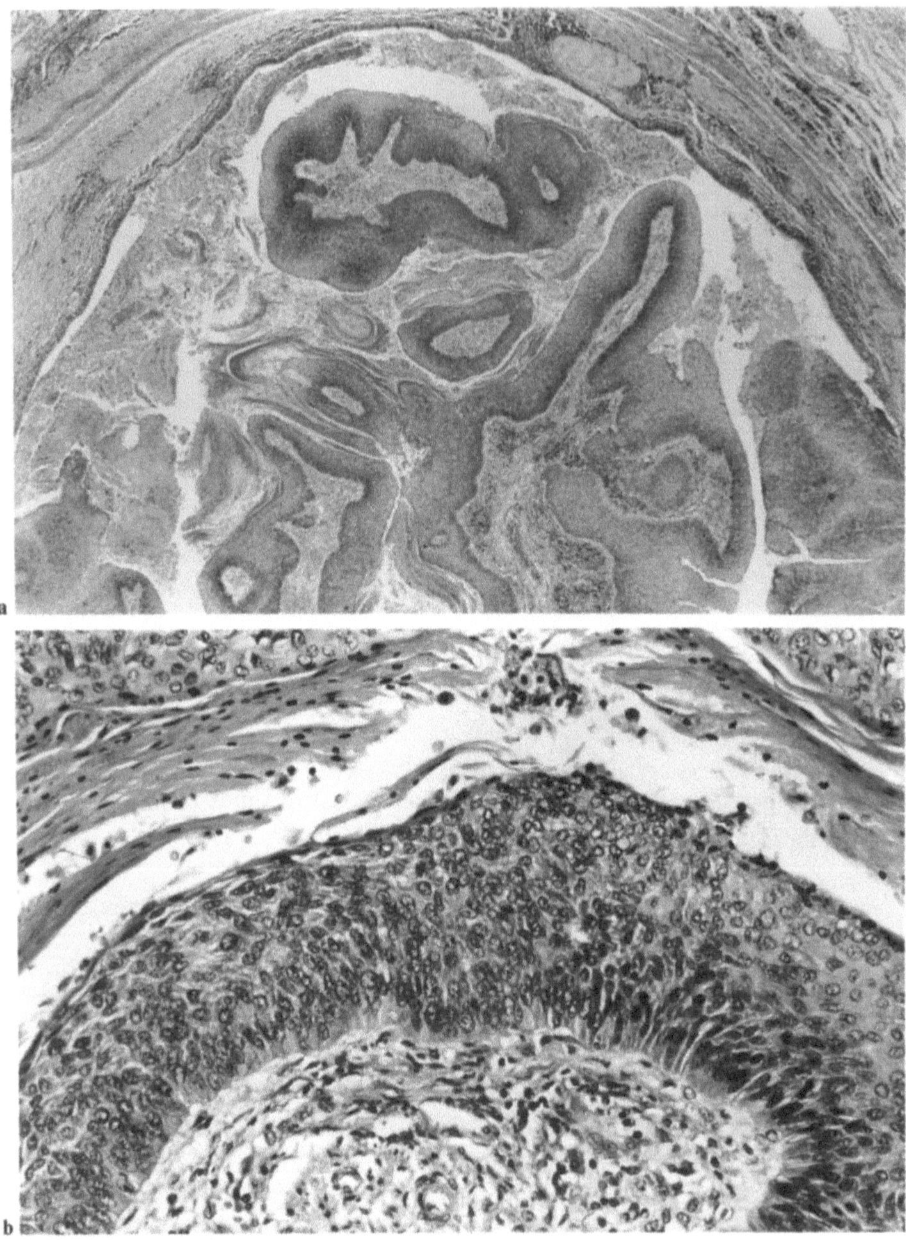

Fig. 2. **a** Papillary squamous cell carcinoma. The bronchial lumen is filled by papillary tumor with extensive squamous carcinoma in situ. An invasive component was also present. **b** A high-power view of the same tumor showing an area of carcinoma in situ

"Transitional" Papillomas

This type of papilloma is often solitary and the epithelium may show any combination of normal bronchial epithelium, metaplastic or transitional epithelium, dysplasia, and carcinoma in situ. Recurrence is frequent and invasive malignancy may supervene.

Papillary Squamous Cell Carcinoma

Endobronchial papillary tumors may show extensive in situ squamous cell carcinoma (Fig. 2). A combination of in situ and invasive malignancy may be present.

Squamous Cell (Epidermoid) Carcinoma

Squamous cell carcinomas most frequently originate in segmental or lobar bronchi and are more common in the upper lobes. Tumors are frequently large at presentation and may undergo central necrosis with cavitation. The essential histological features are stratification of cells with keratinization and intercellular bridges or "prickles." These are formed by retraction of the cytoplasm of adjacent cells be-

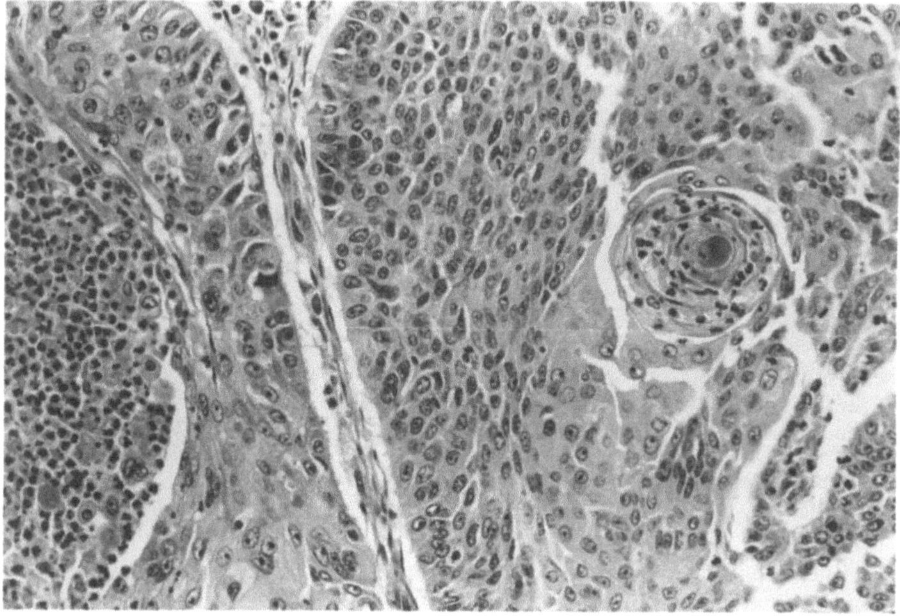

Fig. 3. Moderately well differentiated squamous cell carcinoma. The area of necrosis *on the left* includes atypical keratinized cells, and a keratin pearl is present *on the right*

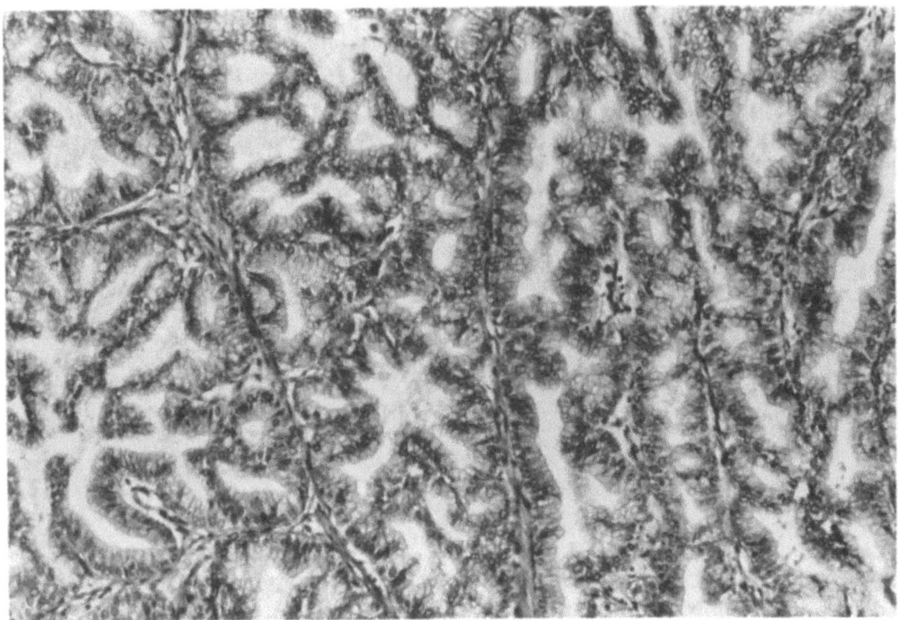

Fig. 4. Well-differentiated adenocarcinoma of acinar type with cells forming a complex glandular pattern

tween cell junctions, making the junctions visible by light microscopy. Squamous cell carcinomas are graded as well, moderately, or poorly differentiated according to the degree and extent of keratinization. In well-differentiated tumors keratin forms pearls or nests (Fig. 3), but in poorly differentiated tumors it may be necessary to search for keratinization of individual cells. The presence of keratin may cause a stromal foreign body granulomatous inflammation.

Adenocarcinoma

In adenocarcinoma, tumor cells form gland-like structures and may have a secretory capacity. The WHO classification separates adenocarcinomas into four groups according to their histological pattern, without regard to their degree of differentiation or cell of origin:

1. Acinar, in which the cells line glandular acini or tubules (Fig. 4).
2. Papillary, in which papillae covered by tumor cells project into irregular spaces (Fig. 5).
3. Bronchioloalveolar (alveolar cell) – a term reserved for well-differentiated peripheral tumors in which malignant cells spread within the existing framework of the lung. They line alveolar spaces without destruction of septa and no significant tumor stroma is formed. Consequently, tumor boundaries are poorly de-

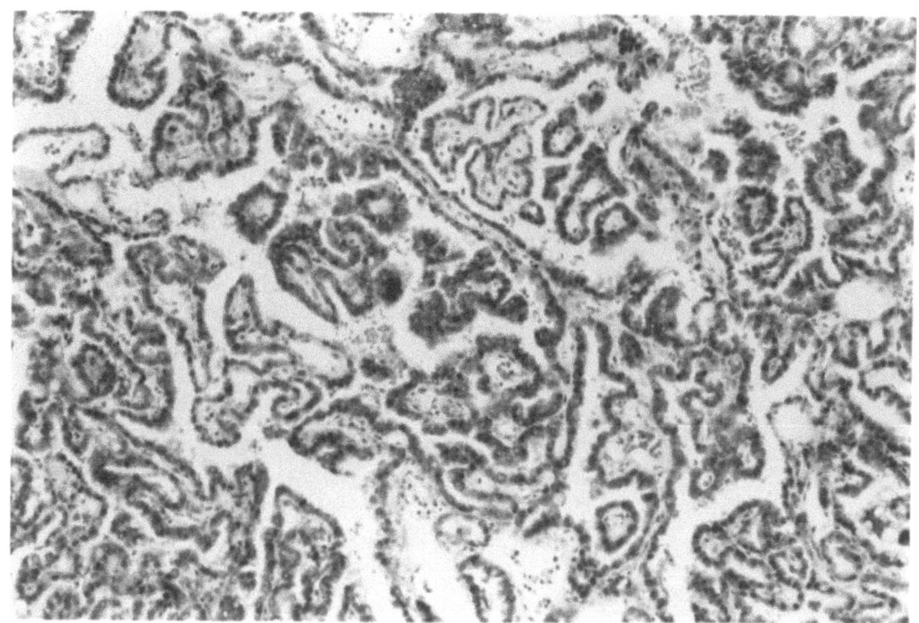

Fig. 5. Papillary adenocarcinoma. Tumor cells cover a narrow connective tissue stalk to form papillary processes

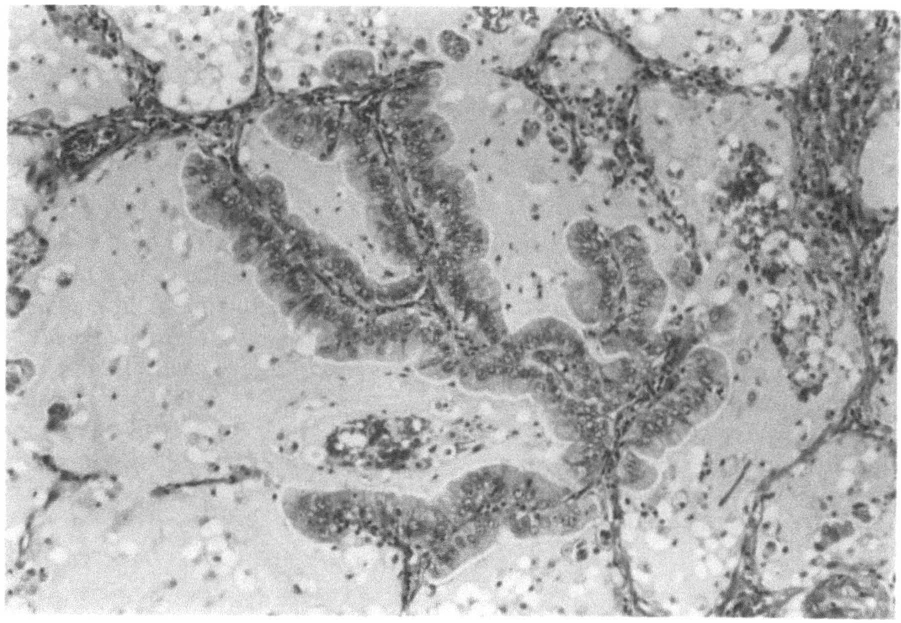

Fig. 6. Bronchioloalveolar carcinoma. Alveolar walls are preserved and some are lined by neoplastic columnar cells

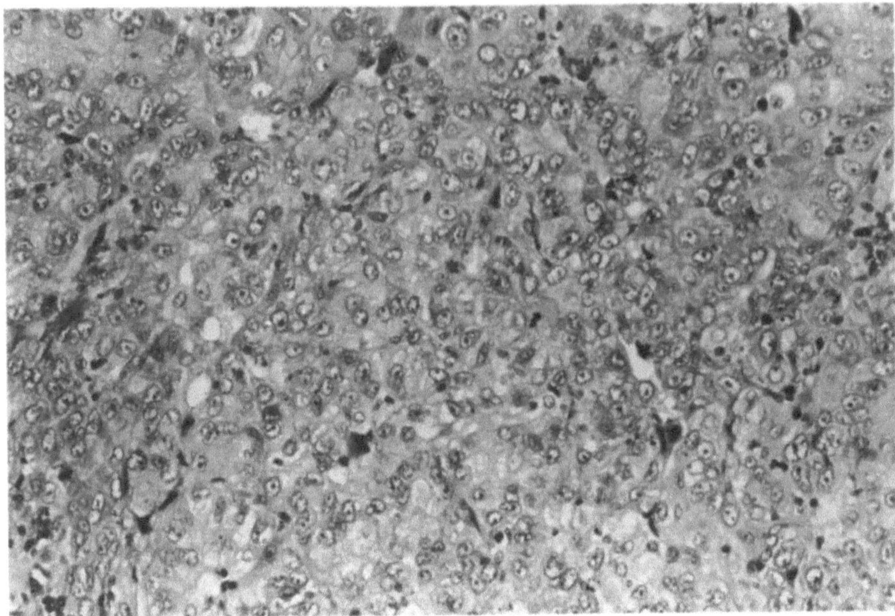

Fig. 7. Poorly differentiated adenocarcinoma (solid carcinoma with mucin production). No convincing evidence of glandular differentiation is apparent but mucin stains were positive

fined and the macroscopic appearances may suggest pneumonic consolidation. Tumors are frequently multifocal and may involve both lungs. This type of tumor may be mimicked by metastatic adenocarcinoma and the term bronchioloalveolar remains contentious (Fig. 6).
4. Solid carcinoma with mucin production. Some adenocarcinomas may appear completely undifferentiated until special stains reveal the presence of mucin (Fig. 7).

Most adenocarcinomas are peripheral, arising from bronchiolar or alveolar epithelium. A small number are central, some possibly of bronchial gland origin. Intra- or extracellular mucin production may be seen in tumors of any pattern. Many show a combination of patterns with a central acinar area, an intermediate papillary area and a peripheral zone resembling bronchioloalveolar carcinoma. A better indication of prognosis is given if a tumor is described as well, moderately, or poorly differentiated and the pattern is regarded as a subsidiary feature. Some adenocarcinomas are associated with preexisting localized or diffuse pulmonary fibrosis, but in some peripheral "scar" carcinomas the fibrosis and elastosis may represent dense stroma induced by the tumor.

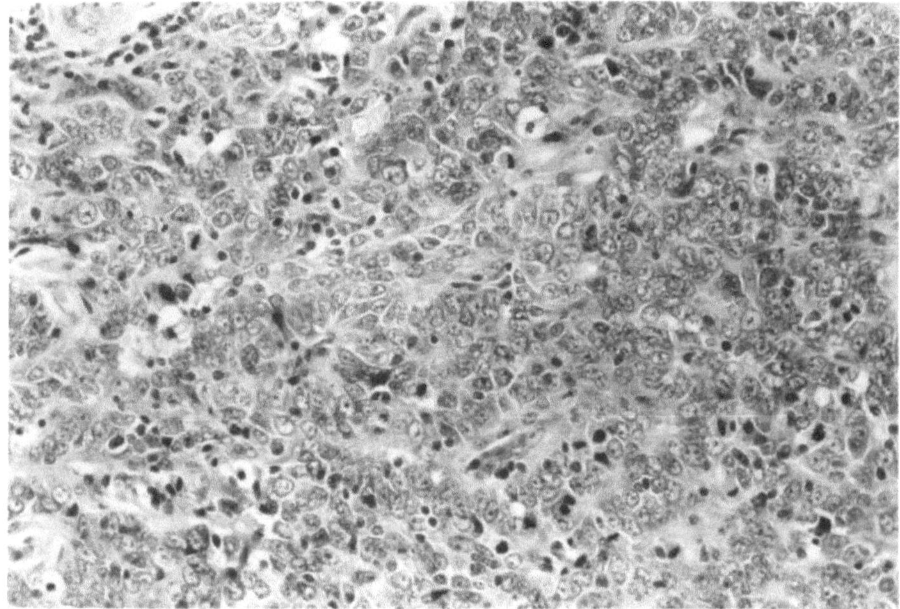

Fig. 8. Large cell undifferentiated carcinoma. This tumor was undifferentiated by both light and electron microscopy

Adenosquamous Carcinoma

Many lung carcinomas show electron microscopic features suggesting both squamous and glandular differentiation. However, tumors showing clear light microscopic evidence of dual differentiation are rare, accounting for about 1% of all carcinomas. Most are peripheral tumors and microscopically show areas with unequivocal evidence of keratinization and intercellular bridges combined with glandular or papillary areas.

Large Cell Undifferentiated Carcinoma

In large cell carcinoma, nuclei are large, round or oval, and vesicular, with a prominent nuclear membrane and nucleolus. The cytoplasm is relatively abundant and cells form solid trabeculae or sheets with no light microscopic features to suggest squamous or glandular differentiation (Fig. 8). Tumors of this type are often peripheral without being clearly related to bronchi.

Two rare variants of large cell carinoma are described:

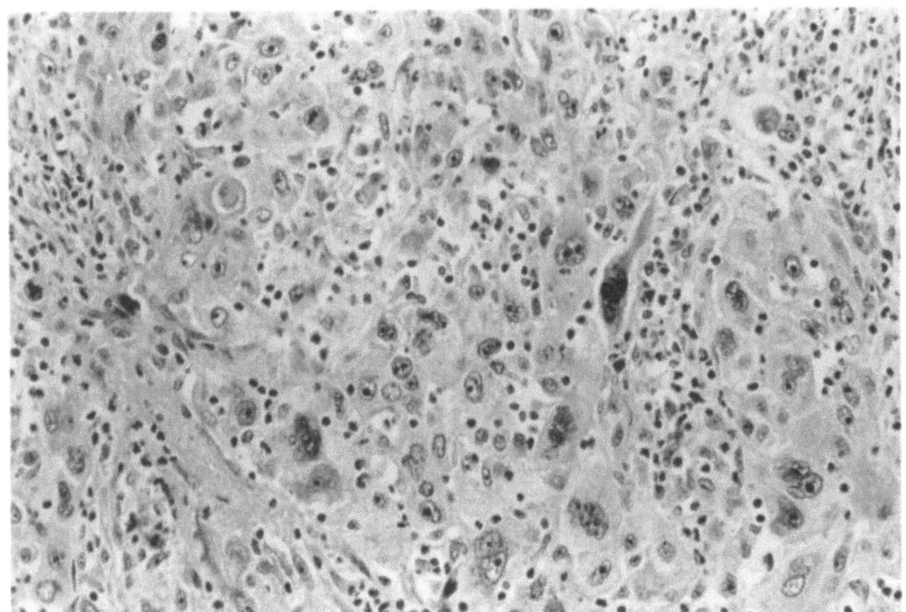

Fig. 9. Giant cell carcinoma. Large multinucleated giant cells with scattered neutrophils, some within the cytoplasm of tumor cells

Giant Cell Carcinoma

Tumor cells are very large and pleomorphic often with two or more nuclei and abundant cytoplasm. They tend to be dissociated without any recognizable pattern and characteristically phagocytize other cells, particularly red cells and neutrophils (Fig. 9). Occasionally areas resembling giant cell carcinoma are seen in poorly differentiated adenocarcinoma and ultrastructurally some giant cell carcinomas show the characteristics of adenocarcinoma.

Clear Cell Carcinoma

If this term is confined to tumors consisting entirely of clear cells, clear cell carcinoma of the lung is an extremely rare entity. The appearance is mainly due to the presence of abundant intracellular glycogen. Every effort should be made to exclude a primary clear cell carcinoma in the kidney or elsewhere. Another tumor likely to cause confusion is the benign clear cell tumor ("sugar" tumor) of the lung.

Strict criteria should be applied before making a diagnosis of large cell carcinoma and its giant cell and clear cell variants:

1. The diagnosis should be made according to light microscopic features. Electron microscopy often reveals features that suggest squamous or glandular differen-

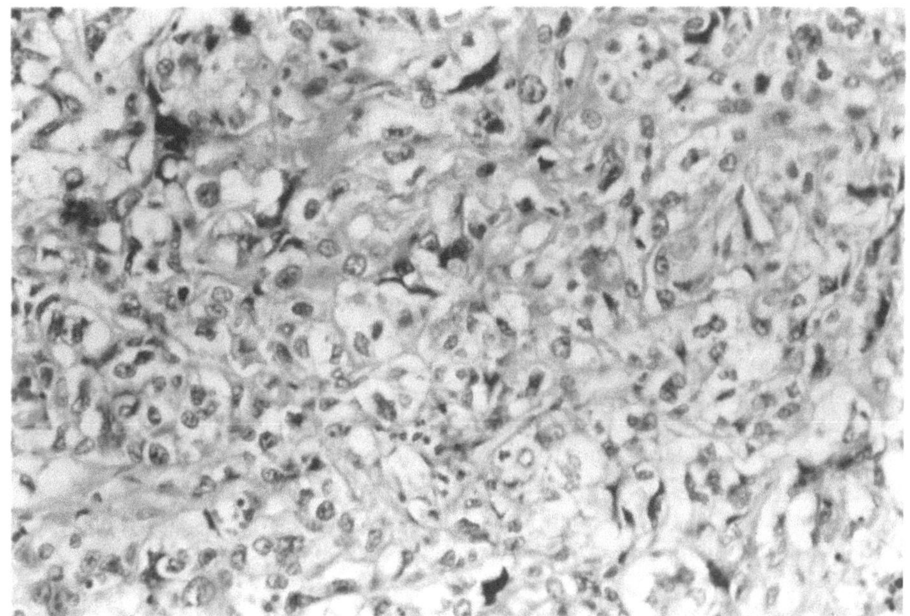

Fig. 10. A clear cell area in an adenocarcinoma

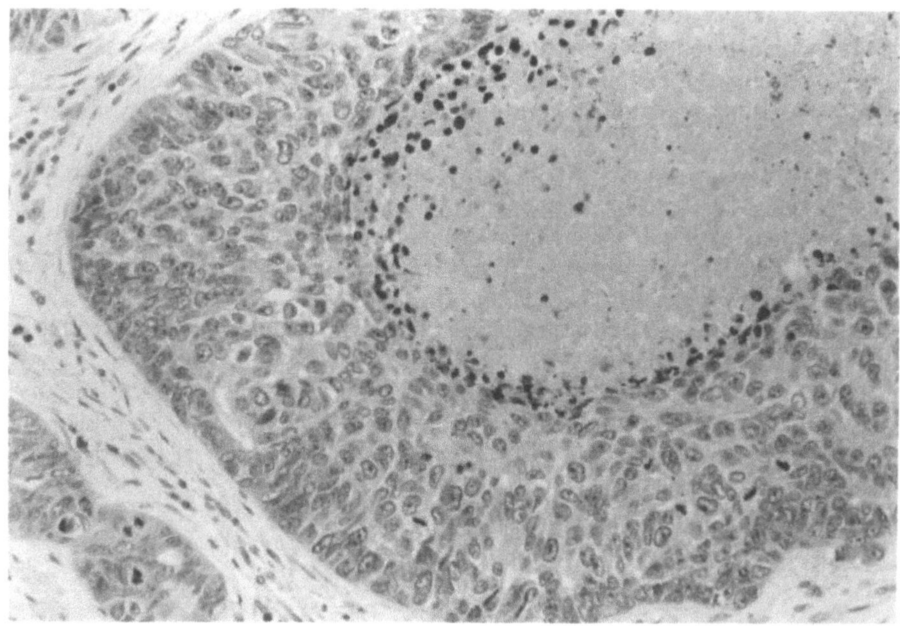

Fig. 11. Large cell undifferentiated carcinoma or poorly differentiated squamous cell carcinoma? Despite the stratification no evidence of keratinization was seen

tiation, or both, but this facility is often not available and the present classification is intended to encourage uniformity based on light microscopy.

2. If any area of the tumor shows clear evidence of differentiation or if mucin stains are positive the tumor is no longer regarded as undifferentiated. Completely undifferentiated areas and clear cell areas may be seen in squamous cell carcinoma and adenocarcinoma (Fig.10) and typical giant cell areas may be seen in adenocarcinomas.

3. In a significant number of tumors keratinization is not apparent but stratification of undifferentiated cells suggests that they are essentially squamous in origin. These tumors are classified as either poorly differentiated squamous cell carcinoma or large cell carcinoma by different pathologists and the terms "large cell carcinoma with stratification" or "squamoid" carcinoma have been suggested as a compromise (Fig.11).

4. Small biopsies are subject to sampling error and a guarded diagnosis should be given until the resected tumor has been adequately sampled. Histopathologists and cytologists should refrain from using the term large cell carcinoma when the diagnosis, based on a small biopsy, is "non-small cell carcinoma with no evidence of differentiation in the small sample examined."

Spindle-Cell Carcinoma and Carcinosarcoma

Although spindle-cell carcinoma is included in the WHO classification as a variant of squamous cell carcinoma, spindle-cell areas may occasionally be seen in both squamous cell carcinomas and adenocarcinomas. These areas merge with more typical carcinomatous areas and represent a pleomorphic component of the tumor. Occasional carcinomas consist entirely of spindle cells and confusion arises with sarcomas (Fig.12).

Carcinosarcomas are clearly biphasic with separation of an epithelial component, usually squamous cell carcinoma, and a sarcomatous stromal component. The latter has a spindle or polygonal cell pattern and may show differentiation to form osteoid, cartilage, or muscle. The two components may metastasize independently. Their histogenesis is unclear but they probably represent complete mesenchymal metaplasia in a carcinoma. Some are polypoid and project into the lumen of a large bronchus (Fig.13).

Pulmonary blastoma is a form of carcinosarcoma which is invariably peripheral, occurs in a somewhat younger age group, and microscopically resembles fetal lung. Branching tubular epithelial structures are present in a stroma resembling primitive mesenchyme (Fig.14).

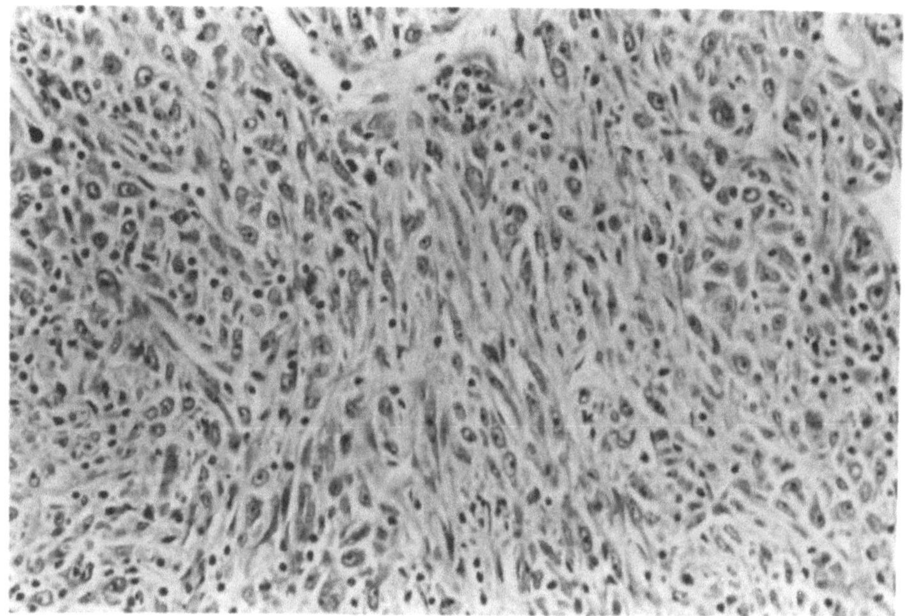

Fig. 12. Spindle-cell carcinoma. This tumor contained no differentiated areas

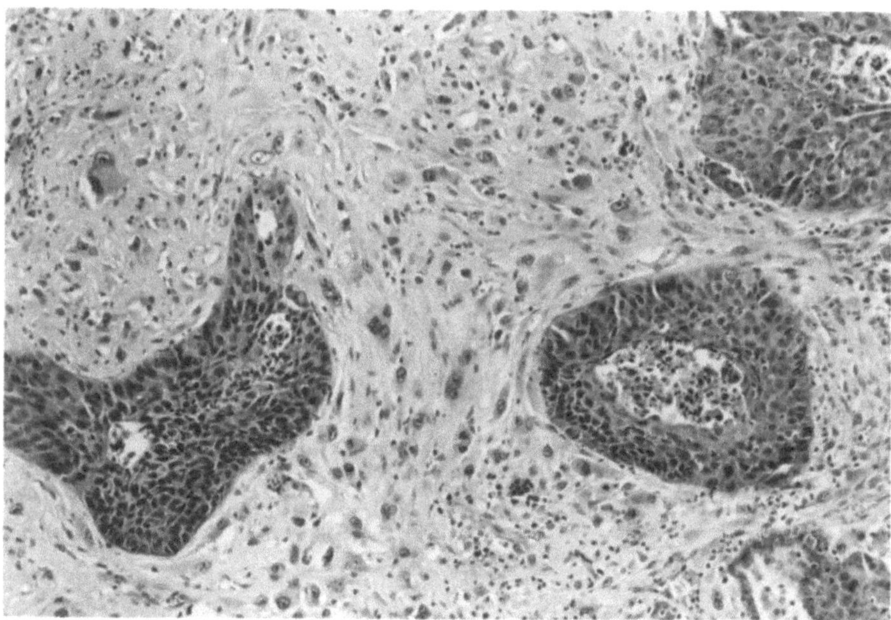

Fig. 13. Carcinosarcoma. Islands of squamous cell carcinoma in a stroma which includes malignant spindle cells and pleomorphic giant cells

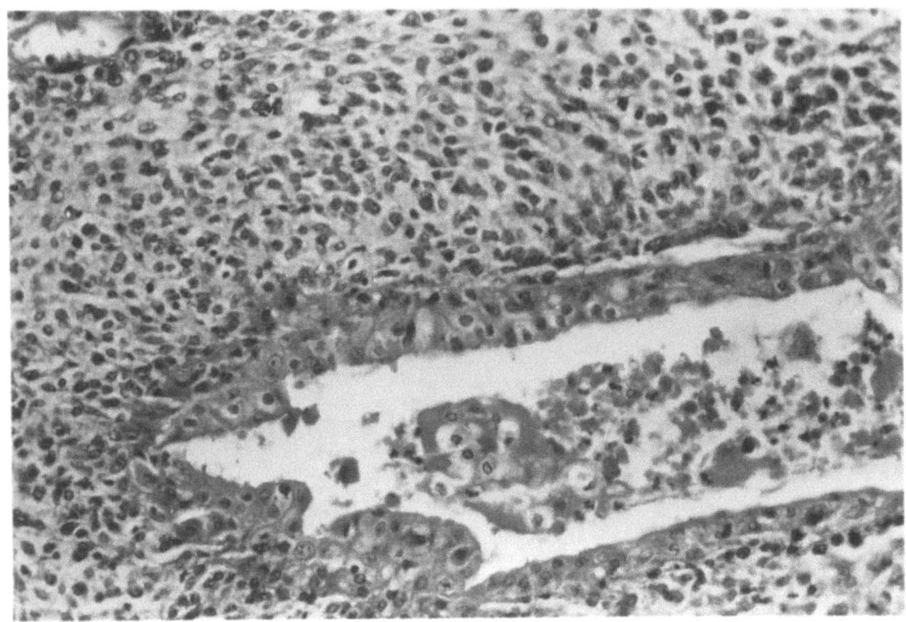

Fig. 14. Pulmonary blastoma. A tubular epithelial component in a stroma of undifferentiated mesenchyme

Small Cell Carcinoma

Differences in behavior and response to treatment make the distinction between small cell carcinoma and non-small cell carcinoma the single most important decision the pathologist must make when examining a lung tumor. Small cell carcinomas usually arise as central tumors and are capable of early hematogenous and lymphatic dissemination. By electron microscopy dense-core neurosecretory granules are evidence of endocrine differentiation and a variety of amines and peptide hormones such as serotonin, bombesin, vasoactive intestinal polypeptide, gastrin, leu-encephalin, and calcitonin can be identified in the cells by immunohistochemical means. Clinical syndromes may be associated with ACTH and ADH production.

The WHO classification recognizes three subtypes of small cell carcinoma:

Oat Cell Type

In this type, previously called "lymphocyte-like," nuclei tend to be two to three times larger than lymphocytes and are round or oval with dense, uniformly distributed nuclear chromatin, often with a stippled appearance. Nucleoli are inconspicuous and cytoplasm is sparse so that adjacent nuclei are often moulded against each other. Cells form cords or nests with little stroma formation and may show

30

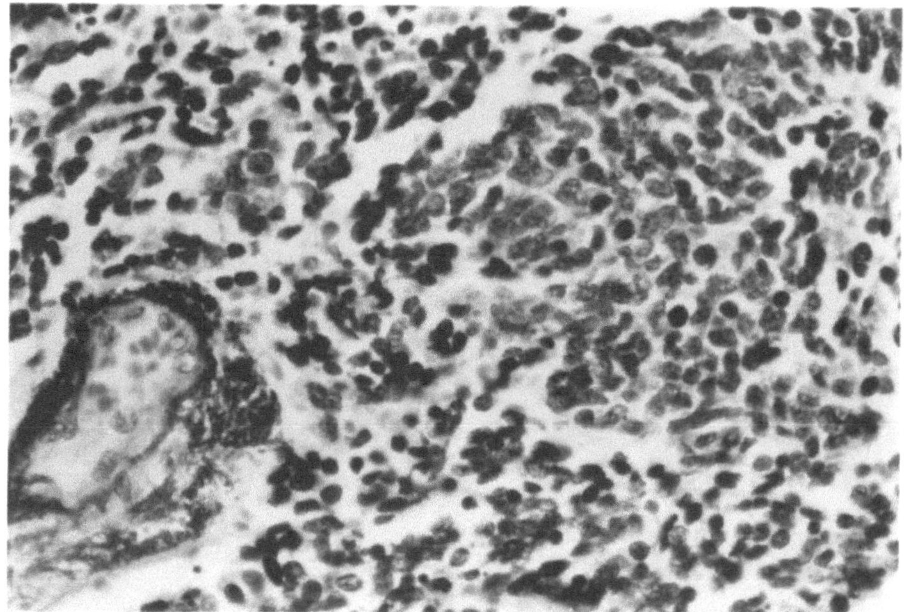

Fig. 15. Small cell carcinoma of oat cell type. Deposits of nucleoprotein are present in the wall of a small vessel

peripheral palisading or rosette formation. A high mitotic rate is accompanied by cell death with nuclear debris among viable cells, and more extensive necrosis leaves surviving cells forming perivascular collars. Hematoxyphilic nuclear material may be deposited in the walls of small vessels (Fig. 15).

Intermediate Cell Type

Nuclear characteristics are similar to the oat cell type but chromatin is less dense, nucleoli may be more prominent, and cells may have significant amounts of cytoplasm (Fig. 16). The polygonal or fusiform cell types of the first WHO classification have now been incorporated into the intermediate cell type and this also makes provision for tumors with a mixture of small and large cells.

Combined Oat Cell Carcinomas

In about 5% of small cell carcinomas there is a definite component of squamous cell carcinoma or adenocarcinoma (Fig. 17). This tendency to differentiate is more pronounced after treatment, and combined tumors are therefore most frequently seen at autopsy.

The diagnosis of small cell carcinoma is often made on the basis of small endoscopic biopsy fragments or cytology. Nuclei tend to be particularly fragile and

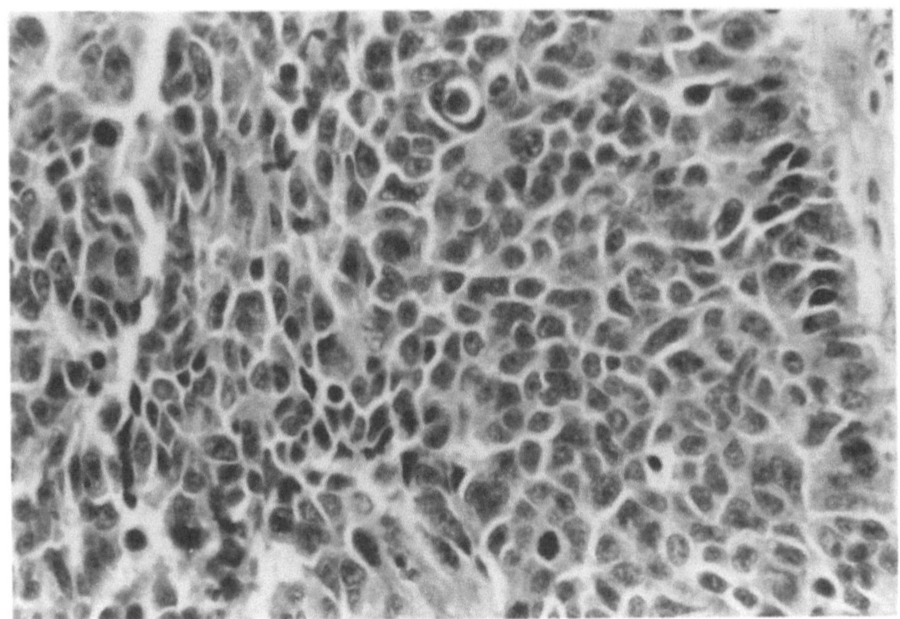

Fig. 16. Small cell carcinoma of intermediate cell type

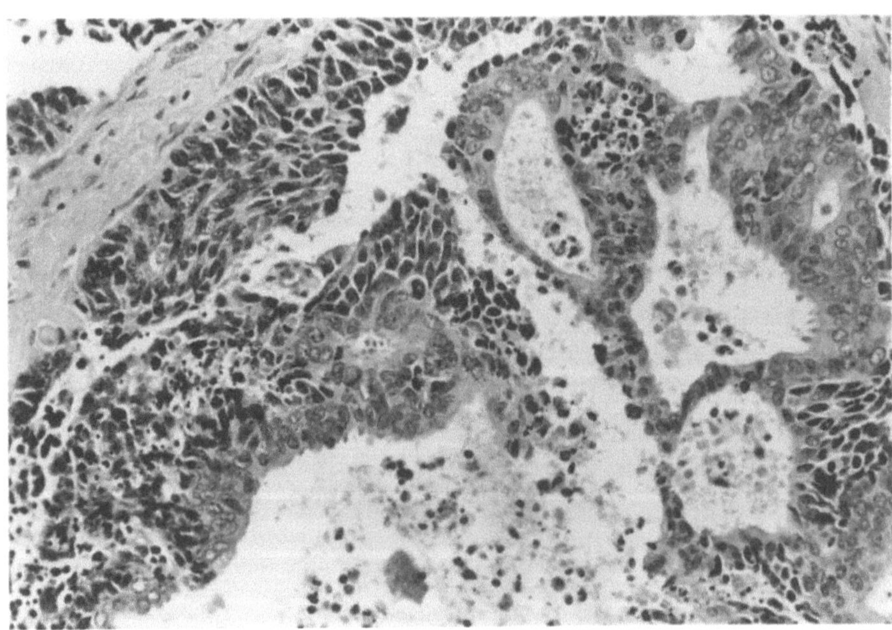

Fig. 17. Small cell carcinoma of combined type. Undifferentiated small cell areas are combined with adenocarcinoma

crush artifact is common, producing a hematoxyphilic smudge. Degeneration, with separation of densely staining, rounded nuclei, frequently blurs morphology and cells from the same tumor may appear different depending on the type of biopsy. Immunohistochemistry may provide a more objective means than routine light microscopy of distinguishing between small cell and non-small cell carcinoma. Specific peptide hormones can be localized and antibodies to neuron-specific enolase and chromogranin are currently being assessed as markers of endocrine differentiation. Monoclonal antibodies raised against small cell carcinoma cell lines may eventually prove useful, but the limitations imposed by small biopsies and formalin fixation remain a problem at present.

Subtyping of small cell carcinoma based on a small sample is subject to a very high interobserver variation. There is no convincing evidence that oat cell or intermediate subtypes respond differently to treatment or have different survival rates. Giant cells, often with two or more nuclei, may be seen in small cell carcinoma. Despite their size, the nuclear characteristics do not appreciably differ and they should not present a diagnostic problem. However, in about 1% of small cell tumors groups of cells with the characteristics of large cell undifferentiated carcinoma may be seen. Although pathologists will vary considerably in the diagnosis of this entity, there is some evidence that combined small cell – large cell carcinoma responds less well to therapy and the survival rate is poor.

For these reasons it has been suggested that small cell carcinoma should be subdivided into:

1. Classic small cell carcinoma – incorporating both oat cell and intermediate cell types
2. Small cell – large cell carcinoma
3. Combined small carcinoma

Tumors of Low Grade Malignancy

Carcinoid Tumors

Bronchial carcinoids originate from bronchial endocrine cells and are capable of producing a variety of amines and peptide hormones. Central carcinoids arise in lobar or segmental bronchi and there is frequently an endobronchial component. Margins are usually well defined and the surface is typically pinkish-tan. The microscopic pattern is varied, with cords, ribbons, or islands of cells separated by a delicate vascular stroma (Fig. 18). Cells have a moderate amount of granular eosinophilic cytoplasm and nuclei are uniform, round or oval, and moderately hyperchromatic. Calcification and ossification may be present in the stroma. Occasional features include mucin production, oncocytic change, with abundant brightly eosinophilic cytoplasm due to the presence of large numbers of mitochondria, and melanin production. Peripheral carcinoids, which are unrelated to bronchi, account for about 10% of tumors and frequently have a spindle-cell pattern.

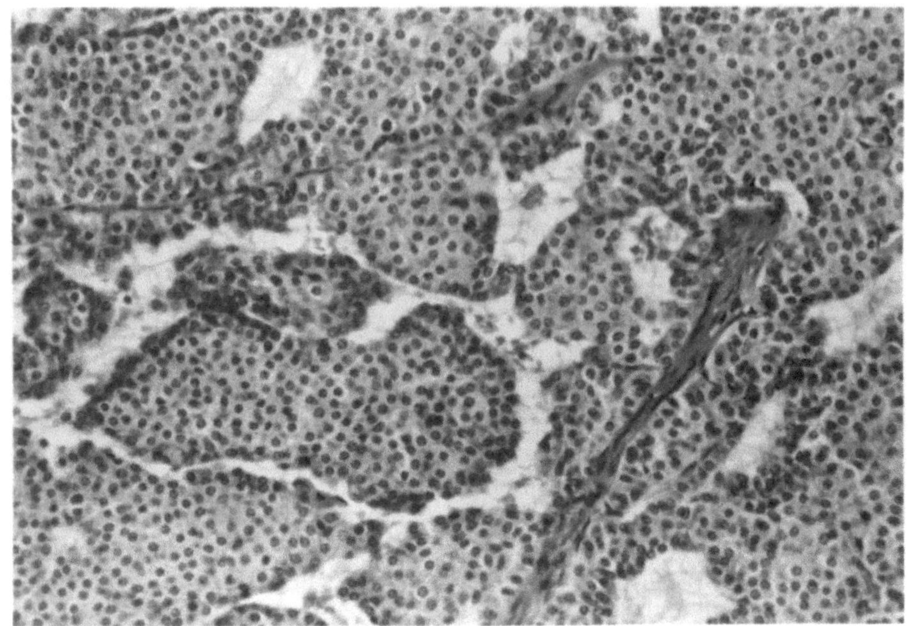

Fig. 18. Bronchial carcinoid tumor with islands of cells separated by a vascular stroma

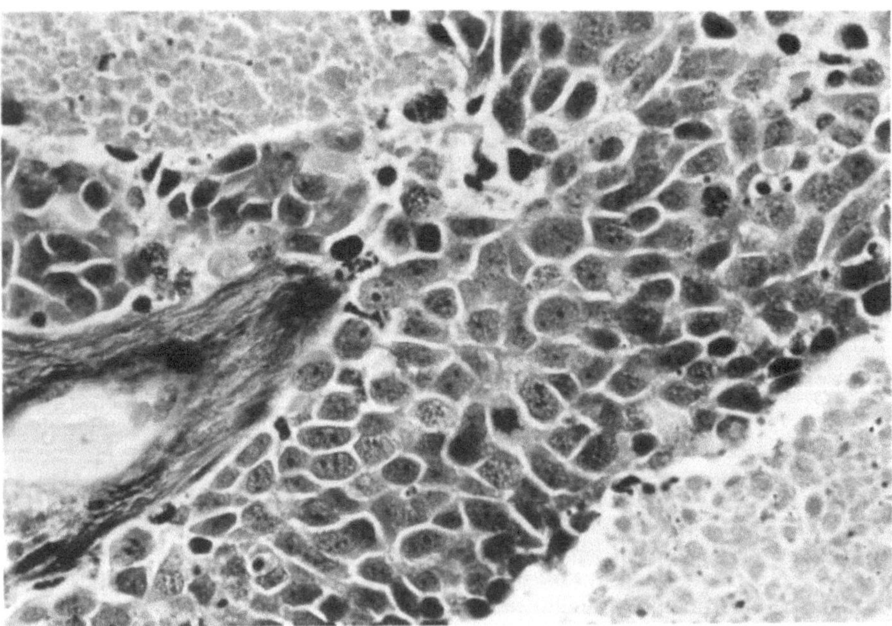

Fig. 19. Undifferentiated carcinoma in which cells have large nuclei, some with prominent nucleoli, and fairly abundant cytoplasm. Staining of vessel walls by nucleoprotein suggests that this should be classified as small cell carcinoma

Although often regarded as benign tumors, carcinoids are locally invasive and a small number recur locally or metastasize, often after a long period. Atypical (malignant) carcinoids are tumors with a recognizable carcinoid pattern but showing increased mitotic activity, nuclear pleomorphism, necrosis or increased cellularity, and disorganization of pattern. These features indicate greater malignant potential.

Some tumors with ultrastructural and immunohistochemical evidence of endocrine differentiation continue to resist classification. The light microscopic features may be intermediate between large cell carcinoma and small cell carcinoma (Fig. 19) or they may combine the features of small cell carcinoma and atypical carcinoid tumor. One possible solution to this problem would be to regard atypical carcinoid tumors as well-differentiated bronchopulmonary neuroendocrine carcinomas and small cell carcinomas as poorly differentiated bronchopulmonary neuroendocrine carcinomas. The spectrum would include a group of intermediate bronchopulmonary neuroendocrine carcinomas, some with large cell morphology, that at present remain unclassifiable. Clearly there is room for new terminology but our eventual understanding of the behavior of these tumors and their response to therapy will depend on clear communication between pathologist and physician.

Tumors of Bronchial Gland Origin

The bronchial seromucous glands may give rise to a range of tumors similar to those seen in the salivary glands. The majority are of adenoid cystic or mucoepidermoid type.

Further Reading

Bolen JW, Thorning D (1982) Histogenetic classification of pulmonary carcinomas. Peripheral adenocarcinoma studied by light microscopy, histochemistry and electron microscopy. Pathol Annu 17: 77–100

Carter D (1978) Pathology of early squamous cell carcinoma of the lung. Pathol Annu 13: 131–147

Carter D (1983) Small-cell carcinoma of the lung. Am J Surg Pathol 7: 787–795

Carter D, Eggleston JC (1980) Tumours of the lower respiratory tract (Atlas of tumour pathology, second series, Fasc. 17). Armed Forces Institute of Pathology, Washington DC

Edwards CW (1984) Alveolar carcinoma: a review. Thorax 39: 166–174

Gould VE, Linnoila RI, Memoli VA, Warren WH (1983) Neuroendocrine cells and neuroendocrine neoplasms of the lung. Path Annu 18: 287–330

Hammond ME, Sanse WT (1985) Large cell neuroendocrine tumours of the lung – clinical significance and histopathologic definition. Cancer 56: 1624–1629

Hirsch FR, Osterlind K, Hansen HH (1983) The prognostic significance of histopathologic subtyping of small cell carcinoma of the lung according to the classification of the World Health Organisation. Cancer 52: 2144–2150

Kimula Y (1978) A histochemical and ultrastructural study of adenocarcinoma of the lung. Am J Surg Pathol 2: 253–264

Matthews MJ (1985) Pathology of small cell lung cancer. Clin Oncol 4: 11-29

Matthews MJ, Mackay B, Lukeman J (1983) The pathology of non-small cell carcinoma of the lung. Semin Oncol 10: 34-55

McDowall EM, Becci PJ, Barrett LA, Trump BF (1978) Morphogenesis and classification of lung cancer. In: Harris CC (ed) Pathogenesis and therapy of lung cancer. Lung biology in health and disease, vol 10. Dekkar, New York pp 445-519

Saccomanno G, Archer VE, Auerback O, Saunder RP, Brennan LM (1973) Development of carcinoma of the lung as reflected in exfoliated cells. Cancer 33: 256-270

Singh G, Katyal SL, Ordonez NG, Dail DH, Negishi Y, Weedn VW, Marcus PB, Weldon-Linne M, Axiotis CA, Alvarez-Fernandez E, Smith WI (1984) Type II pneumocytes in pulmonary tumours. Arch Pathol Lab Med 108: 44-48

Spencer H, Dail DH, Arneaud J (1980) Non-invasive bronchial epthelial papillary tumours. Cancer 45: 1486-1497

Vollmer RT, Birch R, Ogdon L, Crossman JD (1985) Subclassification of small cell cancer of the lung. The southeastern cancer study group experience. Hum Pathol 16: 247-252

Whimster WF (1983) Tumours of the trachea, bronchus, lung and pleura. (Diagnostic tumour bibliographies, no 1) Pitman, London

WHO (1981) Histological typing of lung tumours (International histological classification of tumours No 1) 2nd edn, World Health Organisation, Geneva

Wilson TS, McDowell EM, Marangos PJ, Trump BF (1985) Histochemical studies of dense-core granulated tumours of the lung. Arch Pathol Lab Med 109: 613-620

Woolner EM, Fontana RS, Sanderson DR, Miller WE, Muhm JR, Taylor WF, Uhlenhopp MA (1981) Mayo lung project: evaluation of lung cancer screening through December 1979. Mayo Clin Proc 50: 544-555

Yesner R (1985) Classification of lung cancer histology. New Engl J Med 312: 652-653

5. Histopathology, Ultrastructure, and Cytology

F. R. Hirsch

The first internationally accepted classification of malignant lung tumors was published by the World Health Organization in 1967 and revised in 1981 (Table 1). The aim of the WHO classification of tumors has been to establish a morphologic classification which could be used routinely all over the world. The criteria should be sufficiently consistent to permit any pathologist to classify a given tumor in the same way. Such a classification would be expected to show biological consistency in that tumors similarly classified would have some important biological properties in common. In the following the WHO classification will be reviewed as applied at the Finsen Institute.

Table 1. WHO classification of malignant lung tumors (main types)

Squamous cell carcinoma

Variant

    1. Spindle cell carcinoma

Small cell carcinoma

    1. Oat cell carcinoma
    2. Intermediate cell type
    3. Combined small cell carcinoma

Adenocarcinoma

    1. Acinar adenocarcinoma
    2. Papillary adenocarcinoma
    3. Bronchiolo-alveolar carcinoma
    4. Solid carcinoma with mucus formation

Large cell carcinoma

    1. Solid carcinoma without mucin
    2. Giant cell carcinoma
    3. Clear cell carcinoma

Carcinoids

Mesothelioma

    1. Epithelial
    2. Fibrous (spindle cell)
    3. Biphasic

WHO Classification

General Principles

The classification is based on light microscopic criteria using "standard" staining procedures. Results of electron microscopy (EM) and immunohistochemistry are not included as diagnostic criteria in the WHO classification, but they might in many cases clarify the diagnosis. Consequently these techniques will be dealt with only briefly in the present review.

The grade of differentiation is included in the current classification of the various types of lung tumors. Like in other tumor classifications this grading should be based on the most highly differentiated tissues. If a tumor appears to be without any clearly recognizable component, designations like "undifferentiated" or "anaplastic" are commonly used. In the lung, however, several tumor types are traditionally recognized as being anaplastic in the sense mentioned, but they often still have characteristic shapes or features on the basis of which separate types of anaplastic tumors can be defined. Table 1 gives an overview of the WHO classification.

Squamous Cell Carcinoma

Definitions

A malignant epithelial tumor which by light microscopy has at least one of three differentiating features: individual cell keratinization, pearl formation, or intercellular bridges.

Pathogenesis

Squamous cell carcinomas arise in the basal cells of the bronchial epithelium and progress through varying degrees of dysplasia, carcinoma in situ, and then invasive carcinoma. Most of the tumors (75%–95%) are found in the large bronchi.

Histopathologic Classification

Squamous cell carcinoma is subtyped based on the degree of differentiation and growth pattern:

1. Well differentiated
2. Moderately differentiated
3. Poorly differentiated
4. Spindle cell (squamous) carcinoma

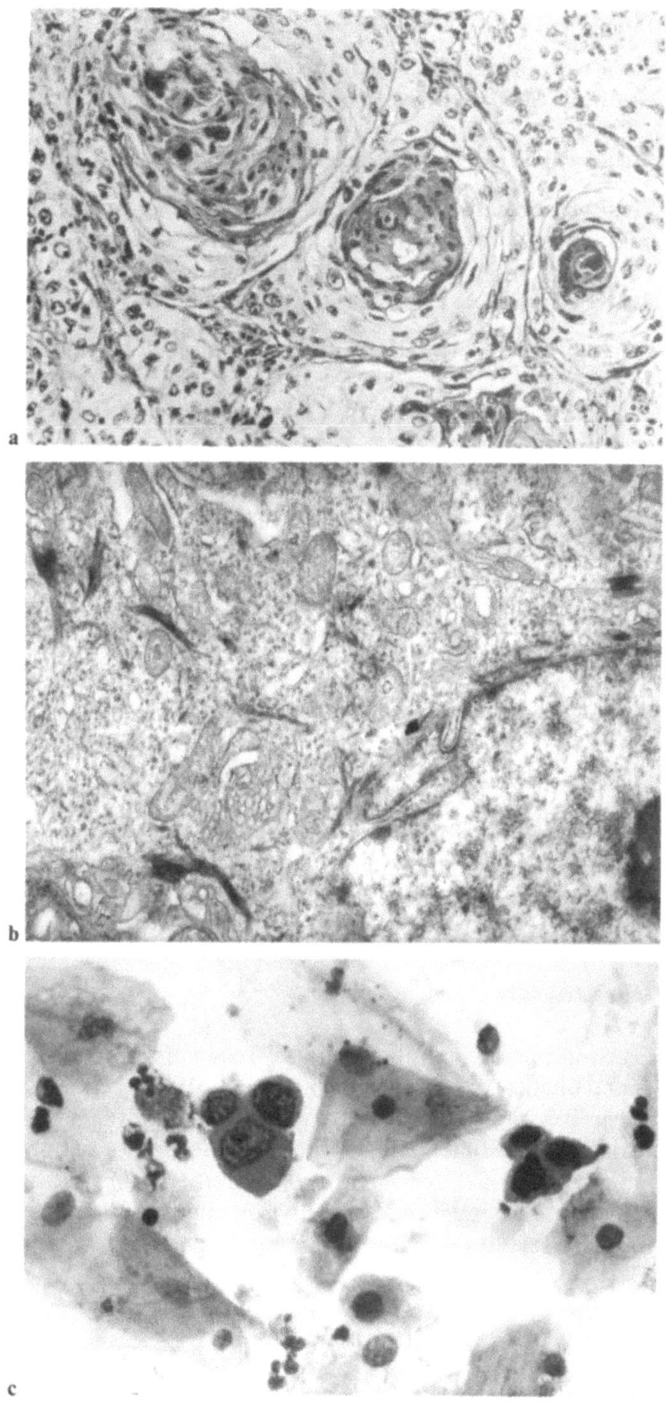

Fig. 1. **a** Squamous cell carcinoma, well differentiated (histology), ×288. **b** Squamous cell carcinoma (EM), ×10224. **c** Squamous cell carcinoma (cytology), ×475

Well-Differentiated Carcinoma

Tumors showing histologic and cellular features such as orderly stratification, obvious intercellular bridges, and keratinization with pearl formation (Fig. 1 a).

Moderately Differentiated Carcinoma

This subtype has features intermediate between well-differentiated and poorly differentiated.

Poorly Differentiated Carcinoma

A tumor fulfilling the criteria for squamous cell carcinoma, i.e., containing keratin and/or bridges, but where these features are sporadically present and the main part of the cells is undifferentiated, or a tumor in which these criteria only are recognized with difficulty.

Many of the tumors of this subtype have extensive intercellular bridges as the only evidence of differentiation. Elastic tissue stains are frequently helpful in revealing the presence of bridges, which can also be well demonstrated by using green filters in the microscope. The individual cells may not be keratinized and pearl formation may not be evident.

Spindle-Cell (Squamous) Carcinoma

A variant of squamous cell carcinoma with a biphasic appearance due to the presence of a component that is identifiable as a squamous cell carcinoma and a spindle cell component derived from it.

The spindle cell component has a sarcoma-like growth pattern. It often exhibits marked cellular pleomorphism and abnormal mitosis. Areas of transition of squamous cell carcinoma into the spindle cell component are demonstrable and provide evidence that the tumor is a variant of squamous cell carcinoma.

Ultrastructure

Electron microscopy demonstrates frequently prominent desmosomes with associated bundles of tonofilaments (Fig. 1 b). When keratin is present within the cytoplasm it is preferentially deposited on the tonofilament bundles. Because of the variations in differentiation which may occur in a tumor it may be of help to examine several different areas by EM rather than base assessment on one single sampling. In this way occasionally squamous carcinomas will be found to contain foci with features of adenocarcinoma.

Cytology

Because of the central location of this tumor compared with most other lung cancer types' tumor cells are more readily sampled in sputum or bronchial washings than the other types.

The size of the individual cells may vary considerably and the nuclei may be anaplastic and pleomorphic as in all carcinomas but are characteristically hyperchromatic with a jagged border (Fig. 1 c). One or several prominent nucleoli may be seen. The cytoplasm is abundant and evidence of keratinization in the cytoplasm is frequently seen. Sometimes the cells fit together to form a squamous "pearl." Subtyping of squamous cell carcinoma should not be based on cytology. There is a tendency of higher degrees of differentiation to be recorded by cytology than by histology because differentiated cells are more likely to be on the surface of the tumor and therefore they more frequently exfoliate into the bronchial lumen.

Small Cell Carcinoma

Definition

A tumor composed of uniform small cells (somewhat larger than lymphocytes) with dense round or oval nuclei, diffuse chromatin, inconspicious nucleoli, and sparse cytoplasm.

Pathogenesis

Small cell lung cancer is most often a centrally located tumor arising from the bronchial epithelium. However, in contrast to the squamous cell carcinoma, which nearly always grows intraluminally, the small cell carcinoma has a marked tendency to invasive submucosal growth; accordingly bronchoscopy is negative or only demonstrates a swollen respiratory mucosa in many cases.

Histopathologic Classification

General Morphologic Features

1. Nuclear characteristics are the most significant diagnostic features. Chromatin is distributed in a uniform, fine, or coarse stippled pattern throughout the entire nucleus. Nucleoli are for the most part small and inconspicuous. Size and shape of the nuclei are of less significance for the diagnosis of small cell carcinoma. Usually the nuclear details are obscure in the cells with hyperchromatic nuclei (Fig. 2).
2. The majority of the cells have meager cytoplasm, resulting in moulding and contouring of adjoining nuclei. In some tumors a moderate amount of cytoplasm may be identified.
3. Mitoses may be numerous in well-preserved tumors but are usually difficult to appreciate in crushed biopsies and autopsy specimens, where the nuclei tend to be hyperchromatic without distinct details.

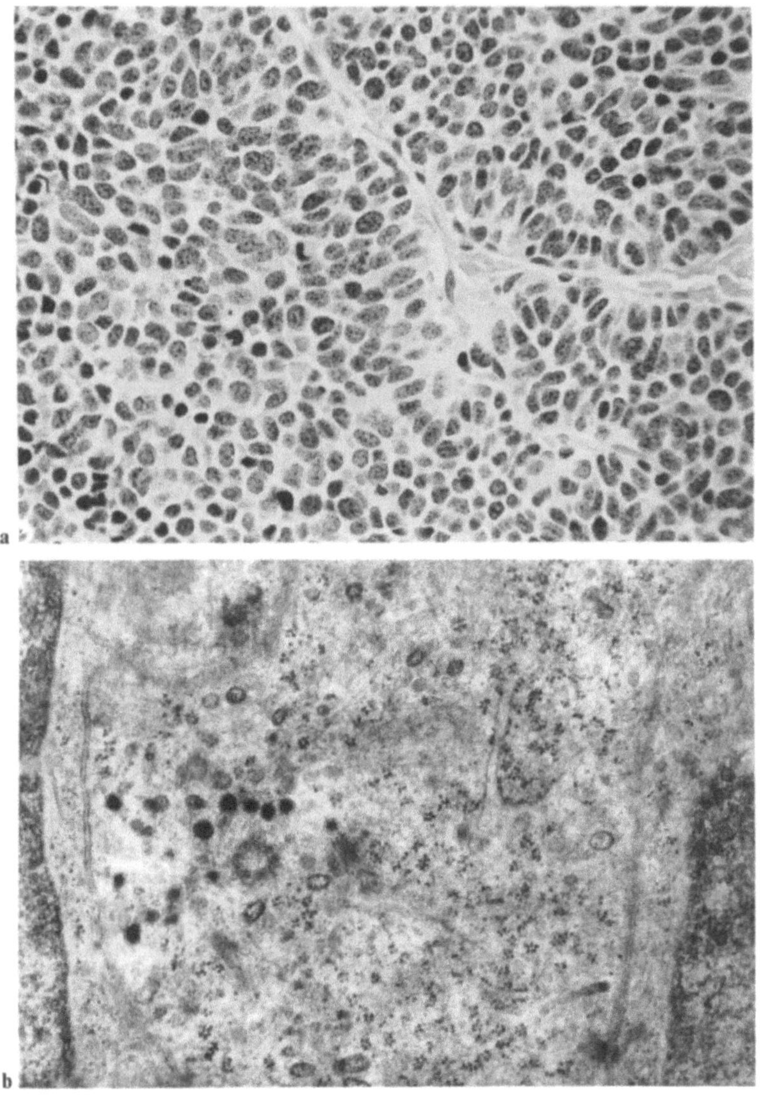

Fig. 2. a Small cell carcinoma (histology), ×240. **b** Small cell carcinoma (EM), ×27600.
c Small cell carcinoma (cytology), ×1024

4. The arrangement of the cells may vary. In some instances neoplastic cells may
   be stratified or arranged in streams or ribbons along the fibrous stroma. Sometimes the cells cuff thin-walled blood vessels, forming a perivascular mantle
   (pseudorosettes).

   Occasionally neoplastic cells form lumina without polarization of nuclei (rosettes), or cuboidal or low columnar cells may form true tubules. The lumina may
sometimes contain scanty mucin production. In a small percentage of small cell

42

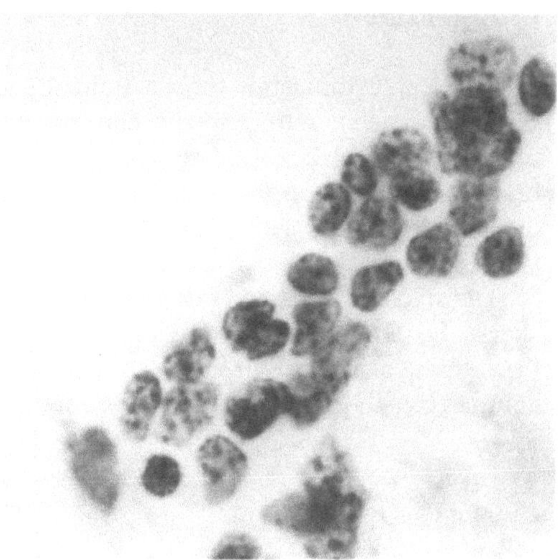

Fig. 2 c

carcinoma of the lung a few discrete foci of squamous differentiation or multi-nucleated giant cells may be identified.

Morphologic subtypes:

Small cell carcinoma is subtyped into three categories:

1. Oat cell carcinoma
2. Intermediate type
3. Combined small cell

Oat Cell Type

This subtype corresponds to the previous "lymphocyte-like" cell type in the WHO classification. The classical oat cells are small cells, round or oval in shape, and arranged in grape-like clusters. The nuclei are dense, hyperchromatic, and devoid of distinguishable characteristics.

Intermediate Subtype

This consists of polygonal/fusiform cells larger than the oat cells with a clearly demonstrable chromatin pattern ("salt and pepper"). Rare prominent acidophilic nucleoli can be demonstrated in these cells. A small cell tumor mixed with large cell elements is categorized as an intermediate subtype of small cell cancer.

Combined Small Cell Carcinoma

As mentioned above some individual foci of malignant squamous cell epithelium and/or glandular structures are included as basal characteristics of a small cell cancer and should not alter a diagnosis of oat cell or intermediate subtype. However, if the structures are consistently found from field to field within the tumor it is classified as a "combined small cell carcinoma."

Ultrastructure

The nuclear/cytoplasmic ratio is typically high in small cell cancer, the profile of the nucleus is smooth, and the chromatin shows minimal clumping in well-preserved areas. The scanty cytoplasm contains few organelles. Adjacent cell membranes are closely opposed and are united by cell junctions that range from focal densities to small, well-formed desmosomes with short tonofilament bundles (Fig.2b).

Dense-core neurosecretory granules are often present but are small and often sparse. In some small cell lung cancers cytoplasmic granules cannot be found, but their absence does not preclude the diagnosis. The granules are smaller and fewer compared with granules found in bronchial carcinoids.

Cytology

The cells make clusters when present in sputum and because of the sparse cytoplasm nuclear molding can often be seen in the adjacent cells. The nuclear characteristics are described above (Fig.2c).

Adenocarcinoma

Definition

A primary malignant tumor with tubular, acinar or papillary growth pattern and/or mucus production.

Pathogenesis

Adenocarcinomas arise from the epithelium of the bronchi and are usually peripherally located. Scar cancers, containing abundant elastic fibers, are often adenocarcinomas.

Histopathologic Classification

1. Acinar adenocarcinoma   Well differentiated
   moderately differentiated
   poorly differentiated
2. Papillary adenocarcinoma   Well differentiated
   moderately differentiated
   poorly differentiated
3. Bronchiolo-alveolar carcinoma
4. Solid carcinoma with mucus formation

Acinar Adenocarcinoma

This subtype presents with a predominance of glandular structures, i.e., acini and tubules with or without papillary or solid areas. Grading by degree of differentiation may be carried out for this subtype (Fig. 3a).

Papillary Adenocarcinoma

Subtype with predominance of papillary structures. Grading by degree of differentiation may be used also for this subtype. The cells tend to be arranged in three-dimensional clusters with communal borders. When psammoma bodies occur in pulmonary adenocarcinomas they most often occur in this subtype.

Bronchiolo-alveolar Carcinoma

An adenocarcinoma in which cylindrical tumor cells grow upon the walls of preexisting alveoli. Separation of papillary from bronchiolo-alveolar carcinoma is especially difficult. Generally the cells of papillary adenocarcinomas are more pleomorphic and anaplastic than those of bronchiolo-alveolar carcinoma.

Solid Carcinoma with Mucus Production

A poorly differentiated adenocarcinoma lacking acini, tubulus and papillae, but with intracytoplasmatic mucin in many tumor cells.

This subtype is characterized by cells having large nuclei, prominent nucleoli, abundant cytoplasm and a compact growth pattern. *Mucin stains* are essential to distinguish these tumors from large cell carcinoma.

Ultrastructure

The adenocarcinoma cells are characterized by canaliculi between the cells, microvilli, and intracytoplasmic secretory granules (Fig. 3b).

Cytology

The tumor cells are usually large with abundant cytoplasm frequently containing mucus vacuoles. Usually the nuclei are large and clear with prominent eosinophilic nucleoli. The nuclei rarely show distinct hyperchromasia and jagged angles characteristic of nuclei of squamous cell carcinoma. Individual cells tend to adhere and form groups or sheets, and sometimes they form acini and central lumina with or without mucin (Fig. 3c).

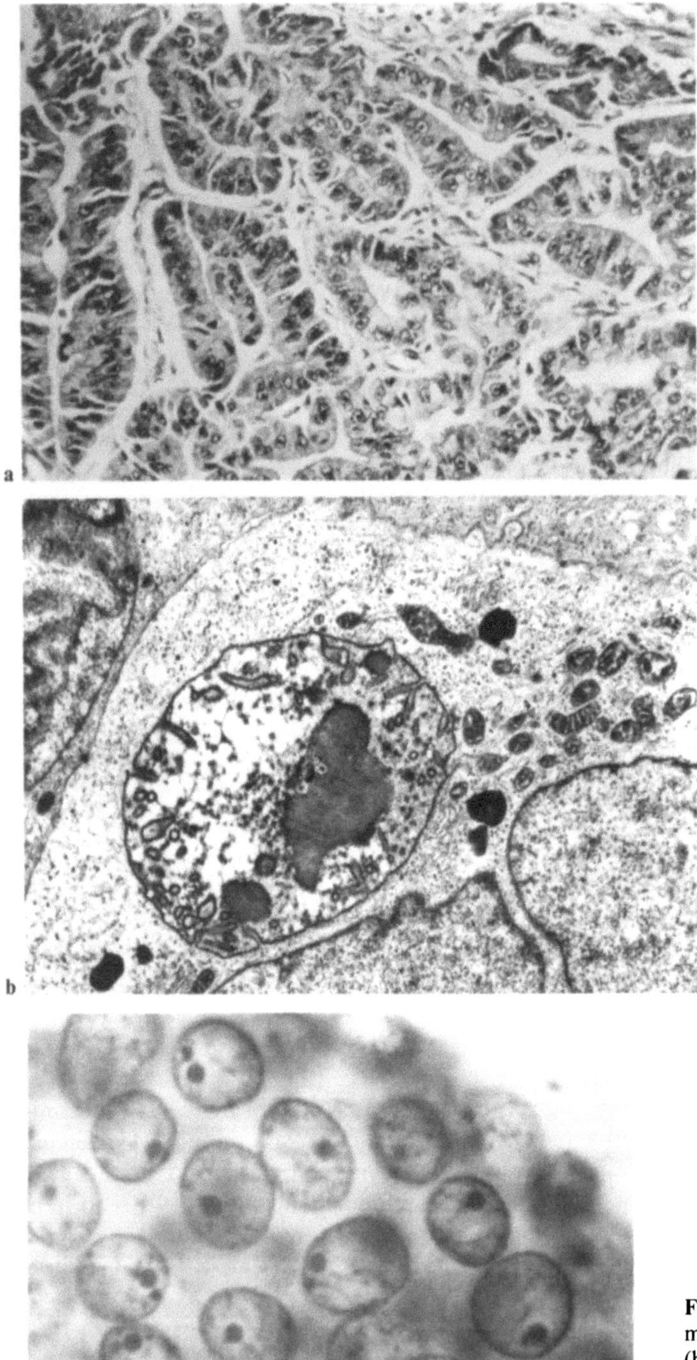

Fig. 3. **a** Adenocarcinoma, well differentiated (histology), ×156. **b** Adenocarcinoma (EM), ×6630. **c** Adenocarcinoma (cytology), ×1560

Large Cell Carcinoma

Definitions

A malignant epithelial tumor with large nuclei, prominent nucleoli, abundant cytoplasm, and usually well defined cell borders, without the characteristic features of squamous cell, small cell, or adenocarcinomas (Fig. 4a).

Pathogenesis

The majority of the tumors classified as large cell carcinoma by light microscopy demonstrate features of adeno- or squamous cell carcinoma when examined ultrastructurally. This could indicate that at least some of these tumors are merely undifferentiated variations of the other types, rather than independent entities.

Histopathologic Classification

Three subtypes of large cell carcinoma are defined:

1. Solid carcinoma *without* mucin production
2. Giant cell carcinoma
3. Clear cell carcinoma

The large cell carcinoma is composed of large polygonal, spindle, or oval cells with abundant cytoplasm. The diagnosis is often made by the exclusion of the other cell types.

Solid Carcinoma Without Mucin

The cells often grow in sheets without organization or desmoplastic reaction. There are large nuclei with prominent nucleoli. The cytoplasm is abundant and often slightly eosinophilic and has well-defined borders without mucus or evidence of keratinization.

Giant Cell Carcinoma

The individual cells may have giant nuclei or may form syncytial multinucleated giant cells. The tumor cells may be extremely bizarre and may appear to contain neutrophil leukocytes in the extraordinary quantities of cytoplasm.

Clear Cell Carcinoma

This variant of large cell carcinoma is composed of elements with clear and foamy cytoplasm without mucin. They may or may not contain glycogen. The large cell carcinoma does not demonstrate any specific growth pattern. The cells tend to be arranged in small nests, clusters, or stratifying sheets. Sometimes the cells grow in an adenomatous fashion.

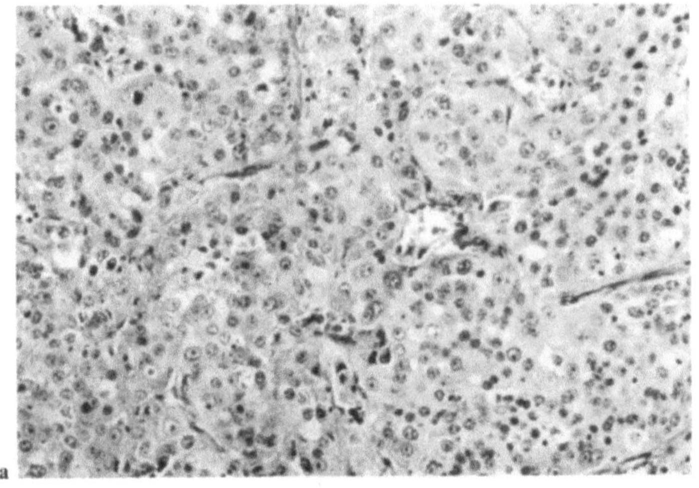

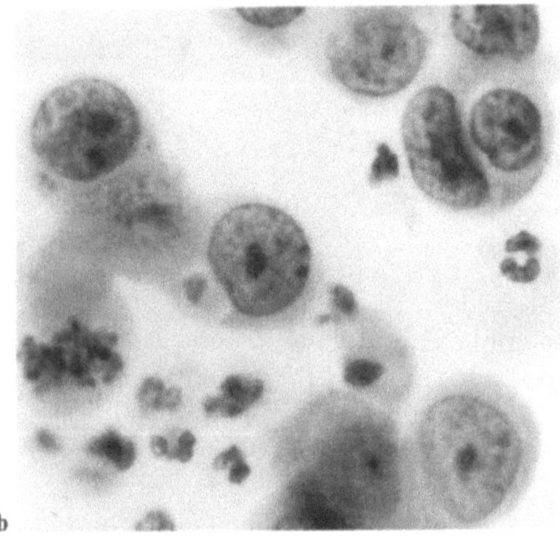

Fig. 4. a Large cell carcinoma (histology), ×154. **b** Large cell carcinoma (EM), ×16940. **c** Large cell carcinoma (cytology), ×1540

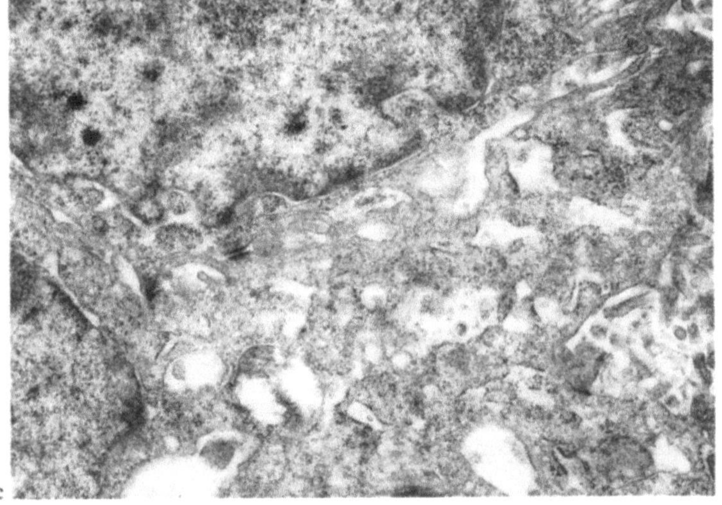

Ultrastructure

It is well recognized that squamous cell carcinomas and adenocarcinomas of the lung, as they dedifferentiate, lose their specific ultrastructural features. Accordingly, a tumor having reached this stage can no longer be subclassified in either category, and at this point the tumor is often called undifferentiated large cell carcinoma. The nucleus is fine and dispersed, and there are moderate to prominent nucleoli. The cells are closely apposed and united by small cell junctions with sparse tonofilaments. Traces of differentiation with microvilli are sometimes seen ultrastructurally but they cannot be seen by light microscopy.

A mixture of large cell and small cell carcinoma is reported in about 10% of small cell lung cancers at presentation, with a considerably increased frequency following cytotoxic treatment (Fig. 4b).

Cytology

Sputum and bronchial washings or brushings of these tumors are frequently interpreted as adenocarcinomas because of the prominent nucleoli present in the neoplastic cells. The individual cells are large polygonal, spindle, or oval with abundant cytoplasm with a large irregular pleomorphic nucleus. Intracytoplasmic hyalin droplets or glycogen may be present. A few isolated cells containing mucin may also be present.

Large cell carcinomas are most frequently diagnosed by needle or surgical lung biopsy or by regional lymph node biopsy. Diagnostic discrepancies occur in bronchial biopsies if representative portions of the tumor are not sampled. Thus, a poorly differentiated adenocarcinoma or squamous cell carcinoma may be interpreted as large cell carcinoma if only undifferentiated portions of a tumor have been biopsied.

A major portion of each tumor categorized as moderately and poorly differentiated squamous cell carcinoma and adenocarcinoma comprises undifferentiated large cell carcinoma cells. When differentiated features are observed the carcinoma can be placed appropriately in either the squamous cell or the adenocarcinoma category. When no specific differentiating features are observed the carcinoma should be classified as a large cell carcinoma.

Giant cells and clear cells are frequently seen also as components of adenocarcinoma and squamous cell carcinoma. Likewise, syncytial multinucleated giant cells are occasionally seen in small cell carcinoma prior to treatment and especially after treatment. Thus, the final classification of these tumors must be based on the possible occurrence of the other features of squamous, adeno-, or small cell carcinoma.

Bronchial Carcinoids

Definition

A low-grade malignant tumor whose cells show the biochemical and ultrastructural features characteristic of both normal cells and tumors of the amine precursor uptake and decarboxylation (APUD) system.

Pathogenesis

Today it is well established that the carcinoids have certain properties in common with other cells in various organs, i.e., (a) the presence of fluorogenic amines and/or the ability to take up amine precursors, (b) the presence within the cells of an aminodecarboxylase, and (c) the presence of specific neurosecretory granules. These features constitute the APUD characteristics. The prevailing hypothesis that these endocrine cells are derived from the neural crest is now being questioned and it is maybe just as conceivable that these tumors are developed from endodermal derived epithelial cells like the other main types of lung cancer.

The majority of bronchial carcinoids are centrally located in the main, lobar, or segmental bronchi, and only 10–15% of the tumors occur in subsegmental and peripheral locations. Dependent upon the location of the tumor within the lung and certain other factors which will be described below, the carcinoids have been regarded by some as consisting of three variants:

1. Central carcinoids
2. Peripheral carcinoids
3. Atypical carcinoids

Central Carcinoid Tumors

These tumors constitute about 90% of all bronchial carcinoids. They typically grow as a polypoid exophytic lesion projecting into the lumen of the bronchus. The overlying mucosa may show changes of squamous metaplasia, but is generally intact. This might explain the low diagnostic yield of exfoliative cytology. The presence of focal mucin within the central carcinoids might together with the intact surface suggest that the tumor originates from the bronchial glands.

Microscopically the cells are arranged in a trabecular or ribbon-like pattern, but quite often also in a mosaic pattern of solid sheets. The cells are uniform with abundant clear or lightly eosinophilic cytoplasm with a granular appearance.

The nuclei are ovoid with a well-defined nuclear membrane and a somewhat vesicular chromatin pattern. Nucleoli are not prominent, and there is a striking uniformity in the cellular appearance. Necrosis, hemorrhage, and mitoses are unusual findings in the classic bronchial carcinoid.

Occasionally mucin or acinar formation are demonstrated. Argyrophilic stains such as Grimelius often demonstrate numerous granules in the cytoplasm, while positive argentaffin stains such as Fontana-Masson stain, are infrequent.

50

Peripheral Carcinoids

The histologic appearance of the peripherally located carcinoids is more variable than that of the centrally located tumors, primarily due to the frequent occurrence of a spindle cell component and the disorderly pattern of the cells.

In tumors with predominance of spindle cell component the tumor might be difficult to separate from the appearance of a mesenchymal tumor. However, the carcinoid cells still retain the typical feature with a slightly eosinophilic cytoplasm, infrequent mitosis (although more frequent than in the central ones), often appreciated organoid growth pattern, positive silver stain, and specific ultrastructural features.

Atypical Carcinoids

An unusual form of bronchial carcinoids is the so-called atypical carcinoid. This particular variety shows increased cellularity, nuclear pleomorphism, increased mitotic activity, and foci of necrosis. These features are generally not associated with carcinoid tumors and can be difficult to distinguish morphologically from a small cell carcinoma of the lung. Since the small cell carcinoma may show a growth pattern similar to that of carcinoids, the individual cell characteristics might be of diagnostic use. The cells of the atypical carcinoid consistently have more abundant cytoplasm and less-marked nuclear abnormality than the small cell tumors.

Ultrastructure

The tumor cells are round with a centrally located nucleus. Adjacent cells are in general closely apposed with few interdigitations of the cell membranes and united by small desmosomes, and bundles of cytoplasmic filaments are associated with the desmosomes. Within the cytoplasm mitochondria are present in moderate number. The most significant feature of bronchial carcinoids is the presence of dense-cored neurosecretory granules. The granules vary in size and are generally numerous, most frequently located in pseudopodal cytoplasmic extensions. The membrane-bound granules have the electron-dense core separated from the membrane by a lucent space.

Cytology

As mentioned the carcinoid cells are infrequently found in cytologic specimens. The cells contain nuclear features of evenly dispersed chromatin or in some cells more hyperchromatic nuclei. The cytoplasm is relatively abundant compared with the small cell carcinoma, which might have a similar nuclear characteristic.

Mesothelioma

Definition

Benign or malignant neoplasm arising from the pleura consisting of mesothelial or fibrous cells – or both.

Pathogenesis

A high incidence of mesothelioma is associated with occupational exposure to asbestos. As described below these tumors may be composed of fibrous and/or epithelial (mesothelial) components. It is likely that this fact reflects the development of tumor components from the surface (mesothelial component) and from the connective tissue (fibrous component). Asbestos has been associated with the diffuse malignant usually mesothelial type of mesotheliomas rather than the localized benign fibrous type.

Classification

The mesotheliomas are classified based on both gross pathology and on histology.

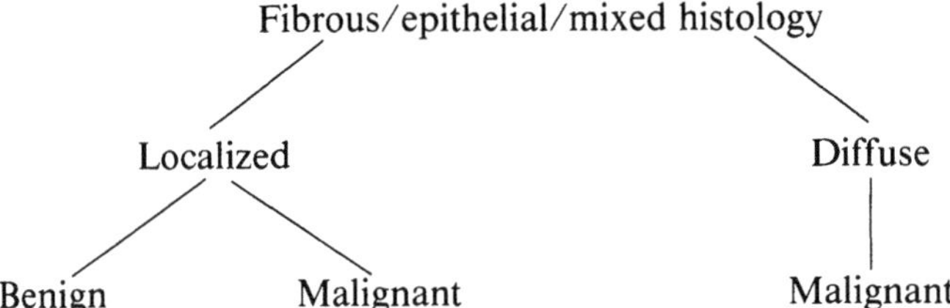

Localized Mesothelioma

These tumors are nearly all of fibrous (spindle cell) type and mostly benign. Malignant localized mesotheliomas are very rare and are typically of the fibrous type.

Diffuse Mesothelioma

These tumors are malignant and involve parietal and visceral surfaces. The histologic appearance varies a great deal. The majority of the tumors are biphasic, i.e., with mixed epithelial/mesenchymal configuration. The epithelial cells may be arranged in a papillary, tubular, cord-like, or sheet-like fashion. The cells often grow in a myxoid stroma. Nuclear appearances vary from those typical of mesothelial cells to highly anaplastic pleomorphic giant cells. They must be distinguished from: (a) reactive mesothelium or (b) adenocarcinoma.

The ability of mesothelial cells to produce hyaluronic acid which is not produced by carcinomas has been used to separate mesothelioma cells from carcinoma cells. Hyaluronic acid can be demonstrated in the tumor and pleural effusions as well. However, the absence of "hyaluronic acid-positive" cells in the pleural effusions cannot exclude the possibility of a mesothelioma. The prescence of strong intracytoplasmic mucicarminophilic or PAS-positive, diastase-resistant material indicates that the neoplasm is probably an adenocarcinoma involving pleura and not a mesothelioma.

Ultrastructure

The characteristic feature of mesothelial cells is the presence of numerous microvilli. They are typically profuse, long, slender, and branching. In most well-differentiated tumors the microvilli may project into acinus-like spaces. With dedifferentiation the cells lose cohesion and polarity, and there is a tendency for microvilli to cover the free surfaces of the cells, resembling the appearance of an adenocarcinoma. Furthermore the cells contain junctional structures, tonofilaments, glycogen granules, and intracellular vacuoles which do not contain mucin.

Cytology

Mesotheliomas shed cells into the pleural fluid in papillary fragments, and loose groups of cells with irregular outside borders corresponding to their long microvilli can be seen by electron microscopy. The nuclear configuration does not demonstrate any specific features compared with other neoplastic cells. The cytoplasm is finely vacuolated in a lace-like fashion. It might be of differential diagnostic value that mesotheliomas rarely shed cells in sputum in contrast to peripheral bronchogenic carcinomas.

Further Reading

Carter D, Eggleston JC (1980) Tumors of the lower respiratory tract. Atlas of tumor pathology. Fascile 17, Armed Forces Institute of Pathology, Washington DC
World Health Organization (1981) Histological typing of lung tumors. 2nd edn Geneva

6. Clinical Features

S. G. Spiro and M. Rørth

The clinical features of lung cancer can be divided into three parts:

1. Intrathoracic (local) symptoms
2. Extrathoracic (metastatic) symptoms
3. Paraneoplastic syndromes

Intrathoracic Symptoms (Table 1)

The intrathoracic manifestations depend on the size and location of the primary tumor. At diagnosis most of the squamous and small cell tumors will be located centrally, while adenocarcinoma tends to present more peripherally.

Coughing is the most frequent primary symptom, being present in 75% of patients. The cough is often unproductive in the early phases. It can be associated with an influenza-like illness or a pneumonia distal to obstruction caused by the tumor. Many patients are heavy smokers, with long-standing symptoms of chronic bronchitis, and thus will have a chronic cough. In such cases, a change in the cough pattern will be an important observation.

Hemoptysis affects 50%–70% of patients, and can be the initial symptom. Even a single occurrence of hemoptysis in a person who has smoked for many years should be investigated.

Chest pain is present in 40% of patients with peripheral tumors, usually adenocarcinoma and large cell carcinoma. It may be caused by pleural or chest wall invasion, but frequently is nothing more than a vague discomfort on the same side as the lesion.

Wheeze and stridor is caused by a tumor narrowing a main airway and therefore is a symptom of the centrally located primary tumor.

Dyspnea is prevalent in more advanced cases and in the multifocal type of bronchioloalveolar carcinoma. However, it can be an early symptom when tumor is superimposed on emphysema. The dyspnea often seems disproportionate to the radiological changes, but ventilation/perfusion scans can show considerable disturbances in perfusion, apparently often caused by a small tumor directly affecting pulmonary blood flow.

Superior vena caval obstruction is caused by extension of the tumor into the mediastinum or by enlarged lymph nodes, usually the right paratracheal chain. It can lead to venous distension on the upper chest wall, shoulders, neck, and face. Mild

Table 1. Clinical features in patients with lung cancer

1. *Thoracic*	Primary tumor
	Cough
	Tightness
	Obstructive dyspnea
	Hemoptysis
	Wheeze
	Intrathoracic spread
	Vascular obstruction
	Superior vena cava syndrome
	(distension of vein, edema)
	Affection of nerves
	Hoarseness (recurrent nerves)
	Dysphagia
	Dyspnea
	Hemidiaphragmatic elevation (phrenic nerves)
	Esophageal compression
	Dysphagia
	Pericardial invasion
	Arrhythmia
	Tamponade
	Cardiac failure
	Lymphatic obstruction
	Dyspnea (effusion)
	Chest wall pain
2. *Extrathoracic*	Lymph nodes
	CNS
	Neurological disorders
	Pain
	Bone/Bone marrow
	Pain
	Anemia
	Bleeding
	Liver
	Pain
	Jaundice
	Fever

to massive edema of the face, neck, and upper thorax can be present. It is most frequently associated with small cell carcinoma. The patient may complain of difficulty in breathing, stridor, dysphagia, blackouts, and severe headaches or coughing. The condition is a medical emergency and requires immediate treatment. Chemotherapy should be used when small cell lung cancer is known or suspected. Radiotherapy is the treatment of choice in non-small cell lung cancer.

Nerve Entrapments

Central tumors can affect the recurrent laryngeal nerve, especially on the left side where the intrathoracic course of this nerve is longer. It can lead to paralysis of the vocal cords with associated hoarseness and a nonexplosive cough. Bronchoscopy will show an immobile abducted vocal cord, and physical examination often reveals absence of, or paradoxical diaphragmatic excursions. The paralysis will significantly worsen the dyspnea in the affected patients. Paravertebral extension can involve the cervical sympathetic nerve and give rise to *Horner's syndrome* (small pupil, ptosis, enophthalmus, and absence of thermal sweating on that half of the face).

Esophagus

Compression and/or invasion of the esophagus leads to dysphagia and sometimes to aspiration, especially if a bronchoesophageal fistule has developed. This can be a serious clinical problem necessitating immediate therapeutic action. It is commonest in small cell lung cancer (SCLC).

Pleura and Chest Wall

Invasion of pleura and chest wall lead to chest *pain*. This symptom is related to peripheral tumors and the pain can be located at any place in the thoracic wall. A typical clinical picture *(Pancoast syndrome)* is associated with tumor extension in the apex of the lung involving the eighth cervical and the first thoracic nerve, the first few ribs, and sometimes sympathetic nerves. Such a patient will typically have pain with extension to the ulnar nerve innervated portion of the arm and sometimes also present with a Horner's syndrome.

Heart and Pericardium

Pericardial invasion may in a few cases lead to cardiac tamponade. Pericardial invasion can also be associated with arrhythmia, or signs of cardiac failure or pericarditis. Often, the early physical signs are rather discrete and pericardial involvement should always be suspected if chest X-ray reveals an increased diameter of the heart. Echocardiography is a very useful diagnostic procedure in such cases.

Lymphatic Vessels

Obstruction of lymphatic vessels and also direct involvement of the pleura may lead to formation of pleural effusion. Clinically, this will lead to obstructive dyspnea.

Extrathoracic Metastatic Symptoms

The common sites of extrathoracic metastatic spread are to the lymph nodes, brain, bones, liver, and suprarenal glands (Table 1).

Lymph Nodes

After spread to the hilum and mediastinal lymph nodes, the commonest lymph nodes to be subsequently involved are the scalene nodes and the glands in the supraclavicular fossi. The neck should be very carefully palpated in every new case of lung cancer. If there is no other site to biopsy, or if it is intended to eliminate the patient from surgery on the grounds of an enlarged lymph node, this can be investigated by needle aspiration cytology. A syringe has its dead space filled with normal saline, and a large (No. 1) needle is attached to the syringe and inserted into the lymph node. Strong suction is then applied and the needle withdrawn and the fluid smeared directly onto a glass slide and fixed immediately. An alternative technique would be to biopsy the lymph node.

Central Nervous System

Cerebral metastases almost always present with neurological symptoms, the commonest symptoms being confusion or signs of a posterior fossa lesion such as inability to walk straight. This is exaggerated if the patient is asked to heel-toe walk. However, any change in neurological status should be investigated with a computed tomography brain scan. Intracranial metastases account for up to 20% of extrathoracic presentations. They must also be suspected in patients with unexplained headaches or personality changes.

Bone Metastases – Bone Marrow

As in the case of epidural metastases, *pain* is the characteristic feature of bone metastases. Bone metastases with clinical symptoms are often found in patients with non-small cell carcinoma, while patients with small cell carcinoma typically have involvement of bone marrow. Bone marrow involvement is generally without clinical symptoms unless the impairment of the production of blood elements is so pronounced that bleeding due to thrombocytopenia and signs of anemia occur. For detection of bone metastases the isotope bone scan is more sensitive than X-rays and the alkaline phosphatase.

Epidural osseous metastases can lead to spinal cord compressing. It is most often located in the thoracic vertebrae, and the principal symptom is pain followed by paralysis of the lower extremities and autonomic functions. Early diagnosis is a necessary condition for a reasonable outcome of treatment.

Liver

More than 25% of patients with small cell carcinoma have liver involvement. Clinically, this can be associated with jaundice and hypochondrial pain. Most often it is, however, not associated with typical clinical symptoms.

Hepatic metastases are suspected either by abnormal liver function tests or by a palpable liver, sometimes with an irregular firm margin. If liver function tests are found to be abnormal, then the liver should be studied with ultrasound techniques, or CT scan, and other causes of abnormal liver function tests should be eliminated. If no other cause for abnormal liver function is found, it should be assumed that the abnormality is due to malignant disease.

Other organs, like the *adrenal* glands and *pancreas,* are often involved when the dissemination of small cell carcinoma is manifest. Clinically, these organs do, however, nearly always preserve their functional ability, and endocrine dysfunction due to direct tumor involvement is extremely rare. Finally, *cutaneous* tumor infiltrates are sometimes seen, especially in small cell carcinoma.

Nonspecific symptoms, such as weight loss, anorexia, and malaise, are associated with a poor prognosis and are often present in conjunction with occult metastases. Bone marrow aspirations and trephine biopsy may also be abnormal in 10%–40% of patients with small cell carcinomas.

Paraneoplastic Manifestations (Table 2)

General

Anorexia and weight loss, weakness, and fatigue are all unspecific symptoms found in patients with bronchogenic carcinoma. As will be discussed later, these manifestations of the disease are of considerable prognostic importance. In general, their cause is unknown. They are conceivably related to production of unknown substances in the tumor. Low-grade fever can also be seen, especially in association with liver involvement.

Neurological Symptoms

Symptoms of neuromuscular origin in patients with lung cancer can be very difficult to interpret, but since these symptoms quite often lead to severe disability, their recognition and possible treatment is of extreme importance. The paraneoplastic symptoms are typically dispersed and bilateral in contrast to the symptoms caused by metastatic lesions in the central nervous system.

Cerebral affection with encephalopatia is characterized by a varying degree of dementia or psychosis. Cerebellar cortical degeneration affects the ability to use the extremities, typically leading to gait disturbances and coordination problems.

Peripheral neuropathy is of sensory nature or combined motor-sensory, never purely motory. Pain and paresthesia are typical clinical manifestations. The causes of these affections of the neurological system are unknown.

Table 2. Paraneoplastic syndromes in lung cancer

1. General	Anorexia
	Weight loss
	Fatigue
	(fever)
2. Neurological	Cortical cerebral atrophy
	Dementia
	Psychic disturbances
	Cortical cerebellar dysfunction
	Gait disturbances
	Dyscoordination
	Peripheral neuropathy
	Pain
	Paresthesia
3. Hypertropic pulmonary osteoarthropathy	Clubbing
	Swelling
	Tenderness
4. Collagen disease (dermatomyositis)	Weakness
	Fatigue
5. Nephrotic syndrome	
6. Coagulation disorders	Thrombotic phenomenons
	Bleeding disorders
7. Myasthenia	Lambert Eaton Syndrome
8. Endocrinological	Hypercalcemia
	Inappropriate secretion of ADH
	Ectopic ACTH/Cushing's syndrome

Hypertrophic Pulmonary Osteoarthropathy

This peculiar paraneoplastic phenomenon occurs in more than 10% of patients with adenocarcinoma of the lung, less frequently with the other cell types. The dominant feature is periostitis of the long bones and clubbing of fingers and toes. Pain, tenderness, and swelling are the symptoms associated with these lesions.

Collagenosis

So-called autoimmune disorders are sometimes associated with malignant disease. *Dermatomyositis* is the most typical example of this. This disease is thought to be caused by immunocomplexes affecting different organs, but the detailed nature of the pathogenesis is still unknown. Dermatomyositis is seen in association with several types of malignancies including lung cancer.

Coagulation Disorders

For unknown reasons, many neoplastic disorders can be accompanied by formation of venous thrombi. These can be migrating and multiple, often involving areas in which no obvious physical reason (tumor presence) for a thrombosis is found. Treatment is difficult, and anticoagulation with anti-vitamin K is often inefficient.

The clinical presentation can be difficult or impossible to distinguish from symptoms caused by metastatic lesions. Malfunction of the complex system of coagulation factors and the balance between these and the thrombolytic systems can also lead to bleeding disorders (e.g., disseminated intravascular coagulation). The cause of these disorders is unknown. No specific relation to any of the subtypes of bronchogenic carcinoma has been found.

Myasthenic Syndrome (Lambert Eaton)

This syndrome is characterized by proximal muscle weakness and fatigue, most pronounced in the pelvic girdle and thigh. In contrast to myasthenia gravis, muscle strength improves with exercise. The syndrome is uncommon (less than 1% of all lung cancer patients) and is nearly always associated with small cell histology.

Endocrine Paraneoplastic Syndromes

Hypercalcemia

Neoplastic disease is the most common cause of hypercalcemia. Hypercalcemia may be seen in patients with solid tumors with bone metastases, but in more than 20% of the cases clinically demonstrable skeletal metastases are absent. One of the major causes of hypercalcemia among the malignancies is bronchogenic carcinoma, especially of the squamous cell type, and also sometimes of the large cell type, while hypercalcemia is uncommon in small cell.

The hypercalcemia without apparent bone involvement is thought to be caused by production in the tumor of humoral substances affecting the breakdown of mineral tissue. The clinical presentation is characterized by neurological symptoms like fatigue, muscle weakness, apathy, disturbances of perception and behavior, and sometimes stupor and coma.

Renal symptoms include polydypsia and renal insufficiency. Furthermore, gastrointestinal symptoms like anorexia, nausea, vomiting, and abdominal pain can be seen.

Hypercalcemia of malignant origin is often characterized by a comparatively insidious onset and, in contrast to cases with hypercalcemia of nonmalignant origin, renal calculi and pancreatitis are seldom seen.

Syndrome of Inappropriate Secretion of Antidiuretic Hormone (SIADH)

The association of hyponatremia and water intoxication with lung cancer was noted in the late 1930s. The syndrome is nearly exclusively (more than 90%) found in patients with small cell carcinoma of the bronchus. Of these patients, 8%–10% develop SIADH with hyponatremia.

The syndrome is due to production in the tumor of ADH or ADH-like substances. The clinical symptoms stem from the water intoxication with hypo-osmolality and hyponatremia, and is characterized by altered mental status, confusion, seizures, and, occasionally, coma.

SIADH has been described to be caused by infections like tuberculosis, and by drugs like cyclophosphamide and vincristine. It is thus important to rule out such conditions before ascribing the etiology to the neoplastic disease. On the other hand, the diagnosis of SIADH in a patient should be followed by a careful search for a tumor of small cell type.

Ectopic Cushing's Syndrome

Small cell carcinomas quite often produce peptide hormones or precursors of such hormones. One of the best-described consequences of this feature is the production of ectopic ACTH. This eventually can lead clinically to so-called Cushing's syndrome. While ACTH production is a rather common phenomenon, clinical signs of hypercorticosteroidism are quite rare. The syndrome is characterized by hypokalemia, hyperglycemia (sometimes requiring insulin), edema, hypertension, and muscle weakness. The "classical" features of Cushing's syndrome, with centripetal obesity, moon face, etc., are very uncommon, probably due to the rapid onset and development of the syndrome, when caused by a malignant disorder. Of the patients who present with Cushing's syndrome, 15%–20% will be found to have a tumor with ectopic ACTH production.

7. Diagnostic Procedures

H. H. Hansen and S. G. Spiro

The Lung

Radiology

Radiological assessment is the cornerstone of the beginning of the diagnosis of malignant disease as it is usually the primary abnormality detected. The plain chest radiograph is the basic tool in the diagnosis and management of patients with lung cancer. There are only a few incidences in which the diagnosis is made and a normal radiograph is obtained.

Detection of lung tumors involves typically two distinct types of patients. Firstly, asymptomatic individuals in which an infiltrate is detected in a screening procedure. The screening procedure can be undertaken as: (a) mass screening for lung cancer of high-risk groups (e.g., male smokers > 45 years), (b) part of a diagnostic workup in general, or (c) from a preoperative evaluation of lung and heart. In such cases, the lesions detected will typically be located in the peripheral lung tissue (more than 50%), while central abnormalities such as increased perihilar density will be indicative of a lung tumor in about 30%. The smallest infiltrate which can be detected by this method is generally about 1 cm in diameter (corresponding to 10^9 tumor cells). In retrospect, however, it is sometimes possible to detect smaller tumors, which initially were overlooked.

With respect to screening, 61% of lung tumors detected by screening were found by X-ray, compared with 19% by sputum cytology in the program of the Mayo Clinic. X-ray screening typically detects peripheral tumors (adenocarcinoma) and sputum cytology central tumors (squamous cell carcinoma). It should be noted that even extensive screening procedures apparently only detect less than 10% of asymptomatic cases of lung cancer.

The radiological picture is typically determined by the extent and location of the tumor itself, and the cause of the radiographic abnormality is not only due to the primary lesion, but also to regional spread and to intrathoracic metastases. The radiological picture reveals some characteristics according to cell type, even though there is a great deal of overlapping. The radiological picture can be indicative for a certain histological type of lung tumor, but a confirmation based on histology of a biopsy, or excised tumor, is always necessary.

A schematic presentation of the characteristics of the different types is given below and in Table 1.

Table 1. Chest X-ray pattern according to histology

	Squamous cell carcinoma	Small cell	Adeno-carcinoma[a]	Large cell
Hilar or perihilar mass	40%	78%	17%	32%
Parenchymal lesion				
<4.0 cm	9%	21%	45%	18%
>4.0 cm	19%	8%	26%	41%
Obstruction, pneumonitis, collapse, or constriction	53%	38%	25%	33%
Peripleural location	31%	32%	74%	65%
Mediastinal enlargement	2%	13%	3%	10%

[a] Bronchioloalveolar carcinomas often have a characteristic appearance with multiple bilateral pulmonary nodules

1. Squamous cell carcinoma is characterized by central location with atelectasis and consolidation in more than 50% of the cases. Hilar enlargement is typical; less than one-third of the patients have peripheral lesions. The tumors are often quite large at presentation; less than one-third have a diameter of less than 4 cm. Cavitation is seen in 5%–10% of the cases, indicating tumor necrosis or lung abscess (Fig. 1).
2. Small cell carcinomas are nearly always located centrally with perihilar infiltration. Typically, one finds consolidation and infiltration peripheral to the central tumor – due to local spread. Enlargement of mediastinal lymph nodes and hilar enlargement is seen more often in this type when compared with other cell types. When peripheral lesions are present, they are often small, i.e., less than 4 cm (Fig. 2).
3. Adenocarcinomas are typically (>75%) located in the peripheral part of the lung as a mass or nodule (Fig. 3). The infiltrate can be uniform or have central lucencies, and is most often located in the upper lobes. At diagnosis, more than two-thirds of the tumors are less than 4 cm in diameter. Bronchoalveolar cell carcinoma is also located in the peripheral lung tissue, often in the vicinity of "scars." It can present itself as a solitary node, like other adenocarcinomas, as lobar infiltrates with consolidation, or as diffuse miliary nodules. The latter presentation can have similarities to tuberculosis (Fig. 4).
4. Undifferentiated large cell carcinoma is often rather big at presentation, and typically located in the lung parenchyma, but hilar and perihilar masses are also quite frequent (Fig. 5).

Carcinomas of the Trachea and Major Bronchi. These tumors can be difficult to see on a plain chest X-ray. Narrowing of the trachea or either main bronchi should be confirmed on the lateral chest X-ray projection. A lateral view should always be obtained in patients with suspected large airway lesions. Some of these patients present with symptoms and signs which are mistaken for asthma. Others complain of hemoptysis, or of bilateral recurrent chest infections.

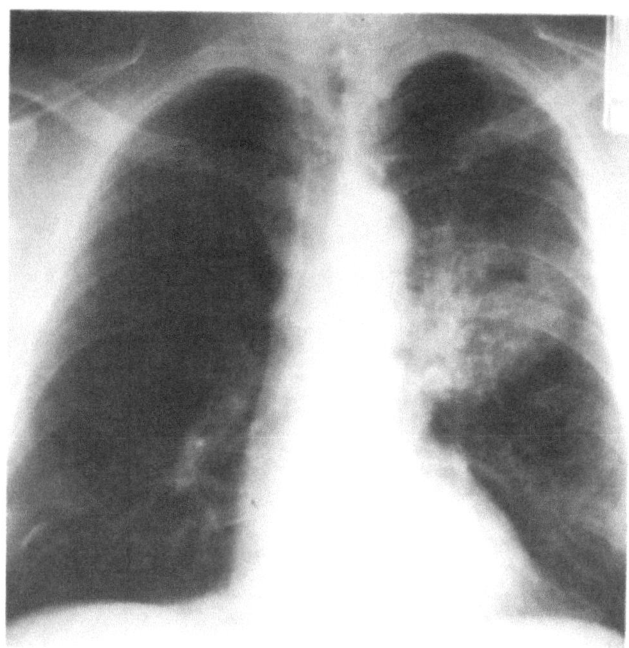

Fig. 1. Chest X-ray of squamous cell carcinoma. Note the cavitation

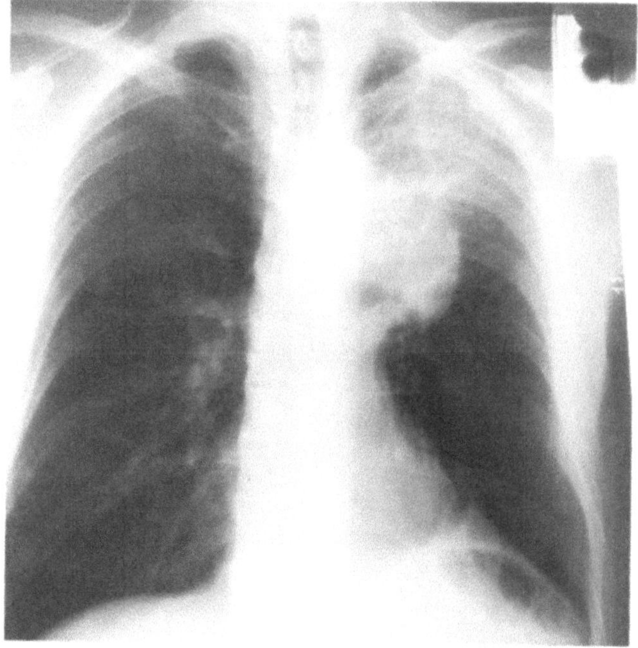

Fig. 2. Chest X-ray of small cell carcinoma

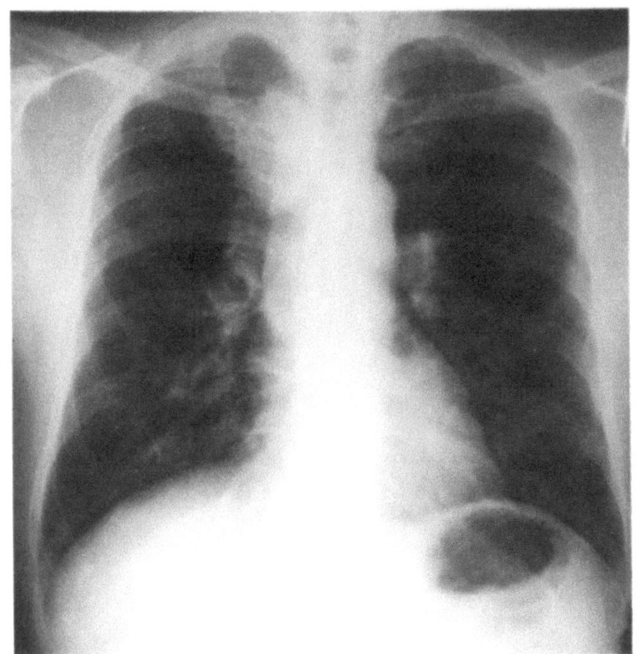

Fig. 3. Chest X-ray of adenocarcinoma

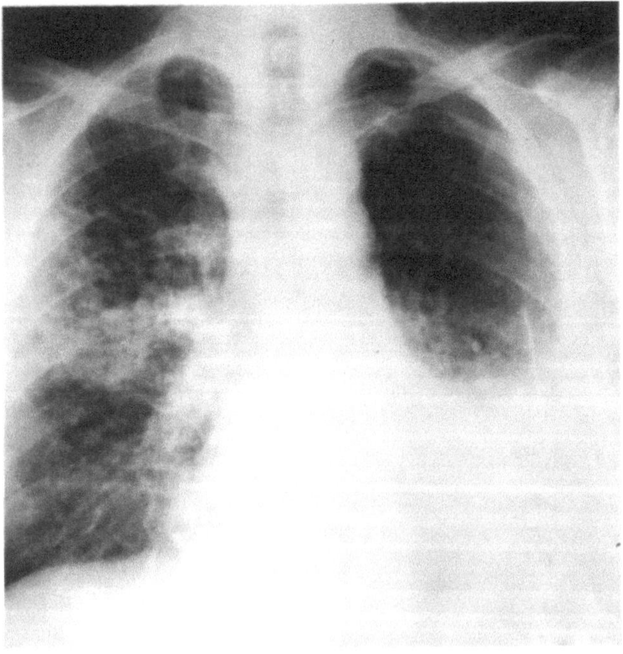

Fig. 4. Chest X-ray of alveolar cell carcinoma

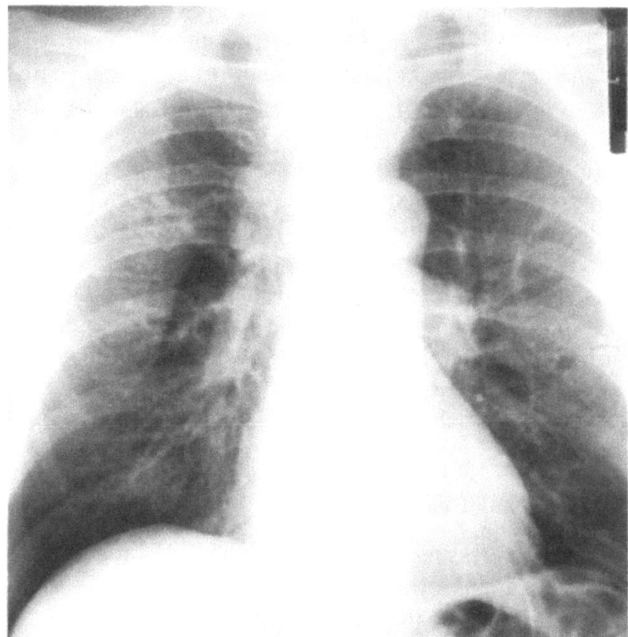

Fig.5. Chest X-ray of undifferentiated large cell carcinoma

Scar Cancer. The cancer developing in an area of tuberculous scarring can cause major diagnostic problems. It is often assumed that the fresh shadow on the chest X-ray is due to a recurrence of pulmonary tuberculosis. The symptoms may even be similar. The presence of calcification in the newly discovered lesion may also mislead the radiologist into thinking the lesion is benign.

Certain interstitial diseases, such as asbestosis and fibrosing alveolitis, are associated with a high incidence of lung cancer. When there is so much intrapulmonary disease present, it can be very difficult to appreciate the development of a new lesion such as a carcinoma. Distortion of the normal anatomy by bronchial obstruction can also be mistaken for progression of the fibrosis.

Pancoast's Tumor. Tumors in the superior sulcus, arising from the subpleural part of the apex, can be difficult to detect on a plain radiograph, even after invasion of the sympathetic nerves, brachial plexus, and ribs has occurred. They occasionally infiltrate these structures before a clear visible mass is present, and the opacification of the apex may be dismissed as being due to pleural thickening. Localized view of the ribs may show destruction, and conventional tomography may be of some assistance.

Among the rarer types, carcinoid tumors are worth mentioning. These are rather slow growing, centrally located tumors, accompanied by atelectasis, consolidation, and hilar mass.

It should be stressed that tumors with diameters of more than 1 cm still can be radiologically occult, i.e., hidden behind normal structures in the thorax. These are typically located in the proximal part of the bronchial tree.

The sensitivity of the standard X-ray of the lungs is limited, and so is the specificity. Of newly diagnosed peripheral nodules, approximately 50% will turn out to be malignant. The radiological features are not specific enough to distinguish between malignant and benign lesions. Only stability (over years) of a radiological lesion in the lung is useful as an indicator of a benign lesion. Features like calcification, often attributed to benign lesions, can also be misleading since malignant tumors may arise next to scars with calcification in granulomas. In general, all nodules should be considered as malignant lesions until otherwise proved.

Atelectasis and/or consolidation of lung tissue is a common feature of pneumonia and tumor lesions. About half of the radiologically diagnosed tumors give rise to these phenomena. In cases where pneumonia is the cause of the X-ray abnormality, a complete clearing is necessary before a diagnosis of malignant tumor can be considered to be ruled out. If the patient does not have symptoms of an infection, he/she should be investigated by bronchoscopy.

Conventional Tomography

With the increasing availability of computed tomography (CT scan), one may ask if there is a place for conventional tomography in the assessment of lung cancer. There is no doubt that it has a part to play, especially, of course, where CT scanning is not available. It is also cheaper and quicker than CT. In recent years the value of tomography has been enhanced by the use of projections in addition to the standard anteroposterior view. The lateral projection often provides much more information than the frontal view. Tomography of the hilae in the oblique position has been shown to be of great use in demonstrating the major airways, the hilar structures, and the mediastinum.

The indications for conventional tomography can be summarized as:

1. To confirm the presence of a lesion in the lung where there is doubt on the plain film
2. To localize the lesion in particular in relation to the major fissures
3. To show nodes at the hilum
4. To show nodes in the mediastinum at:
   a) The subaortic fossa
   b) Subcarinal nodes
   c) Paratracheal nodes
   d) Paraesophageal nodes
5. To demonstrate more adequately than plain X-rays the trachea, main lobar, and segmental bronchi.

Other Radiological Techniques

Computed tomography can detect nodules with a diameter of 3 mm, but the rate of false positivity at that size is in the order of 25%–60%. This means that a therapeutic measure, like surgery, should not be decided on the basis of the findings in a CT scan alone. In the future CT scan of the lungs will play a major role in the staging of lung cancer patients.

Fluoroscopy. As part of some biopsy techniques, fluoroscopy is essential. In the assessment of a high diaphragm, in which phrenic nerve paralysis is suspected, it is also important.

Barium Swallow. A barium-filled esophagus may show indentation at the mediastinal nodes. It is of particular value when the primary lesion is in one of the lower lobes.

Superior Vena Cavography. Injection of contrast medium simultaneously into both arm veins may demonstrate the site of obstruction when there is superior vena cava obstruction (SVCO), and may guide the surgeon or radiotherapist. This technique, however, is rarely used.

Bronchography. This technique has now been replaced in diagnosis by fibre optic bronchoscopy.

Pulmonary Arteriography. This has been used by some to assess the operability of carcinoma of the lung, but most would no longer find it necessary with the development of tomography, CT, and mediastinoscopy.

Ventilation/Perfusion Scanning. Again, this investigation provides little information regarding the lung cancer, although it does highlight the extent of the ventilation, or perfusion, abnormality due to the tumor compressing a large airway vein or artery.

Radioactive Gallium. Gallium 67 is taken up by carcinoma cells in the lung and in the mediastinum, but unfortunately is not specific, and inflammatory foci also take up the isotope. In the mediastinum, however, it may be expected to show the presence or absence of lymph node metastatic deposits. The absence of uptake by lymph nodes has been recommended by some as a criterion to forego mediastinoscopy, which is the usual, final staging procedure before thoracotomy. In practice, separation of the gallium 67 uptake within the mediastinum from an adjacent lung tumor can be difficult, and the technique also lacks the anatomical precision that is available with both CT scanning and mediastinoscopy. Normal uptake of the isotope by the overlying spine and sternum may cause some difficulty in assessment of the mediastinum.

In general, it is thought that if a primary tumor takes up gallium in the lung, and the mediastinal lymph nodes do not, then it would be unnecessary to proceed to mediastinoscopy, but to proceed straight to thoracotomy. However, a positive gallium uptake in the mediastinum should not be taken as diagnostic of tumor, as the false-positive incidence is approximately 15%–30%.

Sputum Cytology

Imaging techniques, however sophisticated, can only indirectly lead to the diagnosis of lung cancer. Before a therapeutic decision is made a definitive morphological diagnosis is mandatory. Preferably, this should be in the form of histological examination of biopsies or resected specimens. In some clinical situations, such a confirmation is not possible, and a cytological diagnosis must suffice. Furthermore, for screening purposes, cytological examinations are useful, provided that their sensitivity and specificity are reasonably good and the methods are simple and convenient. Hence, a great deal of effort has been put into refining techniques to identify and characterize tumor cells from the respiratory tract.

The most obvious source of material for cytological examination is sputum. Material obtained from spontaneous coughing varies considerably in quality, depending on the type of neoplasm and the location of lesions, but also on the technique of sputum production, time of the day, and number of samples examined. The most reproducible results are obtained from morning specimens. The diagnostic yield improves greatly if sputum is sampled on several consecutive days. By increasing the number of sampling days from 1 to 5, the yield of positive material in lung cancer patients increases from less than 50% to more than 80%. Instructions to the patients leading to a deep cough, with deep inhalation and forceful expiration, using the diaphragm, should be implemented. Nose and throat should be cleared before sampling.

Percussion might help some patients to produce useful material. In other cases when sputum production is unsatisfactory, induction can help. This includes the use of saline or mucolytic agents. An aerosol technique, using isotonic saline or Hank's solution, can yield useful material. Finally, it should be noted that sputum examinations can be especially useful in the days after bronchoscopy.

Cytological investigation should be carried out on fresh samples (stored for less than a few hours in room temperature). If a time lapse of more than a few hours between sampling and cytological examination can be anticipated, fixation should take place immediately (e.g., by the use of 50% ethanol and 2% Carbowax).

The usefulness of cytological examination as a diagnostic procedure is heavily dependent on the interpretation by the cytopathologist. By including atypical and suspicious specimens in the term "positive," the sensitivity of the tool is fairly high (around 95%), but at the same time the specificity is reduced considerably.

Realistically, approximately two-thirds of lung cancer patients with central tumor can be diagnosed by cytology examinations of consecutive samples of sputum. As could be expected, the diagnostic yield from sputum is greatest when the tumor is located centrally. Among the centrally located tumors, the diagnostic accuracy is highest for squamous cell carcinoma (67%–85%). The accuracy of the cytopathological results is obviously dependent on the skill of the investigator. One of the most common pitfalls is exfoliated atypical squamous metaplasias, seen in connection with chronic bronchitis or bronchiectasis. Furthermore, the degree of differentiation is important. The best results are obtained when the tumor is well differentiated. The correlation between cytopathological and histopathological diagnosis is shown in Table 2. Of the well-differentiated squamous cell carcinomas, 89% (50% of the poorly differentiated), 70% of the well-differentiated adenocarcinomas (56% of the poorly differentiated), and 87% of the small cell carcinomas were correctly diagnosed from cytological examination of sputum. In other words, if the clinical situation makes a more invasive procedure not feasible, the diagnostic value of a positive sputum examination is generally high enough to form a basis for a therapeutic strategy – especially in small cell carcinomas.

Table 2. Correlation between cytological and histological classification

Cytology	Histology								
	Squamous		Small cell	Adenocarcinoma		Large cell	Adeno-squamous	Unclas-sified	Total
	Well differentiated	Poorly differentiated		Well differentiated	Poorly differentiated				
Squamous									
Well differentiated	73	16	–	–	–	–	–	2	91
Poorly differentiated	6	5	1	–	5	1	1	4	23
Small cell	–	–	34		1		1	4	40
Adeno-carcinoma									
Well differentiated	–	–	–	21	3	–	–	1	25
Poorly differentiated	–	3	1	7	15	3	2	3	34
Large cell	–	–	–	–	1	2	–	1	4
Unclassified	3	8	3	1	2	1	1	5	24
Total	82	32	39	29	27	7	5	20	241

Bronchoscopy

Bronchoscopy is the cornerstone of diagnostic procedures in lung cancer. This is because 80% of lung cancers occur in the proximal airways and are accessible to the bronchoscope. Recently, fiberoptic bronchoscopy has become the most commonly used technique for diagnosing lung cancer, as many patients present with advanced disease, unsuitable for surgery, and physicians therefore carry out the fiberoptic procedure. In general, the yield is higher with fiberoptic bronchoscopy than rigid bronchoscopy. This is because the fiberoptic bronchoscope has greater access to the tracheobronchial tree, particularly in the upper lobes and the apical segments of the lower lobes. For areas directly accessible to both instruments, the yield is identical. The increase in yield is taken from upper lobe lesions not usually biopsiable, although visible to the rigid bronchoscopist.

Most thoracic centers have good working relationships between physicians and surgeons. Most diagnoses of lung cancer made on fiberoptic bronchoscopy, and considered operable, will be rebronchoscoped, using a rigid bronchoscope by the surgeon prior to operation. At bronchoscopy, not only should a diagnosis be made, but the patient's suitability for surgery should be evaluated.

Prior to bronchoscopy, it should be ensured that the patient is fit to undergo this procedure. In general, there is a small transient fall in arterial oxygen pressure during bronchoscopy. Any patient with forced expiratory volume in 1 s (FEV) of less than 1.0 liter should be carefully evaluated. If possible, arterial blood gases should be carried out, and if the arterial PO_2 is 60 mmHg or less, the patient should be given 2 litres oxygen/min by nasal cannula during the bronchoscopy procedure. If in doubt, give oxygen. It is usual to premedicate the patient. All patients should receive atropine 0.6 mg i.m. 30 min before bronchoscopy. Most patients tolerate the procedure better with some sedation as well. Papaverine (20 mg i.m.) 30 min before the procedure is commonly used. If the patient is aged between 65 and 70 years of age, or the FEV is between 750 and 1000 ml, then only 15 mg papaverine should be used. In patients over 70, sedation should only be given if thought safe, but the procedure is generally well tolerated by elderly patients. If during the procedure extreme difficulties are encountered, then diazepam 5–10 mg i.v. will cause transient sedation, which is almost always safe. Postprocedure, these patients should be carefully observed for up to 1 h.

At bronchoscopy, any suspicious lesion should be biopsied at least five times. If sequential biopsies are taken, the yield increases with each biopsy. Following biopsy the tumor should be brushed with a special cytological brush provided. The brushings should be transferred immediately onto a glass slide, and fixed in isopropylalcohol, and examined promptly by an experienced cytologist.

Fiberoptic bronchoscopy is an extremely safe procedure. Hemoptysis, as a result of biopsy, is extremely unusual, provided adequate care is taken. All patients should have a full blood count preoperatively to ensure there is no evidence of unexpected anemia. Any patients undergoing cytotoxic chemotherapy, and being reevaluated by bronchoscopy, should have a hemoglobin of greater than 10 g, a white cell count greater than 3500, and a platelet count greater than 100000 before bronchoscopy is undertaken.

Operative evaluation at bronchoscopy should include careful examination of the carina and the main bronchi to ensure there is no endobronchial compression of these structures. The carina should appear sharp, without any evidence of blunting, and the main bronchi should show no compression along their posterior aspects due to mediastinal lymph nodes, and should move freely and collapse normally when the patient is asked to take a deep breath or cough. The position of the tumor should be carefully recorded on a chart map of the airways, and its distance from the carina should be carefully measured if the tumor is in a main bronchus. An opinion should always be expressed on the bronchoscopy report as to whether the patient appears operable, and if so whether by lobectomy, bilobectomy, sleeve resection, or pneumonectomy.

Bronchoscopy gives a positive biopsy rate higher than 95% for tumors visible through the instrument, and an overall positive rate of 60%–70% for all cases of lung cancer. For squamous cell lung cancer, it is in the region of 90%, and for small cell 80% (the tumor is often submucosal); for adenocarcinomas, the figure is more variable – 80%–95%. Bronchial brushing specimens are as accurate as biopsy specimens in experienced hands.

Transthoracic Lung Biopsy

Even after intensive use of sophisticated endoscopic techniques, it is still sometimes impossible to get diagnostic material for histological confirmation. This is often the case with peripheral lesions, but also when the disease is diffuse, and it is a question of whether it is due to malignant or benign changes. In such cases, a transcutaneous biopsy is an obvious possibility. This procedure has become more and more important in the diagnosis of malignant diseases in the lungs since the introduction of modern transcutaneous needle techniques.

The typical indication for a transcutaneous biopsy procedure is a peripheral lesion in a patient suspected for a lung cancer where bronchoscopy has been negative.

The importance of establishing a histological diagnosis is quite obvious when curative treatment regimen is among the possibilities in the individual cases. But, also in nearly all other cases, the exact diagnosis is important in handling the patient. The selection of the appropriate palliative measures (as, e.g., radiotherapy) at the time of diagnosis or later in the clinical course also often rests on knowledge of the diagnosis.

Information of the prognostic outlook of the individual patient is likewise important, and information on the exact diagnosis and stage of disease is thus required. In general, an aggressive approach to establish a diagnosis is advocated, and this implies the use of invasive diagnostic procedures also in cases where immediate therapeutic consequences might be minimal. Finally, it should be mentioned that the use of transthoracic biopsy techniques can help in establishing whether a lesion is benign or malignant, and thus, in some cases, thoracotomy can be avoided.

The technique applied should be as safe as possible with maximal diagnostic information. In order to fulfill this purpose, transthoracic biopsy should be carried out under guidance of biplane fluoroscopy or CT scan, in order to define exactly where and in what direction the needle should be inserted. Secondly, the diameter and characteristics of the needle should be such that enough material can be sampled for thorough histological investigation. Thirdly, the professionals involved in taking the biopsy, and in the investigation of the biopsy, should be well trained, and this generally again implies that the procedure rests in relatively few hands in a given center or department.

The accuracy of the results from the biopsy procedure has been evaluated by the Johns Hopkins group by comparing biopsy diagnosis with final diagnosis from thoracotomy, clinical course, or autopsy. Malignant diagnosis was established in 87% of the cases (165 of 190). Definite diagnosis of benign tumors in a needle biopsy was only established in 50% of the cases (25 of 50) of patients having a solitary pulmonary mass that later was found to be of benign nature.

With regard to the cell typing of malignant lesions, correct diagnosis can be achieved in 50%–80% of the cases depending on the size of the lesions, the technique applied, and the cell type. Squamous carcinoma and small cell carcinoma seem to be the most reliable cell type diagnosis.

The complications of the procedure are obviously dependent on the technique and skills applied, and on the criteria for patient selection. Contraindications are factors such as a bleeding diathesis (low blood platelets, coagulation disorders), pulmonary hypertension, and suspected vascular lesions at the site of the infiltrate or in the course of the needle. By applying stringent rules and techniques, complications can be held to a minimum. In about 25% of the cases, the pneumothorax evolves, but only in one-fifth of these patients are therapeutic measures like chest tube application necessary. Hemoptysis occurs in about 20% of the cases, but is nearly always limited to blood-tinged sputum for a few hours after the procedure. In the Johns Hopkins series, there were no deaths attributable to the procedure.

In conclusion, the transthoracic needle biopsy is a useful, diagnostic tool, especially to evaluate the nature of peripheral lung infiltrates. Material for histological examination can be collected, but sometimes cytological investigation might suffice.

Pleura

Pleural Fluid

Pleural effusion is seen in many malignant and nonmalignant diseases. Approximately ½ of all cases with pleural effusion develop in patients with malignant diseases. Among patients with lung cancer, approximately 10% of the patients have effusion at diagnosis, but nearly 50% will develop this complication at some time during the clinical course. The presence of pleural effusion will often be suspected from a chest radiogram, but should always be verified either by thoracentesis or by diagnostic aspiration. The pleural fluid should routinely be sent for culture to rule out infections including tuberculosis. Various biochemical tests can be applied to the pleural fluid such as measurements of glucose and protein content, test for "tumor markers" like carcinoembryonic antigen (CEA). All these tests are of minor importance in the routine situation. In the context of lung cancer diagnosis, the cytological investigation is most important. In approximately two-thirds of cases, a cytological diagnosis can be made in patients where malignancy is evidently found.

A further diagnostic tool which can be used for investigation of primary or secondary pleural malignancies is *thoracoscopy*. The technique can be applied in local anesthesia after inflation of air in the pleural space. The patient should thus be able to tolerate a reduction of the lung function caused by pneumothorax of the investigated site. The scope is inserted after a small incision is made, and biopsy can be taken through the scope by guidance of the eye.

Differential diagnosis between diffuse adenocarcinoma and mesothelioma can be very difficult, and can necessitate several biopsies including an electron microscopy examination. Likewise, it can sometimes be difficult to decide whether or not a mesothelioma is truly malignant. The diagnostic accuracy of the thoracoscopy is excellent. Complications of the procedure are limited to the iatrogenic pneumothorax, which sometimes can be difficult to resolve.

Mediastinum

All the common types of lung cancers metastasize to mediastinal lymph nodes. At diagnosis, more than 20% of all lung cancers will have metastases to this region. This is especially typical for small cell and large cell carcinoma. Detection of mediastinal metastases is of obvious importance in the decision process regarding the operability of the patient, and all candidates for radical surgery should undergo extensive investigation of the mediastinum including invasive procedures before a thoracotomy is considered.

Mediastinal masses can only be detected on routine chest roentgenograms when they have reached a considerable size, and the enlarged lymph nodes are often obscured by mediastinal structures, or when the mediastinum is widened by tumor infiltration of prominent great vessels. By using tomography, the sensitivity of the roentgenogram can be increased to 33%-67%, primarily because smaller lesions, e. g., behind the heart, can be visualized.

Positive tomography rarely fails to correlate with positive diagnosis at more invasive investigations, while negative tomograms often do not reliably indicate the absence of mediastinal involvement.

The advent of CT scan has greatly improved the sensitivity of the measures for detecting mediastinal tumors. Almost 90% of the mediastinal tumors can be detected by this tool, and CT scan has been especially efficient in predicting whether or not a mediastinal lesion was resectable. The specificity of CT scan of mediastinum has been recorded to between 60%-90%. The sensitivity can be somewhat improved by using infusion of contrast material to better define vascular structures.

Invasive Techniques

Mediastinoscopy

The modern technique of mediastinoscopy is a safe and direct approach to the mediastinum, and is now a routine procedure as part of the diagnostic workup preoperatively. The mediastinum is approached through a suprasternal incision, whereby the trachea is exposed and the mediastinum can be dissected with a scope through which accessible paratracheal and mediastinal lymph nodes can be removed.

Positive biopsies obtained through a mediastinoscope are present in about 40% of the patients. In contrast to this, only 10%-15% of the patients have scalene or supraclavicular node metastases, earlier used as indications for nonoperativity of lung tumor. As many as 30% of patients with lung cancer presumed to be operable by other diagnostic techniques have been found to have superior mediastinal tumor by a mediastinoscopy. On the other hand, the negative mediastinoscopy in patients with lung cancer indicates a fairly high degree of resectability (between 80%-90%). By subsequent thoracotomy, a false-negative rate of results from mediastinoscopy of between 8% and 12% has been found.

Technique

The modern mediastinoscope is a fiberoptic scope with a blunt-tipped tube for dissection and aspiration. Biopsies are taken by a needle or a forceps. The procedure is most often carried out under general anesthesia, but can also be performed with local anesthesia. The incision is made transversally, just below the thyroid isthmus. The pretracheal fascia is opened inferior to the thyroid and dissection is made by use of the fingers downward along the trachea. The instrument is then introduced and the trachea and the right and left main bronchi plus the paratracheal areas can now be visualized. Tumor masses or lymph nodes can be removed for biopsies. If the biopsy is taken by guidance of the eye, bleeding is minimal and can be easily controlled.

Anterior mediastinotomy is a one-sited approach to the mediastinum, and is especially valuable when the area of the aortic nodes is suspected for involvement of neoplasms. The procedure can be used as a supplement to mediastinoscopy in investigating lesions of the left upper lobe. It can also be used as another site to introduce the mediastinoscope, and is then called anterior mediastinoscopy.

Complications

A review of published data of mortality and morbidity of mediastinoscopy carried out by Jepsen indicated a total of 3 deaths and 99 complications in 7876 patients, corresponding to a mortality rate of 0.038%. The most common complication was bleeding from the innominate artery or azygos vein. Other complications included pneumonia, hemothorax, vocal cord paralysis, perforation of esophagus, mediastinal infection, incision infection, bradycardia, myocardial infarct, stroke, and air embolus.

Mediastinoscopy should only be carried out by an experienced investigator, with access to the help necessary for handling complications, however uncommon these might be.

Distant Metastases

As mentioned earlier, appropriate treatment decisions can only be made after a thorough examination of histological type and extent of disease at the time of diagnosis. In that regard, the detection of distant metastases is highly important. Systemic manifestation of lung cancer is present in more than 50% of the cases at the outset, and the clinical course of lung cancer after apparent curative resection shows that such a figure is an underestimate of the actual degree of dissemination.

The application of the various diagnostic procedures will differ according to the patient's clinical presentation, the histological type of lung cancer, and the yield of the procedure relative to its morbidity, and, finally, but often most important, according to the availability of the various techniques, the skills of the investigator, and the therapeutic implications attached to the results of staging.

The scheme of diagnostic procedures should not be too rigid, but the diagnostic workup for the different types of lung cancer can be generalized to a certain ex-

Table 3. Preferred sites of distant metastases at autopsy in relation to histology (percentages)

Cell type	Liver[a]	Adrenal[a]	Bone[a]	Brain[b]	Other[a]
Squamous cell	30.5	27.4	24.4	13.7	
Small cell	61.9	39.2	37.5	30.5	Abdominal lymph nodes, 56.6
Adenocarcinoma	44.8	42.9	39.9	25.4	
Large cell	39.6	36.4	28.9	29.4	Abdominal lymph nodes, 36.0

[a] Data accumulated from the literature
[b] Data from 247 consecutive patients of the NCI-VA Medical Oncology Service, Washington DC, including all clinical and autopsy incidence

Table 4. Site of distant metastases in relation to histology prior to treatment

Cell type	No. with distant metastases	Percentage with metastases to:					
		Liver	Bone[a]	Brain	Thorax[b]	LN[c]	Skin
Squamous cell	25	8	16	20	36	24	8
Small cell	25	40	72	8	20	8	8
Adenocarcinoma	24	12.5	46	21	29	20	12.5
Large cell	31	6	26	13	38	35	13
Total	105[d]	16	40	15	30	22	10

[a] Excludes direct extension
[b] Refers to contralateral lung and mediastinum and pericardium
[c] Refers to nonregional peripheral lymph nodes
[d] Data from 105 consecutive patients of the NCI-VA Medical Oncology Service, Washington, D.C.

tent depending on preferred site of metastases according to the histology. Preferred sites of distant metastases at autopsy and prior to treatment are depicted in Tables 3 and 4. The limitations of the diagnostic procedures are strikingly shown in the investigation by Matthews, who carried out a careful autopsy investigation of patients dying within 1 month after curative resection. Sixty-three percent of the patients with small cell carcinoma were shown to have distant metastases. The corresponding numbers for squamous, adeno- and large cell carcinoma was 17%, 40%, and 14%. Since these patients represent a special group selected for resection, it is certainly indicative of a high degree of dissemination in lung cancer, especially in small cell lung cancer at presentation.

As indicated in Tables 3 and 4, liver, bone, and brain metastases are the most frequent signs of dissemination. The measures to identify these metastases will be evaluated below.

Detection of Liver Metastases

Evaluation of biochemical valuables, such as transaminases, bilirubin, alkaline phosphatase, and coagulation factors, are routinely used in the follow-up of patients with cancer diseases in order to detect liver metastases. The specificity of these measurements is, however, very low, in that, e.g., cirrhosis of fatty degenerative changes of the liver, and several other diseases, can give positive tests. Furthermore, the number of false-negative results is also quite high. In the presence of verified liver metastases in small cell carcinoma, it was found that alkaline phosphatase was increased in 70% and transaminase in 56%. The more nonspecific lactate dehydrogenase (LDH) was elevated in 79% of the cases. It is thus obvious that biochemical abnormalities are insufficient to determine whether or not a patient has liver metastases. The usefulness of these tests for biochemical screening in a clinical follow-up of patients with cancer has been considerably overestimated, and it is recommended that the application of these techniques, however simple they might be, should be limited.

Other noninvasive diagnostic procedures include imaging techniques like radionuclide scanning. For this purpose a variety of radionuclides has been involved, including [^{99m} Tc] sulfurcolloid and small aggregates of human serum albumin labeled with 99 m-technetium or 131-iodine.

The technique has been widely applied, but in several centers the accuracy has been found to be too low (60%) to justify routine use. The sensitivity is also low since the technique is unable to detect metastases with a diameter of less than 2-3 cm.

The other imaging techniques like CT scan and ultrasonography are better than radionuclide scanning. The development in this imaging technique area has been so rapid that it is not possible to give exact numbers on the accuracy of these techniques at present.

Preliminary data certainly suggest that upper abdominal CT scan can optimize the staging of patients with lung cancer. The role of CT scanning in detection of liver metastases is still not completely clarified. Tumors 1.5-2 cm in diameter should be visible with CT scan, but sometimes the differences in radioopacity between normal tissue and tumor tissue are fairly small. It is possible that use of special contrast material will be able to improve the diagnostic yield of CT scan of the liver. Furthermore, the practical applicability of the scanning technique will increase as the techniques for guided fine needle biopsies, coupled to the imaging technique, are developed.

Ultrasonography has already proved very valuable in the diagnosis of liver lesions. With the present-day technique, ultrasonography is easy to combine with needle biopsies. By decreasing the diameter of the needles (fine needle technique) it has been possible to reduce the number of complications considerably. Fine needle biopsies do, however, only provide material for cytological examinations. If histological confirmation is needed, a larger needle can be used.

False-positive results from ultrasonography, due to inhomogeneous echoarchitecture of the liver, can be seen in 5%-15% of the cases. This stresses the need for cytohistological confirmation of the ultrasonic diagnosis. The overall diagnostic accuracy of ultrasonically guided biopsies is near to 90%, and the predictive value of positive results is more than 95%.

The complication rate is very low, but it is nevertheless recommended that patients with bleeding diathesis, or high risk of cholascos, should be biopsied under careful observation.

Imaging techniques are useful in describing the extent of tumor, but the presence or absence of malignancy should always be verified by morphological proof.

This can be achieved by combining the imaging technique with needle biopsy, but another and also very useful approach is to use *peritoneoscopy* with liver biopsy under visual guidance. This technique was introduced in the diagnostic workup of cancer patients when it was realized that percutaneous liver biopsy with the Menghini technique was unsatisfactory, giving a sensitivity of only 45%, if 25 or more nodules were scattered throughout the liver, and substantially less with lesser degrees of involvement. Peritoneoscopy can be carried out in local anesthesia with inflation of room air or carbon dioxide in the peritoneal cavity. Biopsies can then be taken percutaneously under visual guidance through a small incision in the appropriate area. The advantage of peritoneoscopy is obviously the direct visualization of the liver surface, and the possibility to see where, exactly, the biopsy is taken, and also to control possible bleeding after biopsy. The disadvantage is the inability to depict changes which might prevail deep in the liver tissue. Sometimes the technique might be impossible to carry out because of adhesions in the peritoneal cavity, which is especially the case after previous abdominal surgery in this region.

Peritoneoscopy has especially been used in the staging of patients with small cell carcinoma. By using this technique in almost 200 patients with this cell type, hepatic metastases were detected in more than 20% of the patients. In addition, 9% had macroscopic signs of liver metastases, which could not be biopsied for technical reasons, or because of bleeding diathesis. Usually, the liver metastases are visualized on the surface of the liver, but in 10% of the patients with liver biopsy, the metastases are not visible on the exposed surface of the liver.

Comparisons of the different techniques for evaluating the liver are being carried out. Today, the two best methods for detecting hepatic metastases are peritoneoscopy with visually guided biopsy and ultrasonography with needle biopsy. A comparison between these two methods should form the basis for a decision on which method to recommend for future routine use in the diagnostic workup of lung cancer patients.

Detection of Bone and Bone Marrow Metastases

The skeletal system consists, in principle, of two organs, namely the bone marrow and the osseous tissue. These two organs are obviously intimately connected, but in terms of seeding of metastases there seem to be distinct differences. Clinically, metastases to the osseous tissue are characterized by pain, while metastases to the bone marrow primarily affect the hematopoietic tissue, which clinically may lead to thrombopenia or anemia, but seldom pain. In terms of the lung cancer types, small cell carcinoma has a high propensity for bone marrow involvement compared with the other types, especially squamous cell carcinoma. This type, on the other hand, when disseminated, fairly often involves the osseous tissue.

Evaluation of bone marrow should be part of the diagnostic workup for lung cancer patients, especially in small cell carcinoma, but also in the other types especially if myelosuppressive drugs are going to be part of the therapy.

The bone marrow can only be evaluated by an invasive procedure like a needle biopsy from the iliac crest, or aspiration of bone marrow from the sternum. The needle biopsy techniques applying Jamshidi or Radner needles are now preferred by most centers. The needle biopsy should be combined with aspiration, so that the information can be maximal. Imprints from the biopsy, marrow aspiration with smears, and blood specimens should be performed.

With regard to the frequencies of metastases in the bone marrow, a number of studies have confirmed the high propensity of small cell carcinoma to metastasize in this way. The numbers vary, however, from 17% to 50% positive, probably reflecting the differences in patient selection.

At the Finsen Institute, where the patient material is unselected, i.e., all cases from a certain area of Denmark are referred, bone marrow involvement was found in 22.5% of the patients with small cell cancer. The number of positive tests could be increased by approximately 10% when using *bilateral* aspiration, and biopsy from the iliac crest.

The osseous part of the bones can be evaluated by scans and X-ray, and also by biopsy techniques as outlined above. The bones are obviously in principle easy to evaluate by X-ray, but it should be stressed that the bone lesion seldom can be demonstrated before the bone decalcification occurs to an extent of 50%–75%, and that the size of the lesion exceeds 1–1.5 cm in diameter before it can be visualized. For these reasons, roentgenography is far too insensitive to be used for screening or surveying purposes. It is, however, desirable in cases of bony symptoms (pain) or in order to confirm tumor involvement in areas positive of bone scans to perform X-ray of an appropriate part of the skeleton. In a differential diagnosis between benign and malignant causes of abnormalities in bone scans, X-ray is obviously needed. Less than 50% of the patients with skeletal involvement proved by biopsies have primarily positive findings on skeletal X-rays.

The realization of the limited sensitivity of the skeletal roentgenograms has stimulated the search for techniques applying bone-seeking radioisotopes with gamma-emmision making external imaging possible. The first isotopes used were ^{85}Sr and ^{18}F. The applications of these isotopes in the clinic were limited by the high exposure level (^{85}Sr), short half-life (^{87}mSr), or unavailability (^{18}F). Today, the isotope normally used is [^{99m}Tc] pertechnetat, coupled to polyphosphate. The phosphate compound makes the complex seeking the bone, since the phosphate is incorporated in newly formed bone tissue. The radioisotope thus becomes located in the lesions whenever new bone formation takes place.

It is important to stress that bone scintigrams used in this way actually depict the rebuilding of osseous material secondary to a lesion and as such the recorded lesions are obviously not specific for malignant processes. The scans are positive in 69% of patients with bone marrow involvement, probably reflecting an indirect action of cancer cells in the bone marrow on bone formation processes rather than direct osseous involvement.

In some cases, with clearly osteolytic lesions in the bones, the scans are negative due to the fact that the new formation of bone is inhibited for some reason.

Finally, it should be mentioned that the interpretation of bone scans can be difficult and interobserver variability is definitely a problem which should be kept in mind. For these reasons, we feel that the bone scintigrams add little useful information to the diagnostic workup in lung cancer patients.

Detection of Central Nervous System Metastases

Among the lung cancers, small cell lung cancer is the most frequent disease with brain metastases, including an especially high incidence of metastases in the cerebellar and pituitary region. However, CNS metastases in the other types also occur in a significant number.

The occurrence of metastases to the central nervous system has been an increasing clinical problem in the management of lung cancer patients due most of all to a longer survival, especially of patients with small cell carcinoma. Already, at time of primary diagnosis, however, there is a considerable number of patients who have symptomatic or asymptomatic brain metastases.

In order to detect CNS metastases, the clinician has the following techniques at hand:

A thorough clinical neurological examination, lumbar puncture with investigation of the cerebrospinal fluid, brain scintigram, CT scan, and myelography.

Clinical examination carried out by an experienced neuro-oncologist has been shown to carry a high degree of specificity. In patients with neurological disturbances indicating a focal lesion, and without known arteriosclerotic disease, a malignancy should always be suspected.

Even in the absence of focal findings, CNS affection should be considered when the patient presents with symptoms like headache, gait disturbances, dizziness, and unexplained vomiting.

Scanning techniques applying [^{99m}Tc] pertechnetate are still used as a visualizing technique. Their limitation lies in the lack of sensitivity, especially in the posterior cranial fossa, where the background radioactivity is fairly high, and the possibility of detecting metastases are, therefore, low. But, also the specificity is limited. Brain scanning will probably gradually be replaced by CT scan, as this technique becomes more widespread and more specific. By using contrast medium in the vascular system during the CT scan of the brain, a high sensitivity and specificity can be obtained. The exact magnitude of these variables must await the finalizing of ongoing studies.

In patients where the propensity of cerebral metastases is high, i.e., patients with small cell carcinoma, CT scan with contrast should be considered as a screening method for detection of asymptomatic metastases. In a series of 81 patients in Copenhagen with small cell lung cancer who were thought to have disease restricted to the thoracic cavity, asymptomatic metastases were detected in 6.

The corresponding figures for other types of lung cancer are lower, but still unknown. In patients with no neurological symptoms the routine use of the CT scan is probably not rewarding.

Investigation of the CNS in cases suspected for lesions in the system should include a lumbar puncture with investigation of the cerebrospinal fluid for tumor cells (cytology) and protein content. The presence of tumor cells in the CNS indicates meningeal carcinomatosis, a complication seen more frequently as the patients survive for a longer time. In order to define larger lesions in the spinal medulla, myelography should be applied.

Metastases from lung cancer are the most frequent cause of spinal cord compression among the malignant diseases. The lesion is most often located in the vertebrae, i.e., extradurally in the bone. Metastases within the spinal cord are extremely rare.

Detection of Other Metastases

Cutaneous and subcutaneous metastases are generally easily detected by clinical examination. Lesions of this kind should always be biopsied or aspirated with a fine needle in order to verify the malignant nature.

Lymph nodes can also sometimes be readily accessible (cervical, axillary), and should in such cases again be cytological or histologically verified as metastases. Lymph nodes in mediastinum or retroperitoneum can be visualized on CT scan.

The value of CT scan and ultrasound, in the overall diagnostic workup and staging of the lung cancer patient, are still under debate but it seems likely that especially CT scan of thorax, brain, and abdomen can be of immense importance, delineating the presence and the size of metastatic lesions in areas otherwise not easily accessible for diagnostic procedures. Already, preliminary data available suggest that the extent of disease can be heavily underestimated by routine investigations, while a CT scan gives a much more precise picture.

The *pancreas* and the *adrenals* can harbor metastatic lesions, especially in patients with small cell carcinoma. CT scan is probably going to be the method of choice in defining metastatic lesions in these organs. Radioisotopes, used for scintigrams, have been of some value, but they are generally not specific enough and the imaging takes too long a time to be of clinical importance.

Finally, it should be mentioned that a great deal of research effort is currently put into the development of scanning techniques applying monoclonal antibodies. Modern techniques of producing monoclonal antibodies make it possible to produce antibodies with known characteristics in large quantities. By coupling these antibodies to gamma-emitters, it is possible that a new scintigram technique can be developed. Technical problems, lack of specificity and stability of the products, and several other problems make this attempt purely experimental for the time being.

8. Staging

P. Goldstraw

Systems of cancer staging provide a shorthand description of an individual tumor, thus easing communication between clinicians and allowing comparison of treatment results. To have any relevance such systems must relate to prognosis and hence help in decisions regarding treatment. It is widely acknowledged that for many cancers prognosis is concerned with the degree to which the local tumor has invaded adjacent structures, the extent to which it has metastasized along regional lymphatic channels, and the presence or absence of distant metastases. Such features may be described utilizing a TNM (tumor, nodal involvement, metastases) classification, in which advancing T categories relate to the increasing presence of adverse prognostic features of the primary tumor, advancing N categories to more extensive metastasis along regional lymphatics, and M categories to the absence or presence of distant metastases. Many such classifications are in use for a great range of cancers, including lung cancer; the one most widely adopted is that of the American Joint Committee for Cancer Staging and End Results Reporting. This is based on a recommendation by the UICC and was applied to lung cancer for the first time in 1973 by Mountain and colleagues [1]. They studied 2000 proven cases of lung cancer in which for each case 111 items of information were assessed for their prognostic significance. Those features found to be significant for the primary tumor were: its size, its position within the bronchial tree, local extension to surrounding structures, and the presence of such complicating features as collapse and consolidation, or pleural effusion. To a degree they present alternatives in the assessment of peripheral or central tumors. The features found to be significant when studying regional lymphatic spread were its presence or absence and whether such spread is limited to the lung with involvement of intrapulmonary or hilar glands or is more extensive, including mediastinal node metastases. When considering distant metastases the most important feature is whether they are present or absent, but the system allows for more detailed documentation of the number of metastases and the organs involved. This staging system has recently been refined [2] and will be used increasingly, and hence is the system utilized throughout this chapter (Tables 1 and 2).

Clearly staging becomes more precise as investigations proceed and more information becomes available. Clinical staging (cTNM) permits the incorporation of information from all investigations prior to treatment. If treatment entails thoracotomy, then further staging information is obtainable to permit a surgical/evaluative classification (sTNM). If resection is undertaken, then once a detailed histological assessment is available, a postsurgical pathological staging (pTNM) is possible, taking account of the additional information. Such staging categories

Table 1. Definitions for staging bronchogenic carcinoma (American Joint Committee on Cancer 1983)

Primary tumor (T) determinant

TX   Tumor proven by the presence of malignant cells in bronchopulmonary secretions but not visualized roentgenographically or bronchoscopically; or any tumor that cannot be assessed as in a retreatment staging

T0   No evidence of primary tumor

TIS   Carcinoma in situ

T1   A tumor that is 3.0 cm or less in greatest dimension, surrounded by lung or visceral pleura, and without evidence of invasion proximal to a lobar bronchus at bronchoscopy[a]

T2   A tumor more than 3.0 cm in greatest dimension, or a tumor of any size that either invades the visceral pleura or has associated atelectasis or obstructive pneumonitis extending to the hilar region. At bronchoscopy, the proximal extent of demonstrable tumor must be within a lobar bronchus or at least 2.0 cm distal to the carina. Any associated atelectasis or obstructive pneumonitis must involve less than an entire lung

T3   A tumor of any size with direct extension into the chest wall (including superior sulcus tumors), diaphragm, or the mediastinal pleura or pericardium, without involving the heart, great vessels, trachea, esophagus, or vertebral body; or a tumor in the main bronchus within 2 cm of the carina without involving the carina

T4   A tumor of any size with invasion of the mediastinum or involving heart, great vessels, trachea, esophagus, vertebral body, or carina, or presence of malignant pleural effusion[b]

Nodal involvement (N) determinant

N0   No demonstrable metastasis to regional lymph nodes

N1   Metastasis to lymph nodes in the peribronchial or the ipsilateral hilar region, or both, including direct extension

N2   Metastasis to ipsilateral mediastinal lymph nodes and subcarinal lymph nodes

N3   Metastasis to contralateral mediastinal lymph nodes, contralateral hilar lymph nodes, ipsilateral or contralateral scalene or spuraclavicular lymph nodes

Distant metastasis (M) determinant

M0   No (known) distant metastasis

M1   Distant metastasis present: specify site(s)

---

[a] The uncommon superficial tumor of any size with its invasive component limited to the bronchial wall which may extend proximal to the main bronchus is classified as T1.

[b] Most pleural effusions associated with lung cancer are due to tumor. There are, however, a few patients in whom cytopathological examination of pleural fluid (on more than one specimen) is negative for tumor, and the fluid is nonbloody and is not an exudate. In such cases for which these elements and clinical judgement dictate that the effusion is not related to the tumor, the patient should be staged T1, T2, or T3, excluding effusion as a staging element

Table 2. Stage grouping of TNM subsets. These TNM categories may be studied individually or grouped together to form stages 1, 2, 3a, 3b, or 4

Occult carcinoma	TX	N0	M0
Stage 0	TIS	Carcinoma in situ	
Stage I	T1	N0	M0
	T2	N0	
Stage II	T1	N1	M0
	T2	N1	
Stage IIIa	T3	N0	M0
	T3	N1	
	T1–3	N2	
Stage IIIb	Any T	N3	M0
	T4	Any N	M0
Stage IV	Any T	Any N	M1

should not be altered in the light of subsequent information. Whatever treatment is given, as follow-up proceeds staging may alter. If further treatment becomes necessary a reevaluation stage (rTNM) may include additional investigations. Should death occur and an autopsy be performed, a final staging (aTNM) can be done.

The investigations required to arrive at a clinical staging (cTNM) will vary and may not all be available. Once a stage has been arrived at for each TNM category, there is little point in extending investigations further. The TNM stage has unfortunately little relevance for the great majority of patients with small cell lung cancer (SCLC), and the methods discussed here relate to the other cell types - squamous, adeno, and large cell cancers - collectively termed non-small cell lung cancer (NSCLC). This method is depicted in diagrammatical form in Fig. 1.

T Stage

Clinical history and examination may suggest T3 status with symptoms or signs of chest wall invasion or T4 status with features suggesting mediastinal invasion. Invasion of the lateral chest wall produces the characteristic, persistent, progressive pain located to the area of invasion. If invasion occurs at the lung apex, as with a Pancoast type of tumor, there are associated symptoms and signs due to involvement of the brachial plexus, the sympathetic chain, and subclavian vessels. Mediastinal invasion may be evident by its effects on the recurrent laryngeal or phrenic nerves, or compression of viscera such as the superior vena cava, esophagus, or trachea. Such involvement of mediastinal structures, sometimes the result of a T4 tumor, is more commonly due to the presence of mediastinal glands, an N2 or N3 status.

Plain chest radiographs may determine the size of a peripheral tumor or disclose clinically unsuspected rib erosion. With central tumors the degree of associated collapse/consolidation may permit T staging. Elevation of the hemidiaphragm may indicate a T4 tumor if screening confirms paradoxical motion. Any pleural effusion confers T4 status but aspiration and cytology are necessary to detect malignant cells. Occasionally, if cytology is negative and the aspirate non-bloody, the clinician may consider the effusion not to arise from the tumor and stage the tumor T1, T2, or T3. Bronchoscopy is necessary to establish tissue diagnosis and permits the T staging of central tumors.

Computed tomography (CT) may suggest mediastinal invasion not suspected on a routine radiograph. The specificity of such a finding, however, is only 85%, and hence alone it should not contraindicate resection.

Mediastinal exploration will be discussed in greater detail under N stage. It may also disclose invasion unsuspected by other investigations, especially with upper lobe tumors. It is a valuable investigation if contemplating pulmonary resection.

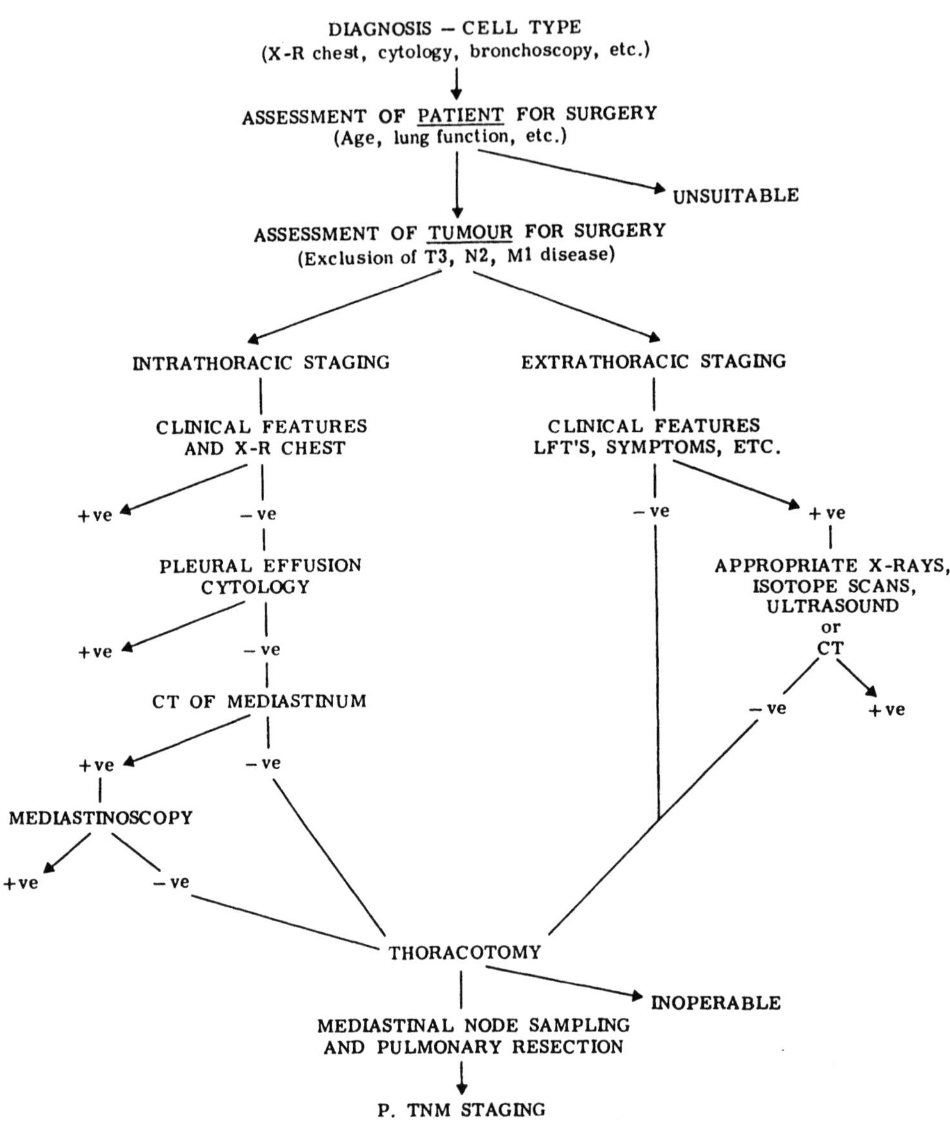

Fig. 1. Investigative sequence in the intrathoracic staging of non-small cell lung cancer

N Stage

Hilar gland involvement, N1 status, cannot be detected clinically, and its assessment on routine chest radiographs is poor. As more sophisticated radiographic techniques are utilized, such as conventional tomography or CT, the number of abnormalities detected will increase, but their interpretation may prove difficult. In these radiographic techniques the definition of abnormality is based upon an arbitrary size criterion, with most reports assuming a 1–1.5-cm diameter as the upper limit of normality. Nodes may, however, have enlarged due to previous inflammatory changes such as tuberculosis or may swell in response to infection associated with the tumor. Conversely, small nodes may contain metastatic deposits. Not surprisingly, therefore, the specificity (true negative/true negative + false positive) and sensitivity (true positive/true positive + false negative) of CT scan examinations will fall below that which is ideal and often move in a reciprocal fashion. Fortunately N1 status has little influence on management in NSCLC since even in its presence, surgery remains the treatment of choice. It does require more extensive resections, often pneumonectomy, but unless the patient's lung function is so marginal as to permit lobectomy but not pneumonectomy, then this staging has no preoperative significance.

Mediastinal node involvement is, in contrast, crucial to the decision regarding surgery. The great majority of patients with ipsilateral mediastinal node involvement, N2 disease, and all of those with contralateral involvement, N3 disease, are inoperable. Occasionally mediastinal gland involvement will be evident clinically or visible on a chest radiograph. In these circumstances histological confirmation of their involvement is unnecessary, unless tissue diagnosis is required after less invasive tests such as sputum cytology or bronchoscopy.

As with hilar glands the use of more sophisticated imaging techniques – conventional tomography, gallium, or CT – will increase sensitivity at the cost of specificity. Hence, if positive, such tests require confirmation by surgical exploration of the mediastinum. These tests may, if negative, permit the avoidance of mediastinal exploration, but this presumes that each scanner and radiologist is evaluated during a period in which routine mediastinoscopy is employed. The routine preoperative use of mediastinoscopy removes any value from these elaborate imaging techniques.

Preoperative evaluation of the mediastinum by cervical mediastinoscopy will detect unsuspected N2 disease in approximately 25% of subjects otherwise considered suitable for surgery. Such a technique is known to improve resectability rates to around 95%, especially for upper lobe tumors [3]. It is less able to detect mediastinal involvement by invasion or glandular metastases in the case of lower lobe tumors, since that involvement may be beyond the reach of the mediastinoscope. This subject will be discussed in the section on surgery. The lymphatic drainage of the left upper lobe is influenced by the interposition of the aortic arch, and it has been shown that for tumors in this location left anterior mediastinotomy is a valuable supplement to cervical mediastinoscopy, detecting invasion or mediastinal gland involvement in 15%–30% of subjects having a normal cervical exploration. The technical aspects of these explorative procedures are beyond the scope of this chapter.

Noninvasive Assessment of the Mediastinum

Although it is clearly advisable that mediastinoscopy should be the routine preoperative final staging assessment, noninvasive tests have been assessed thoroughly in recent years. As stated above, both gallium and CT scanning will increase the sensitivity of identifying abnormality compared with less sophisticated techniques. However, the role of CT scanning and gallium are still somewhat uncertain [4]. Several studies are available comparing CT staging of the mediastinum to mediastinoscopy and pTNM staging. Studies using the first generation CT scanners with 18-20-s scanning times claimed a low incidence for the sensitivity of mediastinal adenopathy (44%-75%). However, using newer models with a 2-3-s scanning time, the sensitivity has improved to 80%-94%. Gallium scanning, having a similar sensitivity to CT scanning, also has a comparable incidence of false-positive scans requiring mandatory mediastinoscopy following a positive scan.

The available data for CT scanning followed by biopsy or thoracotomy allow certain helpful conclusions:

1. The predicted value of a negative CT scan (specificity data) is of the order of 90%-95%, and in these cases a mediastinoscopy may be omitted before thoracotomy. The availability of a CT scanner will avoid mediastinoscopy in some cases.
2. Similarly, when CT shows the mediastinum to be normal but suggests that the hilum is abnormal, mediastinal exploration may also be omitted before thoracotomy.
3. The predictive value of a positive scan is much more variable (50%-100%), and therefore mediastinal exploration should be performed. However, in these cases the surgeon should particularly attempt to examine the abnormality seen on the CT scan. If mediastinoscopy is normal, thoracotomy should be done.

Thus, if CT scanning is not available to a thoracic unit, all patients with an apparently normal mediastinum on plain and lateral PA chest X-rays should be subjected to mediastinoscopy [5]. In this way those patients with occult mediastinal disease will be identified and be staged as N2 or N3 disease.

The appreciation of N2 status contraindicates thoracotomy in the vast majority of patients. Surgery may still be justified in a small minority with well-differentiated squamous carcinoma, in which involvement of the mediastinal glands is limited to the microscopic, intracapsular involvement of the ipsilateral, low, paratracheal glands. In such peculiar circumstances complete resection is possible in 65% with 5-year survival figures of 18% [6]. Even in such a favorable subgroup, however, glandular metastases are usually more extensive than predicted at mediastinoscopy.

M Stage

The presence of distant metastases is often suspected clinically. The recent onset of bone pain is highly suggestive, and this point should be specifically sought in questioning. Patients are notorious in rationalizing such pain to "lumbago" or "arthritis". There may have been a recent change in personality, sometimes associated with memory loss, features more apparent to relatives than clinicians. Unexplained weight loss (> 3 kg in the previous 6 months) is suggestive of occult metastases and makes a more detailed search for metastases worthwhile.

Clinical examination may reveal evidence of metastasis, with local bone tenderness, neurological deficit, palpable irregular hepatomegaly, or supraclavicular glands. A full blood count showing an unexplained anemia (Hb < 10 g%) or liver function tests with abnormal alkaline phosphatase or serum calcium are additional nonspecific indicators of occult metastases, and then more elaborate tests are justified.

In the absence of clinical features to suggest metastases or of the nonspecific indicators of occult metastases, radioisotope scans are of no value and are as likely to be misleading as helpful in the search for occult metastases. In the presence of such features, however, isotope scans of brain, liver, and bone are worthwhile. Gallium scanning is similarly important, if this technique is available.

The role of CT scanning in detecting occult metastases has yet to be evaluated, but it is probable that it will prove to be the most sensitive test presently available. The specificity of this technique is as yet unknown. Early results suggest that CT scanning will identify occult metastases in the chest or abdomen in 10% of patients otherwise fit for surgery. The pick-up rate in the brain is likely to be considerably lower, < 5%. In only 2%–5% of subjects will CT of the brain or abdomen provide the only evidence of metastases to contraindicate surgery [7].

Staging at Thoracotomy

If thoracotomy is done, careful restaging is essential to arrive at sTNM prior to undertaking resection. In addition to checking on cTNM, the maneuvre also allows the most precise estimate on subsequent pTNM. Features of the tumor influencing T staging should be noted, and a systematic evaluation of nodal secondaries performed. The latter should include excision biopsy of mediastinal lymph node stations so that each is identified for the pathologist. It is quite impossible for the pathologist to differentiate nodes attached to a resection specimen as hilar or mediastinal. The numbering of mediastinal gland stations using an arbitrary system such as that of Naruke [8] avoids confusion over nomenclature. Any glands left attached to the specimen should therefore be N1. In 25% of cases such routine examination of mediastinal nodes will reveal N2 disease unsuspected on preoperative staging. Such patients may well benefit from resection, with 5-year survival figures of 40%.

It is important that any pathologist examining resection specimens appreciates those features of the tumor and attached nodes which will influence pTNM staging.

Autopsy Staging

This final assessment of tumor staging requires a diligent postmortem by a pathologist familiar with TNM staging (aTNM). In addition to assessing the tumor's characteristics and regional lymph node metastases, a thorough examination for distant metastases requires the routine examination of the brain, contralateral lung, abdominal viscera, and bones. All organs should be sliced with no greater thickness than 1 cm.

Relevance to Small Cell Lung Cancer

The TNM system has no relevance in SCLC other than for a tiny, fortunate minority whose lesions remain sufficiently localized to justify surgery. Some of these cases will be identified after resection of an asymptomatic peripheral pulmonary nodule. With the use of fine needle biopsy to obtain preoperative tissue diagnosis, this group is declining. Preoperative staging in SCLC should be especially rigorous and include CT scanning of brain, chest, and abdomen, bone isotope scan, and bilateral iliac crest marrow trephine biopsy. The role of mediastinoscopy in localized SCLC with a normal mediastinum on CT scanning is uncertain, but it would seem a reasonable final staging investigation.

For the great majority of sufferers with SCLC, staging is academic and usually restricted to limited versus extensive disease. Limited disease is defined as the tumor confined to one hemithorax and the ipsilateral supraclavicular fossa. Mediastinal gland involvement will be present in as many as 94% of these cases. Staging into the two categories is usually accomplished by a history, examination, and chest radiograph. Patients with limited disease comprise one-third of all cases, but this figure falls with any intensification of staging procedures.

References

1. Mountain CF, Carr DT, Anderson WAD (1974) A system for the clinical staging of lung cancer. AJR 120: 130–138
2. Mountain CF (1986) A new international staging system for lung cancer. IV World Conference on Lung Cancer. Chest (suppl) 89: 225–233
3. Pearson FG (1968) An evaluation of mediastinoscopy in the management of presumably operable bronchial carcinoma. J Thorac Cardiovasc Surg 55: 617–625
4. Goldstraw P (1986) CT scanning in the preoperative assessment of non-small cell lung cancer. In: Hansen HH (ed) Lung cancer: basic and clinical aspects. Martinus Nijhoff, Boston, pp 183–199
5. Goldstraw P, Kurzer M, Edwards D (1983) Preoperative staging of lung cancer: accuracy of computed tomography versus mediastinoscopy. Thorax 38: 10–15
6. Pearson FG, Delarue NC, Ilves R, Todd TRJ, Cooper JD (1982) Significance of positive superior mediastinal nodes identified at mediastinoscopy in patients with resectable cancer of the lung. J Thorac Cardiovasc Surg 83: 1–11
7. Grant D, Edwards D, Goldstraw P (1986) Preoperative CT staging in lung cancer. Abstract 155, Annual Meeting, Royal College of Radiologists, Sheffield, England
8. Naruke T, Suemasu K, Ishikawa S (1978) Lymph node mapping and curability at various levels of metastasis in resected lung cancer. J Thorac Cardiovasc Surg 76: 832–839

9. Staging and Prognosis

H. H. Hansen, F. R. Hirsch, and M. Rørth

The presence, the location, and the number of metastases in patients with cancer are important predictive parameters for the clinical course. They also have decisive therapeutic implications especially if local modes of therapy such as surgery or radiotherapy are included.

With respect to lung cancer various staging systems have been used mainly in connection with surgery, where the TNM system is the most commonly used. The TNM system describes the localization and the size of the primary tumor including possible local invasion while N is used to describe the degree of nodal involvement and M to inform about the presence of distant metastases.

Information concerning the anatomy of the primary site, local lymph node involvement, and metastatic sites is important for optimal staging, and for lung cancer these factors vary considerably from one histologic type to another.

Staging can be subdivided into five categories:

1. Clinical diagnostic staging
2. Surgical resection – pathologic staging
3. Surgical evaluative staging
4. Retreatment staging
5. Autopsy staging

The rules for classification according to the system used at the Finsen Institute, which is in accordance with those for the American Joint Committee for lung cancer, are as follows:

Clinical-Diagnostic Staging. This is based on the anatomic extent of the disease detected by examination before thoracotomy or the implementation of other treatment. Such an examination may include a medical history, physical examination, routine and special roentgenograms, endoscopic examinations including bronchoscopy, esophagoscopy, mediastinoscopy, thoracentesis, or thoracoscopy, and any other examinations, including those used to demonstrate the presence of extrathoracic metastasis.

Postsurgical Resection-Pathologic Staging. The surgical pathology report and all other available data should be used to assign a postsurgical treatment classification to those patients who have had a resection.

Surgical-Evaluative Staging. This should be based on all the data obtained for the clinical-diagnostic classification and on information obtained at the exploratory thoracotomy, including biopsy but not including the information obtained by complete examination of a therapeutically resected specimen.

Retreatment Staging. In the course of follow-up examinations, a patient may manifest evidence of progressive disease indicating treatment failure. Before initiating further treatment, the extent of tumor should be reassessed carefully, using all available information, and the patient should again be staged.

Autopsy Staging. In case of death of a lung cancer patient, the extent of the cancer found at autopsy may be recorded by the TNM system and an autopsy stage may be reported.

With respect to the TNM classification one can either use the UICC staging system (Table 1) or the American Joint Committee TNM system. They vary only in minor areas from each other. An overall data form as suggested by the American Joint Committee on cancer staging of lung cancer is given in Table 2.

With the TNM classification as background it is possible to stage lung cancer patients in various groups, which include (a) *occult stage:* TX, N0, M0, (b) *stage 1:* TIS = carcinoma in situ, N0, M0, (c) *stage 2:* T2, N1, M0, and (d) *stage 3* (Table 2).

The definitions of the stages are as follows:

Occult Stage: TX, N0, M0. An occult carcinoma with bronchopulmonary secretions containing malignant cells but without other evidence of tumor, metastasis to the regional lymph nodes, or distant metastasis.

Stage 1: Tis, N0, M0. Carcinoma in situ. T1, N0, M0; T1, N1, M0; T2, N0, M0. A tumor that can be classified T1 without any metastases or with metastases to the lymph nodes in the peribronchial or ipsilateral hilar region only, or a tumor that can be classified T2 without any metastases to nodes or distant organs. (Note: TX, N1, M0 is also theoretically possible, but such a clinical diagnosis would be difficult if not impossible to make. If such a diagnosis is made, it would be included in stage 1).

Stage 2: T2, N1, M0. A tumor classified as T2 with metastases to the lymph nodes in the peribronchial or ipsilateral hilar region only.

Stage 3: T3 with any N or M; N2 with any T or M; M1 with any T or N. Any tumor more extensive than T2, any tumor with metastases to the lymph nodes in the mediastinum or any tumor with distant metastases. (Note: Staging grouping is significant for all cell types listed under histopathology except undifferentiated small cell carcinoma in which there is a poor correlation between TNM stage and survival rates. The anatomic extent of small cell cancers may, however, be recorded by the TNM system for future reference.)

The correlation between the stage and survival is quite evident when one analyzes the survival by clinical diagnostic stage data in details for the various cell types such as squamous cell carcinoma, adenocarcinoma, and large cell carcinoma as shown in Fig. 1 and 2.

For unresectable patients, a more simplified staging system is usually used with division of patients between localized (limited disease, LD) or extensive disease (ED). This staging system was first used by the VA Lung Cancer Group in the United States and it remains the most widely used for staging patients who are not candidates for surgery. Limited disease is defined as tumor confined to one hemithorax with or without local extension including mediastinal and supraclavicular lymph nodes, while extensive disease is defined as demonstrable tumor beyond

Table 1. UICC classification

Rules for classification
The classification applies only to carcinoma.
There should be histological verification of the disease to permit division of cases by histological type. Any unconfirmed cases must be reported separately.
Information derived from surgical exploration prior to definitive treatment is admissible for clinical classification, the fact to be stated.
The following are the minimum requirements for assessment of the T, N, and M categories. If these cannot be met, the symbol TX, NX, or MX will be used.

T categories: Clinical examination, radiography, and endoscopy
N categories: Clinical examination, radiography, and endoscopy
M categories: Clinical examination and radiography

Anatomical Sites
1. Trachea   162.0
2. Main bronchus   162.2
3. Upper lobe   162.3
4. Middle lobe   162.4
5. Lower lobe   162.5

Regional lymph nodes
The regional lymph nodes are the intrathoracic nodes.

TNM pretreatment clinical classification
T   Primary tumor
Tis   Preinvasive carcinoma (carcinoma in situ)
T0   No evidence of primary tumor
T1   Tumor 3 cm or less in its greatest dimension, surrounded by lung or visceral pleura and with no evidence of invasion proximal to lobar bronchus on bronchoscopy
T2   Tumor more than 3 cm in its greatest dimension or tumor of any size which, with its associated atelectasis or obstructive pneumonitis, extends to the hilar region.
       At bronchoscopy the proximal extent of demonstrable tumor must be at least 2 cm distal to the carina. Any associated atelectasis or obstructive pneumonitis must involve less than an entire lung and there must be no pleural effusion
T3   Tumor of any size with direct extension to adjacent structures such as the chest wall, diaphragm, or mediastinum and its contents or tumor at bronchoscopy less than 2 cm distal to the carina or tumor associated with atelectasis or obstructive pneumonitis of an entire lung or pleural effusion
TX   Any tumor that cannot be assessed or tumor proven by the presence of malignant cells in bronchopulmonary secretions but not visualized by radiography or bronchoscopy
N   Regional lymph nodes
N0   No evidence of regional lymph node involvement
N1   Evidence of involvement of peribronchial and/or homolateral hilar lymph nodes, including direct extension of the primary tumor
N2   Evidence of involvement of mediastinal lymph nodes
NX   The minimum requirements to assess the regional lymph nodes cannot be met
M   Distant metastases
M0   No evidence of distant metastases
M1   Evidence of distant metastases
MX   The minimum requirements to assess the presence of distant metastases cannot be met

The category M1 may be subdivided according to the following notation:

Pulmonary	PUL		Bone marrow	MAR
Osseous	OSS		Pleura	PLE
Hepatic	HEP		Skin	SKI
Brain	BRA		Eye	EYE
Lymph nodes	LYM		Other	OTH

Table 2. Data form as suggested by the American Joint Committee for Staging

TNM Classification

Primary Tumor

Size	*Intra-bronchial Location*	*Extra-pulmonary Extension*	*Atelectasis or Pneumonitis*	*Pleural Effusion*	*TNM Classi-fication*
Positive bronchopulmonary secretions without demonstrable tumor or cannot be assessed				☐	TX
No evidence of primary tumor				☐	T0
Carcinoma *in situ*				☐	Tis
3 cm or less ☐	Not proximal to lobar bronchus ☐	None ☐	None or peripheral only ☐	None ☐	T1
More than 3 cm ☐	≥ 2 cm distal to carina ☐	None ☐	Extends to hilar region but < entire lung ☐	None ☐	T2
Any size ☐	< 2 cm distal to carina ☐	Chest wall, diaphragm, or mediastinum ☐	Involves entire lung ☐	Present ☐	T3

Regional Nodes

No demonstrable metastasis to regional lymph nodes	☐	N0
Metastasis to peribronchial or ipsilateral hilar nodes	☐	N1
Metastasis to mediastinal lymph nodes	☐	N2

Distant Metastasis

No (known) distant metastasis	☐	M0
Distant metastasis present (specify)	☐	M1

these limits. The VALG staging system was originally proposed because of its suitability for radiotherapy, which was the main modality of nonsurgical therapy at the time when the system was introduced. Both in untreated and treated patients there is a clear correlation between staging as mentioned above and survival.

In addition to the prognostic value of the major histopathologic classifications, it has also been shown that grading of the tumor influences survival, with the best survival occurring for patients with well-differentiated or moderately well differentiated squamous cell and adenocarcinoma, compared with more undifferentiat-

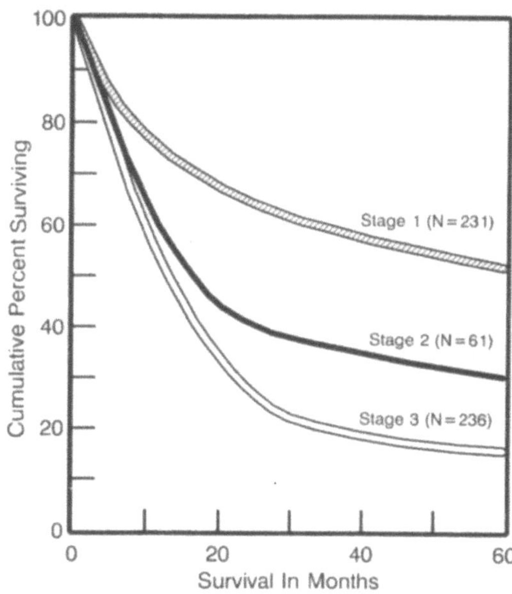

Fig. 1. Survival of patients with squamous cell carcinoma of lung by clinical diagnostic stage. (Reproduced by permission of the American Joint Committee for Cancer Staging and End Results Reporting)

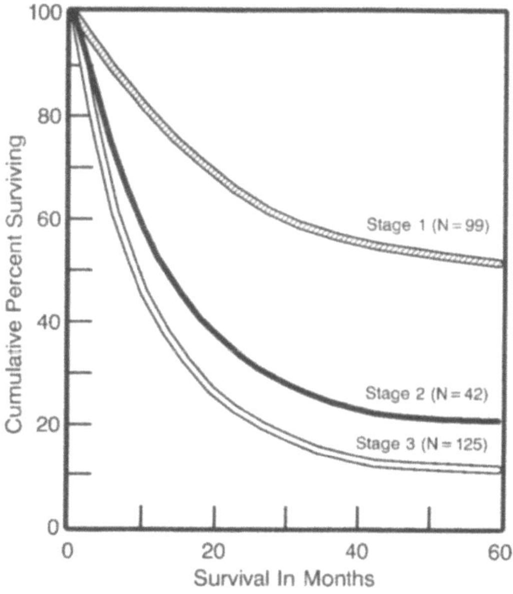

Fig. 2. Survival of patients with adenocarcinoma and undifferentiated large cell carcinoma of lung by clinical diagnostic stage. (Reproduced by permission of the American Joint Committee for Cancer Staging and End Results Reporting)

ed epidermoid and adenocarcinomatous tumor. Another major factor influencing survival is the performance status of the patients. Several systems for recording a patient's activity and symptoms are used and are more or less equivalent as follows:

Performance	WHO scale	Karnofsky scale
Normal activity	0	90–100
Symptomatic but ambulatory, cares for self	1	70– 80
Ambulatory more than 50% of time, occasionally needs assistance	2	50– 60
Ambulatory 50% or less of time, nursing care need	3	30– 40
Bedridden, may need hospitalization	4	10– 20

Overall one can conclude that it is important to stage cases with lung cancer for several reasons: (a) to aid in the selection of the most effective treatment, (b) to assist in determining prognosis, (c) to make possible meaningful comparison of end results reported from different sources, and (d) to help evaluate the effectiveness of the treatment including the reasons for failure.

10. Treatment at the Finsen Institute

H. H. Hansen, F. R. Hirsch, and M. Rørth

The treatment of lung cancer should be considered in accordance with the histo-pathologic type of lung cancer and the stage of disease.

For practical reasons, the treatment will be presented for the following three categories of patients: group 1, patients with squamous cell, large cell carcinoma, and adenocarcinoma ("non-small cell" lung cancer); group 2, small cell lung cancer; and group 3, mesothelioma.

Treatment of Squamous Cell, Adeno-, and Large Cell Carcinoma

Surgery

The primary *curative* treatment for the above-mentioned cell type is surgery. A success of surgical treatment for lung cancer is highly dependent on the appropriate selection of patients. The criteria for this selection relate to the biologic nature of the tumor, the anatomic extent of disease, and the patient's physiologic status. Candidates for definitive resection include only patients with stage I and stage II disease, and a small group of patients with stage III, where the disease is confined to the ipsilateral hemithorax, and in whom complete resection is considered technically feasible.

In addition, evaluation of the pulmonary function is mandatory before surgical resection is undertaken in order to be sure that the patient has sufficient lung function after resection. An adequate evaluation should thus indicate the patients who are at high risk for simple thoracotomy, but also estimate the maximum tolerated extent of pulmonary resection possible, and predict the postresection ventilatory capacity.

Of the tests used to evaluate the function of the airways, the flow volume relationship, the forced expiratory volume in 1s (FEV_1), and the forced vital capacity (FVC) are considered the most reliable. The function of the alveolar capillary surface can be evaluated by measuring the carbon monoxide capacity and the blood gases while the ventilation/perfusion of the given area of the lung can be evaluated by the use of radioactive isotopes. If the pCO_2 is elevated at rest, chest surgery cannot be recommended, while decrease in pO_2 is not inconsistent with surgery, as pO_2 often increases after the intervention.

If the FVC is equal to 2.5 liters or more, the patient has essentially normal lung function and can tolerate a pneumonectomy. If the FVC is below 2.5 liters, a ventilation and perfusion scan should be performed in order to ensure a normal ventilation/perfusion relationship in the nonaffected lung and maintain the levels of blood gases within a normal range. If the calculated FEV_1 after operation is less than 1.0 liters, the patient is considered to have severe ventilatory impairment, and surgical resection of lung tissue cannot be considered.

The extent of the resection should be carefully planned preoperatively on the basis of the foregoing evaluation, even though final selection of the operative procedures must take place at the time of exploration. A procedure that encompasses all existent neoplastic tissue, and provides the maximum conservation of lung tissue, is usually the procedure of choice. It is well established that the surgical mortality is increasing with more radical procedures; however, potential for cure should not be compromised strictly by accommodating a conservative policy.

The choice of surgical procedure is usually indicated by the location of tumor involvement as determined by interoperative microscopic ventilatory reserve. The following general guidelines hold true in most situations:

1. *A wedge or segmental resection* will be selected for patients with small peripheral tumors (<2 cm in greatest diameter), with no evidence of extension or metastases (T1,N0,M0, stage I disease). In some of these patients, the preoperative diagnosis of cancer may be doubtful. A conservative resection for this extent of disease is particularly applicable in a patient whose pulmonary status is severely compromised.
2. *A lobectomy* is usually the choice for a patient with a centrally located tumor mass, completely contained within the lobe. The lobar bronchus may be involved, but there must be an adequate tumor-free margin for resection. There may be lymph node extension or metastases that are limited to the first level of lobar lymphatic drainage that can be totally encompassed by an en bloc dissection. These tumors are usually classified as stage I disease or stage II disease.
3. *Pneumonectomy* is the procedure of choice for all physiologically able patients having more extensive disease than described above. This will include tumors extending to the orifice of the lobar bronchus and tumors originating within or extending to the main stem bronchus. Further, when the primary tumor involves more than one lobe, pneumonectomy is generally undertaken. Extended pneumonectomy is recommended in the presence of mediastinal lymph node involvement stage III N-2 disease (a) if the involvement is limited to the node of the ipsilateral tracheobronchial angle or subcarinal space, (b) the histopathologic evaluation of the nodes at mediastinoscopy and thoracotomy shows that the capsules of the nodes are intact with no perinodal disease, (c) the histopathologic classification is squamous cell carcinoma.
4. *Radical pneumonectomy,* defined as resection with intrapericardial ligation of vessels, is applicable in selected patients where the disease extends proximally to the major vessels, but in which technical resection remains possible.
5. *Sleeve lobectomy* is not considered an elective alternative to pneumonectomy in physiologically competent patients as it compromises complete removal of all potentially involved lymphatics. However, this procedure may be selected as an alternative to no surgery for patients with limited pulmonary reserve having tumor involving the lobar and the adjacent main bronchus.

A special group of stage III groups consists of patients with "superior sulcus tumor," located in the upper lobe with invasion direct into the parietal pleura, and invasion of intracostal muscle or ribs. They usually present with painful apical syndrome or with a true Pancoast syndrome which include a lytic lesion of the adjacent bony chest wall and/or a Horner's syndrome. In this particular category of patients, preoperative radiotherapy is usually applied in a dose of 3000 rad in 3 weeks, followed by lobectomy or more extended resection.

The results of surgery for non-small cell cancer is given according to stage in Figs. 1 and 2. It is noteworthy that the best results can be obtained for squamous cell carcinoma in particular, when one is comparing stage II and III of this histologic cell type with adenocarcinoma and undifferentiated large cell carcinoma.

Adjuvant Therapy to Surgery

The results of surgical treatment of lung cancer have essentially been unchanged during the past 2 decades, for which reasons a lot of interest has been focused on the use of adjuvant therapy such as radiotherapy, chemotherapy, and immunotherapy given either pre- or postoperatively. Numerous prospective randomized trials have been performed even combining three or four modalities of therapy, but the results have been very disappointing. With a few exceptions, such as the use of preoperative radiotherapy in cases with superior sulcus tumors (see above), there is at present no evidence which can substantiate the routine use of either of these modalities in combination with surgery.

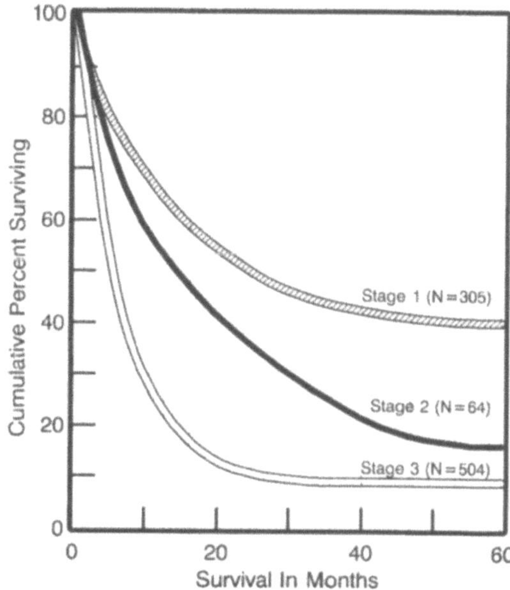

Fig. 1. Survival of patients with resected squamous cell carcinoma of lung by postsurgical treatment stage of disease. (Reproduced by permission of the AJC for Cancer Staging and End Results Reporting)

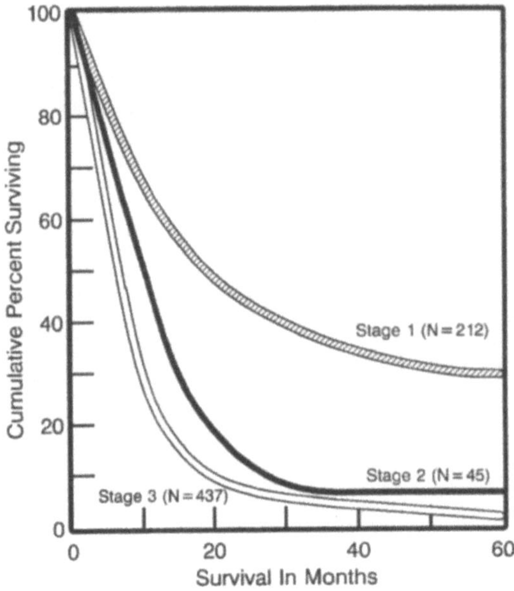

Fig. 2. Survival of patient with resected adenocarcinoma and undifferentiated large cell carcinoma of lung by postsurgical treatment stage of disease. (Reproduced by permission of the AJC for Cancer Staging and End Results Reporting)

Radiotherapy

Introduction

Despite the fact that lung cancer patients have been treated with radiotherapy since the late 1940s, the exact role of this modality remains controversial. The reason for this situation is caused by factors such as: (a) lack of sufficient number of adequately controlled randomized trials, (b) lack of separation of the major histologic types of lung cancer, (c) lack of updated results from a number of clinical trials, and (d) lack of detailed analysis of clinical prognostic variables.

Furthermore, analysis of the data is hampered by varying standards of staging of initial disease, definition of the physical status of patients, criteria for assessment of early response to therapy, and the use of varying techniques with different modes of delivering the radiation therapy.

In the following, we will briefly present how radiotherapy at present is administered to patients with lung cancer, in particular, the "non-small cell" type, at the Finsen Institute. Before deciding on whether to use radiotherapy or not, it is important to assess the potential value of the treatment, not only in conventional terms of survival, which is usually short, but also in terms of palliation of existing symptoms and the general quality of life. It has to be remembered that radiotherapy is or may be accompanied by considerable morbidity, even when used by skilled persons.

The aim of radiotherapy is usually to deliver a tumoricidal radiation dose to the primary tumor including local regional areas of spread. The volume will therefore include the primary mass, hilar and mediastinal lymph node areas, and a margin for the microscopic extension of the tumor. A compromise has to be reached between the dose necessary to sterilize this large volume, the patient's tolerance, and the radiobiologic tolerance of associated intrathoracic structures. In practice, this means irradiating the smallest possible volume of normal lung tissue not exceeding the spinal tolerance.

Treatment Planning

Detailed clinical, bronchoscopic, and radiologic information concerning the location and regional spread of the primary tumor is necessary to determine the anatomic volume to be treated. Usually, a treatment simulator machine is used to determine the proximal and distant extent, and the width of the volume to be used. Various field arrangements can be used depending on the shape and position of the high-dose volume relative to the spinal cord.

Usually, megavoltage equipment is used with a 4- to 10-million-volt (MeV) energy linear accelerator, or cobalt-60. This energy gives a relatively low entrance skin dose, and adequate penetration to the deeper tissues with excellent collimation of the beam, thus permitting very little scatter to the adjacent normal tissues. Dose inhomogeneity can be avoided by the use of wedge filters as compensators, and the dose calculation is corrected for greater transmission through aerated normal lung. Sensitive normal structures such as the spinal cord and the larynx can be shielded to avoid excessive irradiation. Port films obtained on the treatment machine should be used to verify final beam positions. Various doses and fractionation schedules are used in the treatment of lung cancer. Despite extensive literature and some firmly held opinions, optimal conditions have not been universally established. At present, we are using 5000 rad in 25 daily fractions when more "radical" radiotherapy is given. In other cases, a "split-course" technique is used, which consists of 2000 rad in 5 daily fractions, repeated after a 4-week gap. The latter is considered more practical because within a short period it is possible to establish whether or not the tumor is radiosensitive, and prompt administration allows for the presenting symptoms to be rapidly relieved.

When considering the indication for "radical" radiotherapy, the small proportion of possible candidates can be divided into the following groups: (a) stage I patients in whom there is a medical contraindication to thoracotomy. It should be emphasized, though, that an attempt to give curative irradiation will compromise the patient's pulmonary reserve considerably. (b) Stage II lung cancer found unresectable at thoracotomy.

Again, however, it should be stressed that large clinical trials, demonstrating whether or not the use of radiotherapy in the above-mentioned situations improves median or long-term survival, are still lacking.

Palliative Radiotherapy

For the majority of patients with "non-small cell" lung cancer, the extent of disease makes the prospects of cure by any available treatment method unrealistic. The majority of patients with extrathoracic disease at presentation have a life expectancy of between 3 and 4 months. In most cases, the presence of advanced local disease or metastases will give rise to distressing symptoms. In this group of patients, the use of radiotherapy might improve the quality of the remaining life period. Radiotherapy must be given at a minimum cost both in terms of radiation-associated morbidity and general inconvenience to the patient. Successful palliation of symptoms is almost always caused by tumor regression, and it is therefore necessary to use a dose and technique which reliably produce tumor response. The general philosophy of palliative radiation is aimed at growth restraint, rather than at tumor sterilizations, and uses relatively large volumes with a corresponding reduction in the dose of irradiation.

Numerous doses and fractionation schedules are in use, e.g., 3000 rad in 10 fractions over 2 weeks, 2000 rad in 5 fractions over 1 week, and a single fraction of 750-1000 rad. At present we have found the schedule of 2000 rad in 5 fractions over 1 week to be the most convenient with the least morbidity.

Radiotherapy of Intrathoracic Disease

Hemoptysis and cough, perhaps the most common distressing symptoms, are easily controlled by radiotherapy. Up to 75% of patients treated will experience some degree of relief. Dyspnea caused by bronchial obstruction can be improved in about half the patients, depending on the site and duration. In cases where mediastinal lymph node enlargement causes compression of the esophagus, the dysphagia can be relieved in 80% of the patients.

The syndrome of superior vena cava obstruction should also be relieved by radiotherapy, even in the presence of metastatic disease. More than half of the patients will experience relief. In our experience, there is no reason to combine radiotherapy with the use of steroids or the use of chemotherapy.

Local pain due to chest wall or rib involvement can be partially relieved in a large fraction of patients, while pain due to brachial plexus involvement in apical lesions is much less responsive to radiation.

Radiotherapy of Extrathoracic Disease

Radiotherapy is often widely used in treating metastatic lesions secondary to lung cancer, e.g., in the brain, spinal cord, and bones.

Central nervous system irradiation is usually given as whole brain irradiation with a dose of 3000 rad in 10 fractions over 2 weeks, which achieves a good short-lasting (median 2-3 months) palliation in 75% of all cases. The application of corticosteroids (e.g., prednisone 100 mg or dexamethasone 16 mg daily) will further give symptomatic benefit by reducing the intracranial pressure and edema surrounding the intracerebral deposit.

Spinal cord compression is observed in 8%-10% of all patients with lung cancer. If it occurs, laminectomy remains the treatment of choice for obtaining a rapid decompression because of the rather low radiosensitivity of "non-small cell" lung cancer, while radiotherapy is primarily reserved for patients with slowly evolving or stable compression syndromes, or for situations where the general conditions preclude the possibility of surgical intervention. In the latter group of patients, the prognosis is extremely poor, often 2-3 months, but in order to relieve the pain and diminish the neurologic symptoms the use of radiotherapy is advisable. A dose of 3000 rad in 10 daily fractions is most commonly used.

The effectiveness of radiotherapy in pain relief in patients with bone metastases secondary to lung cancer is well known. About 30%–50% of the patients can be pain free or have a considerable improvement in pain in non-weight-bearing areas where the risk of subsequent pathologic fracture is minimal. Single fractions of radiotherapy may be sufficient, e.g., 800 rad; otherwise the simple course of low-dose irradiation, e.g., 400 rad daily × 5, is sufficient.

Sequelae of Radiotherapy

Among the most commonly observed side effects are radiation esophagitis, which develops usually 5–10 days following the completion of treatment. The symptoms include dysphagia, and some symptomatic relief can be obtained by modifying the diet slightly, while the use of topical anesthetics can also be of some help.

The frequency with which symptomatic esophagitis develops is dose related. At doses in excess of 5500 rad, 40%–50% of all patients developed this complication.

More delayed side effects include pneumonitis and pulmonary fibrosis. Between 5% and 15% of patients receiving high-dose chest radiotherapy become breathless and develop an accompanying nonproductive cough 2–6 months after radiotherapy. A chest X-ray will frequently demonstrate soft irregular shadowing in the irradiated zone. The syndrome is usually self-limiting, and symptomatic relief may be obtained by administering steroids systemically.

The frequency and severity of pulmonary fibrosis is usually related to the radiation dose in the lung and to the volume of the lung encompassed in the high-dose area. Assessment of the physiological changes demonstrates severe abnormalities which are usually a result of the postradiation fibrosis, the tumor, and preexisting lung disease.

Another complication which is rarely seen is radiation myelitis, radiation myolopathy, and radiation-induced pericarditis. The two latter complications are seen in less than 5% of all cases.

Chemotherapy in "Non-Small Cell" Lung Cancer

Chemotherapy has no established role in the routine treatment of non-small lung cancer. In more recent studies, combination chemotherapy with, e.g., vindesine plus *cis*-platinum or etoposide plus *cis*-platinum, have been reported to give objective remissions with more than 50% reduction of tumors in 20%–40% of previously untreated patients. Complete remissions are rare. In some studies, a modest prolongation of survival can be achieved comparing responding patients with nonresponding patients. Highest response rates can be obtained in patients with adenocarcinoma and epidermoid carcinoma, while large cell carcinoma is a very unresponsive tumor. At the present time, chemotherapy in patients with non-small cell lung cancer should be considered as an experimental treatment form. In patients with poor prognostic features, such as low performance status, extensive disease, massive weight loss, high age, previous therapy, the likelihood for tumor regression is very low. Accordingly, treatment with cytostatic agents should only be instituted in highly selective unresectable cases, and after the patients have been informed completely about the limitations of the treatment. Again, it is preferable if the patient can be included in a controlled clinical trial usually in a multicenter setup.

Small Cell Carcinoma of the Lung

Following the introduction of combination chemotherapy, the treatment of patients with small cell lung cancer (SCLC) has undergone major changes in the 1970s. These changes resulted in a four- to fivefold prolongation of the median survival of all small cell lung cancer patients, including a long-term disease-free survival of over 3 years duration in 8%–10%. Considerable progress has thus taken place, but there is still no standardized therapy for small cell carcinoma. Efforts are continuing at many centers and in national and international groups in order to gather increasing knowledge of the special biologic features of small cell carcinoma, including alternative therapies in the hope that this neoplasm can be converted into a more readily curable disease. The treatment of SCLC is therefore continuously evolving. The treatment of most SCLC patients, through a systematic approach using clinical trials, is the means by which this evolution will maximize the success of this quest.

Before initiating treatment it is important to have the purpose of the treatment in mind. In the elderly patients, the palliative part of the treatment might be the most important, while in the younger patients, long-term survival, if possible, cure, is usually the main goal of the treatment, in spite of the occurrence of severe toxic effects of the treatment in periods. Accordingly, it is important to have the patients carefully evaluated with respect to main prognostic factors before instituting treatment.

The known prognostic factors for SCLC are listed in Table 1. Currently, the two most important prognostic factors are pretreatment performance status and extent of disease. With respect to age and sex, patients < 60 years of age appear to do better than those > 60, and females appear to have better prognosis than males. Additionally, a pretreatment weight loss of more than 3 kg appears to impart a significantly adverse prognosis.

Table 1. Prognostic factors in small cell carcinoma

Stage of disease: localized versus extensive
Performance status
Pretreatment weight loss
Sex
Age
Histopathologic subclassification[a]
CNS metastases
Bone metastases
Liver metastases

[a] Prognosis is especially poor for the intermediate type with large cell elements

The prognostic value of the histopathologic subclassification of small cell carcinoma, according to the WHO classification of 1981, is still somewhat confusing, with disagreement on the impact of subhistology. This may be a reflection of the lack of consistency in different pathologic findings, rather than a genuine difference in the biology of the oat cell type versus the intermediate type of SCLC. It is noteworthy that recently a specially poor prognosis has been demonstrated for patients with small cell lung cancer characterized before treatment as having tumors with both small and large cell components. These tumors were previously classified in the mixed histologies, but are now included in the intermediate type subgroup.

Chemotherapy

The ideal therapeutic goal in small cell lung cancer is the most effective treatment for producing the highest percentage of long-term disease-free survivors (cures) with the lowest possible morbidity. Multiple agents have been shown to possess antitumor activity in small cell lung cancer, and a list of these is shown in Table 2. Many studies of combination chemotherapy, usually derived from the active single agents, have been carried out during the past decade. The most active combinations have included such compounds as vincristine, etoposide (VP-16-213), cyclophosphamide, doxorubicin (Adriamycin), CCNU, and methotrexate. Among the most commonly used and highly active are the following: (a) vincristine, etoposide, and cyclophosphamide; (b) CCNU, vincristine, cyclophosphamide and etoposide; and (c) cyclophosphamide, doxorubicin, and vincristine. Examples of the latter regimens are given in Table 3, including the actual doses and schedules of the various compounds.

Generally, it is clear that drug combinations with three or four drugs are superior to single agents in treating the disease, and that the best results are currently

Table 2. Active single agents in small cell carcinoma

Epidodophyllotoxin derivatives
Tenoposide (VM-26)
Etoposide (VP-16)
Alkylating agents
Cyclophosphamide (cytoxan, endoxan)
Isophosphamide
Hexamethylmelamine
Vinca alkaloids
Vincristine
Vindesine
Platinum derivatives
cis-Platinum
Carboplatin
Nitrosourea derivatives
CCNU
Doxorubicin
Methotrexate

Table 3. Combination chemotherapy of small cell carcinoma: commonly used regimens

1. Cyclophosphamide 1000 mg/m^2 i.v. q. 4 weeks, day 1
   CCNU 70 mg/m^2 p.o. q. 4 weeks, day 1
   Vincristine 1.3 mg/m^2 i.v. (maximally 2 mg) q. 4 weeks, day 1,
     except first 4 weeks, when administered weekly
   Etoposide (VP-16) 75 mg/m^2 p.o. days 2, 3, 4, 5 in each cycle q. 4 weeks
2. Cyclophosphamide 750 mg/m^2 i.v. q. 3 weeks
   Doxorubicin 50 mg/m^2 i.v. q. 3 weeks
   Vincristine 1.3 mg/m^2 i.v. q. 3 weeks
3. Cyclophosphamide 1000 mg/m^2 i.v. day 1 q. 3 weeks
   Doxorubicin 45 mg/m^2 i.v. day 1 q. 3 weeks
   Etoposide (VP-16) 50 mg/m^2 daily i.v. on days 1–5 q. 3 weeks

achieved when using three or more agents. It also appears that more aggressive chemotherapeutic regimens produce slightly better response rates with longer median duration of response and apparently an increased number of patients with long-term disease-free status. The exact dosages and schedules obviously depend on the various combinations used and the tolerable toxicity of the individual compounds and their interactions. Compounds which act synergistically are likely to play an important role.

Currently, in order to deliver maximum therapy, it is necessary to achieve a certain level of toxicity, i.e., a constant and predictable decrease in hematologic parameters. Infectious episodes during periods of granulocytopenia will, therefore, occur. With most combination chemotherapeutic regimens, the major part of the treatment can take place on an outpatient basis.

When given aggressively, the above-mentioned regimens will result in a response rate in excess of 80% for both stages of small cell lung cancer, and it can thus be used in the acute treatment of superior vena cava syndrome. Even with the most conservative evaluation and interpretation of staging results, combination chemotherapy produces complete responses in more than 30%–40% of patients with limited disease and in more than 15%–20% of patients with extensive disease. Provided an adequate staging procedure has been done, the median survival for patients with limited disease should be 14 or more months, and the median duration of survival for patients with extensive disease should be 8 or more months. Approximately 15%–20% of patients with limited disease and less than 5% of those with extensive disease will achieve a long-term disease-free survival of more than 2 years. All studies done so far indicate that patients who achieve a complete response (CR) have a significantly longer survival than patients with a partial response, and that only patients achieving a CR have the potential for long-term disease-free survival.

In all studies it has also been uniformly found that patients with limited disease live significantly longer than those presenting with extensive disease. An example of survival data comparing limited and extensive disease, based on data from Finsen, is given in Fig. 3.

With respect to the duration of treatment it is still uncertain for how long a time one has to treat in order to achieve optimal results and, particularly, what the duration of treatment should be in order to achieve cures. The majority of clinical

106

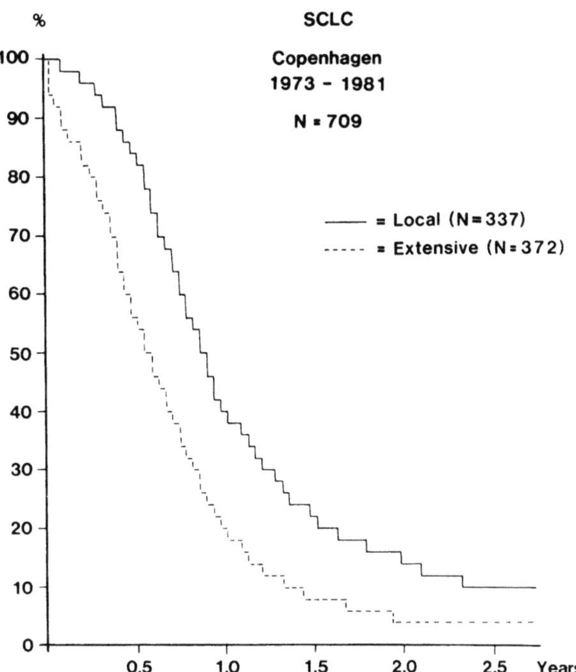

Fig. 3. Survival of 709 consecutive patients with small cell carcinoma of lung according to extent of disease

trials are presently maintaining chemotherapy for periods varying from 6 to 12 months, with longer periods being used in patients showing a response. At our own institution, we treat, at present, responding patients for periods of 10–12 months, discontinuing the treatment at that time if careful reevaluation, including bronchoscopy, peritoneoscopy with liver biopsy, and bilateral bone marrow examination, indicates a CR.

A number of trials and centers are focusing on varieties of options to improve the present systemic therapy. These issues include (a) the use of alternating (non-cross-resistant) combination chemotherapy, (b) scheduling of drug administration in order to take advantage of the cell cycle changes induced by the initial therapy, (c) incorporation of new agents with high activity in the combination chemotherapy regimens, (d) the use of intensive high-dose chemotherapy with or without bone marrow transplantation, (e) the simultaneous use of synergistic compounds, and (f) immunotherapy. All these methods are investigated, but they cannot at present be recommended as routine in the management of patients with small cell lung cancer.

As mentioned above, the initial treatment usually produces response and symptomatic improvement in 80%–90% of patients; however, the largest group of patients relapse within a period of 10–12 months. The first relapse may be local or may occur in metastatic sites, the liver, bone, or brain. The subsequent treatment will depend on the location of this relapse. If a peripheral relapse is occurring, one would tend to change the chemotherapy, including other active agents not used in the initial treatment.

The results with the latter combinations are, however, generally disappointing, with response rates of less than 30%-35%, and a median duration of response of 2-3 months. If the recurrence is exclusively local, palliative radiotherapy can be instituted, but, again, the results are disappointing with respect to survival. It should be stressed, however, that the palliative effect is often very good, even when using radiotherapy in relatively low doses as given at our institute with a fractionation of 400 rad daily × 5, with an interval of 3 weeks, after which the second series of radiotherapy with the same schedule and dose can be given if a positive effect of the first treatment has been observed.

Radiotherapy

Small cell carcinoma of the lung is known to be the most radiosensitive of all lung cancers, but the role of radiotherapy in the management of this disease still remains to be defined. At present, radiotherapy is mainly used either for prophylactic brain irradiation in an attempt to reduce the incidence of CNS metastases, or in combination with chemotherapy in the management of patients presenting with intrathoracic limited disease.

The role of radiotherapy to the primary tumor and regional lymph nodes, in the overall management of small cell carcinoma, remains to be clarified. Several studies, including some of our own studies at the Finsen Institute, have addressed this question, using various types of combination chemotherapy and radiotherapy in various schedules and doses. Many of the studies are ongoing, and detailed information and conclusive data are still lacking. Based on our own study, with a follow-up of 5 years, the use of combined modality therapy does not appear to be superior to chemotherapy alone. At present, we are therefore not using radiotherapy to the primary tumor in the overall management of patients with small cell carcinoma. Combined mode of therapy may no doubt decrease the incidence and delay the time of local recurrences; however, it apparently also increases the morbidity.

The optimal way of combining radiotherapy and chemotherapy is uncertain at present. Many studies are focusing on methods reducing the considerable toxicity of such treatment including esophagitis, pneumonitis, and myelotoxicity. The schedule and the dose of radiotherapy to be used for the long-term local control of disease remain uncertain, and are likely to be dependent on the chemotherapy used. Technologic advances, however, are likely to have considerable impact on the ability to use combined-modality therapy. One would expect that the use of CT scan, especially in the planning of treatment, will result in a reduction of the field size, and thereby minimize the radiation damage to normal lung tissue and to the surrounding normal tissues.

As to prophylactic cranial irradiation, this has been used because CNS metastases are now recognized as a frequent complication to small cell carcinoma. Involvement of the CNS is seen in more than 10% of the patients initially, and it occurs in more than 50% of all cases according to autopsy data. The incidence of CNS metastases increases with longer survival as a result of improved systemic therapy.

A number of randomized studies have focused on the use of prophylactic irradiation, and a number of reviews have been published. At present it appears that prophylactic brain irradiation, if used, should be limited exclusively to patients achieving a complete remission within 2-3 months after initiation of therapy. The most commonly used schedule for prophylactic brain irradiation is a total of 3000 rad given as a whole brain irradiation in a period of 3 weeks.

More recently, reports have been published describing possible late-occurring CNS side effects of CNS irradiation, including cerebral atrophy, which should caution the general use of CNS prophylactic irradiation.

Surgery

Within the past few decades, small cell carcinoma of the lung has been recognized as a widely disseminated disease in most cases. Thus, initial surgery with a curative intent has essentially ceased, with the exception of the small group of patients (less than 1%) who present initially with a small isolated T1, N0, M0 lesion. This is also the case for the rare patients with initial T2, N0, M0 or T1, N1, M0 disease, provided surgery is followed by combination chemotherapy.

Mesothelioma

As mentioned earlier, mesothelioma is classified into localized or diffuse types. The therapy is in accordance with these classifications, with surgery being indicated for the former, but not for the latter. Surgery should consist of a thoracotomy with resection of the pleural tumor. The results vary considerably from institution to institution. The 5-year survival is usually recorded as being about 40%.

With respect to diffuse mesothelioma, it constitutes between 50% and 60% of all malignant epitheliomas in the pleural cavity. The treatment remains of an experimental investigational nature, and the results of radiotherapy, given either with application of intrapleural 98-gold or external irradiation, are disappointing. The results are similarly disappointing with chemotherapy, both with single agents and combination chemotherapy, and the routine use of the latter treatment modalities thus cannot be recommended.

Further Reading

Aisner J (1985) Lung Cancer. Churchill Livingstone, London
Carter D, Eggleston JC (1980) Tumors of the lower respiratory tract. Atlas of tumor pathology. Fascicle 17. Armed Forces Institute of Pathology, Washington DC
Hansen HH, Rørth M (1980) Lung Cancer 1980. Excerpta Medica, Amsterdam
Ishikawa S, Hayataka Y, Suemasu K (1980) Lung Cancer 1982. Excerpta Medica, Amsterdam
Straus MJ (1983) Lung Cancer. Clinical diagnosis and treatment, 2nd edn. Grune and Stratton, New York
WHO (1981) World Health Organization: Histological typing of lung tumors, 2nd edn. Geneva

11. Surgical Treatment in Non-Small Cell Carcinoma of the Lung: The Memorial Sloan-Kettering Experience

N. Martini, M. S. Bains, P. McCormack, L. R. Kaiser, M. E. Burt,
and A. H. Pomerantz

Carcinoma of the lung remains the most common cancer in men in the United States. It has been the most common cause of cancer death in men and its incidence is still rising. Unfortunately, since 1985 it has now become also the most common cause of cancer death in women. The American Cancer Society projected for 1986 that 149 000 new cases of lung cancer would be detected in the United States alone, and of these 130 100 would die of their disease. It has also predicted that 41 100 cases of cancer death due to lung cancer would occur for women, 1200 more than the breast cancer death anticipated in women in 1986 [1].

Despite this high incidence, the overall curability of lung cancer has remained low. Currently, overall 5-year survival ranges from 10% to 13% [1]. Survival without treatment is rarely possible and most untreated patients die within 1 year of diagnosis, with a median survival of less than 6 months.

Cigarette smoking remains the most important risk factor influencing the incidence of lung cancer in the United States. Eighty-five to 90% of all lung cancers are found in smokers. Despite this fact, not enough is being done in either government or private sectors to effect reduction of the use of tobacco in the adult population. Although advertisement in newspapers and television media is no longer permitted, billboard advertising is still encouraged by individual tobacco companies. The American Medical Association only recently recommended the banning of all advertisement regarding cigarette consumption in the United States.

The frequency of the various histologic types of lung carcinoma seen at the Memorial Sloan-Kettering Cancer Center (MSKCC) is also changing (Fig. 1). Today, adenocarcinoma has become the most frequent histologic type of lung cancer, and is responsible for 50% of all lung cancers. Epidermoid or squamous cell carcinoma represents only 30% of all lung cancers, and oat cell or small cell carcinoma 15%, with large cell carcinoma making up less than 5%. This predominance of adenocarcinoma is also noted in several cancer institutes in the United States [2, 3, 4] but not in others.

Prognosis in carcinoma of the lung is influenced by the stage of the disease at presentation, which in turn determines its resectability. Because of this fact, it has become important to carefully to stage all carcinomas of the lung at the time of their initial clinical presentation. Since 1972 the American Joint Committee's TNM staging system has been used throughout the United States and Canada [5]. Curative treatment requires the effective control of the primary tumor before metastases develop. Except for small cell carcinoma, surgery remains the most effective mode of treatment, provided the tumor is resectable and the risks of the procedure are low.

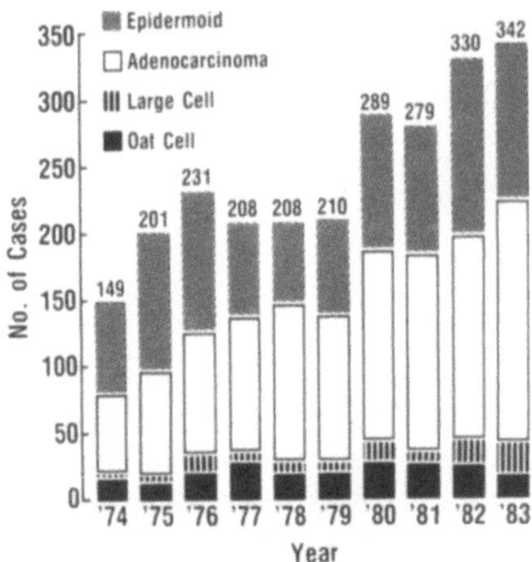

Fig. 1. Yearly accrual of carcinoma of the lung at Memorial Sloan Kettering Cancer Center by histology

Despite the increasing incidence of lung cancer, there are as yet no new methods to detect lung cancer at an early stage. The only two methods of early detection remain chest roentgenography and sputum cytologic examination. There are as yet no serologic tumor markers that are clinically applicable to detect early lung cancer.

Occult Carcinomas of the Lung

Few patients are found to have lung carcinoma before it becomes radiographically apparent. These patients represent 1.5% of our clinical case experience in primary lung cancer at Memorial Hospital [2]. These are individuals who participate in early lung cancer detection programs and submit sputum cytologic examinations on a routine basis, or patients who present to Institutions with hemoptysis in the absence of any abnormal findings on routine chest roentgenograms. Occult carcinomas presenting in this fashion, need a careful investigation to localize the site of the cancer. The fact that the patient has a normal chest roentgenogram and a positive sputum cytology does not necessarily indicate that the patient has lung carcinoma, let alone an early lung carcinoma [6]. A careful head and neck examination is essential. In our experience, patients who present with a positive sputum cytology in the absence of radiologic findings are noted to have a carcinoma in the head and neck region in one out of three instances. If the head and neck examination is normal, then a careful diagnostic bronchoscopy is performed. With the use of the modern fiberoptic bronchoscope it has become possible to extend the inspection of the tracheobronchial tree from the main stem and lobar bronchi to segmental and subsegmental bronchi to sixth- and sometimes seventh-generation bronchi. By this method alone with careful and diligent inspection of the tracheobronchial tree in patients with radiologically occult carcinomas, one can usually identify the site of the lung carcinoma. If the lesion is located centrally in a main or a lobar bronchus, it is readily visualized and a biopsy easily obtained. However, in many instances the tracheobronchial tree appears entirely normal at bronchoscopy. In these instances, a meticulous sampling of each segmental bronchus by endobronchial brushing and cytologic analysis becomes necessary. Careful attention to detail to avoid cross contamination has resulted in localizing these peripheral tumors in nearly all instances. Following localization, the treatment of choice for a radiologically occult carcinoma of the lung is surgical extirpation of the primary tumor by lobectomy or pneumonectomy. Since most occult carcinomas are relatively central in position, lesser resections usually are not possible. Unfortunately, despite early detection and localization, one out of three patients presenting with radiologically occult carcinomas are found at operation to have advanced disease with lymphatic metastases or extension to parietal pleura and mediastinum [6].

The detection of radiologically occult lung carcinomas is uncommon. The case yields from lung cancer screening programs directed at detecting this presumably earliest stage of disease have been extremely low. Of 10 040 male cigarette smokers 45 years of age or older screened in our own prospective study of early lung cancer detection, all were evaluated by chest radiography and half were randomized for additional sputum cytologic analysis, the so-called dual screening group. For the entire screened population, 53 confirmed lung cancers were found, a yield of 0.5%. Of these, 23 were detected in the roentgenogram only group, and 30 in the dual screen group [7]. Of 4968 patients in the dual screen group, 7 cases of proven radiographically occult lung carcinoma in the in situ or microinvasive stage were detected, a yield of less than 0.2%. Nationwide, less than half of 1% of all lung cancers seen are detected in the radiographically occult stage. Over the past 35 years at Memorial Sloan-Kettering Cancer Center we have been able to accumulate 65 patients with radiologically occult carcinomas of the lung. Of these, 90% have been epidermoid carcinomas. Few were adenocarcinomas and to date we have not observed a small cell carcinoma at a radiologically occult stage. Fiberoptic bronchoscopy localized these lesions in nearly all instances.

More sophisticated techniques of in vivo fluorescent staining of mucosal malignancy with hematoporphyrin derivative may further enhance the sensitivity and specificity of bronchoscopic localization. Parenterally administered hematoporphyrin derivative has been shown to be taken up selectively by malignant endobronchial cells, which can then be visualized bronchoscopically by laser-stimulated fluorescence. This technique has proven helpful in identifying and localizing occult malignancy that is not apparent to the naked eye at broncoscopy [8]. This method allows detection of the earliest forms of carcinoma in situ together with atypical squamous metaplasia. In addition, photodynamic therapy using trans-bronchoscopic laser-induced photoexcitation of hematoporphyrin derinative has been shown effective by Hayata et al. in eradicating occult endobronchial lung cancer, though long-term experience to date has been limited [9].

The treatment of choice of radiologically occult lung carcinoma is surgical resection. The median survival of these patients is very long and presently holds at 9 years. Importantly, we have not observed a single case of recurrence of the original lung carcinoma following resection of a radiographically occult stage I lung cancer, despite periods of follow-up extending to 25 years. Unfortunately, the risk of developing other carcinomas in this group of patients remains a threat to long-term suvival. In our experience 45% of these patients develop new carcinomas, the majority of which are new airway carcinomas. It is essential, therefore, that a continued surveillance of these patients be carried out at 6- to 12-month intervals indefinitely.

Treatment of T1 N0 M0 and T2 N0 M0 Tumors

The more common form of early lung carcinoma seen by most physicians is the one that is referred to as stage 1 carcinoma. Many of these are detected on routine chest roentgenograms in patients that present for unrelated medical conditions. For instance, some present for management of their inguinal hernia, others for abdominal pain and cholecystitis, or for management of their diabetes. A routine chest roentgenogram is done as part of their investigational workup and detects a discrete peripheral lesion, a so-called coin lesion of the lung. If the patient is fortunate enough to have taken chest roentgenograms a year or two earlier, these are used to compare the interval change between the films, and the accuracy of detecting an early carcinoma is enhanced. In this setting, lesions that are more than 1 cm in diameter, perticularly in individuals who have been smokers and are 50 years of age or older, are suspected to be early lung carcinomas until proven otherwise and are promptly acted upon. In our experience patients with peripheral tumors in the T1 N0 M0 stage, namely tumors that are less than 3 cm in diameter, confined to lung parenchyma without evidence of regional lymphatic metastases, extension to chest wall, diaphragm, pleura, or distant metastases, have a 5-year disease-free survival of 83% when treated by primary sugical resection [10]. Tumors greater than 3 cm in diameter still confined to lung without metastases when treated by surgical resection also have a very favourable prognosis with an anticipated 5-year survival free of disease in 2 out of 3 patients, or 65% of instances. The overall 5-year survival in stage 1 carcinoma of lung T1 or T2 in size is currently 72% at 5 years. It is essential, however, that at the time of the surgical resection for carcinoma of the lung that a meticulous and systematic lymph node dissection and evaluation of the mediastinum be carried out, lest lymphatic metastases in those sites are overlooked. It is in so doing that the patient is assured of a correct post-surgical or pathological staging of his carcinoma and that his expectations of survival for many years are indeed extremely favorable (Fig. 2). Patients with this favorable prognosis following resection are also at high risk to develop second carcinomas and, in our experience, 1 out of 3 or 33% of these patients develop second primary malignancies. Therefore it is imperative that the follow-up of patients with early lung cancer despite treatment remains continuous with periodic radiographic and clinical evaluations at 6- to 12-month intervals. We do not routinely follow our postoperative patients with sputum cytology in the absence of symptoms of productive cough or hemoptysis. This is in accord with the NCI cooperative early lung cancer detection programme which has determined chest roentgen-

114

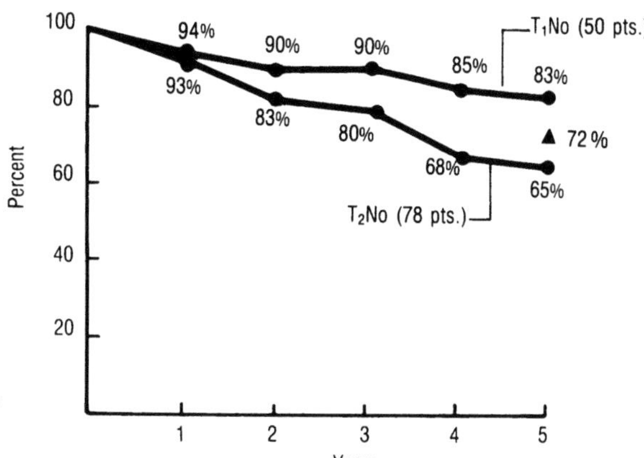

Fig. 2. Survival of resected T1N0 and T2N0, non-small cell carcinoma of the lung

ography to be the most sensitive method currently available for detecting lung cancer. Sputum cytology, on the other hand, was found to be a less sensitive but more specific index of disease [11, 12].

Treatment of T1N1 and T2N1 Tumors

An intermediate group of patients with carcinoma of the lung also present with moderately localized disease amenable to potentially curative resection. This group includes patients who have their primary tumor confined to the lung but with the presence of peribronchial or hilar lymph node metastases. This group of patients are classified to have N1 disease without mediastinal lymph node metastases or distant organ involvement. In this group are the T1 N1 and the T2 N1 tumors. N1 nodes include the hilar, interlobar, lobar, segmental, and more peripheral lymph nodes exclusive of mediastinal lymph node involvement. These N1 nodes correspond to nodal levels greater than or equal to ten in our standardized map of pulmonary lymphatic drainage (Fig. 3). The treatment of choice in this group of patients is again surgical resection of their primary tumor, with a systematic mediastinal lymph node dissection to ensure the absence of lymphatic metastases in the mediastinum. Half of these patients following resection are anticipated to remain free of disease 5 or more years from treatment [13].

In a recent retrospective review from our institution of 78 patients with N1 disease treated by resection, the 5-year survival was 49% for the entire group, 56% for T1 N1 patients, and 48% for the T2 N1 patients (Fig. 4). The incidence of recurrence both locally and distally was high. Fifty percent of these patients have succumbed to local, regional, or distant recurrence in the course of their follow-up. Adjuvant therapy in the form of postoperative radiation therapy and/or chemotherapy has been tried in this group of patients, but there is as yet no evidence that either mode of adjuvant treatment influences overall survival. The main reason is

115

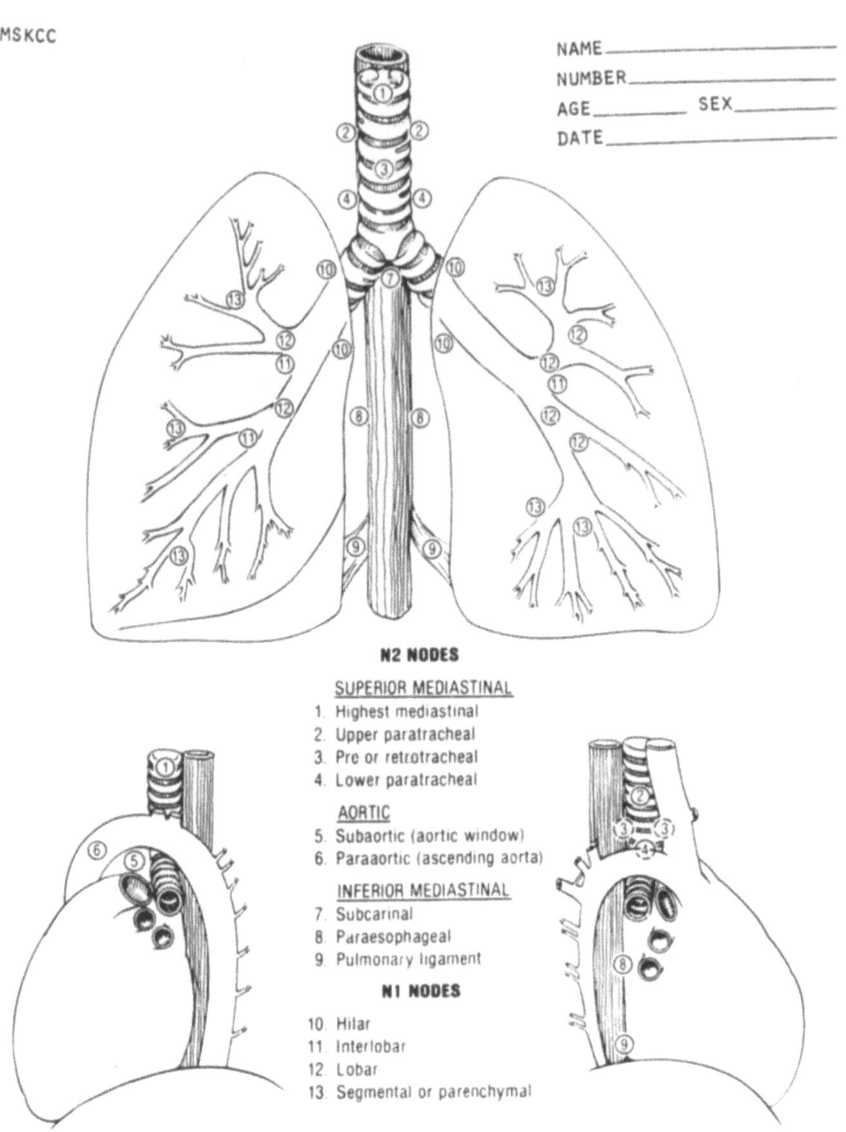

Fig. 3. Lymph node map [38]

that patients with N1 disease represent less than 5% of the lung cancer population, and no single institution accumulates enough case material to be able to assess the value of specific adjuvant treatment regimens in this patient group. Multi-institutional cooperative studies are necessary to evaluate adjuvant treatment.

Clearly some form of adjuvant treatment would seem necessary in this group, to salvage the 50% who develop recurrence. Within this small group of patients, no specific survival advantage was noted between those with epidermoid carcinomas and those with adenocarcinomas of the lung [13]. Recurrence was more fre-

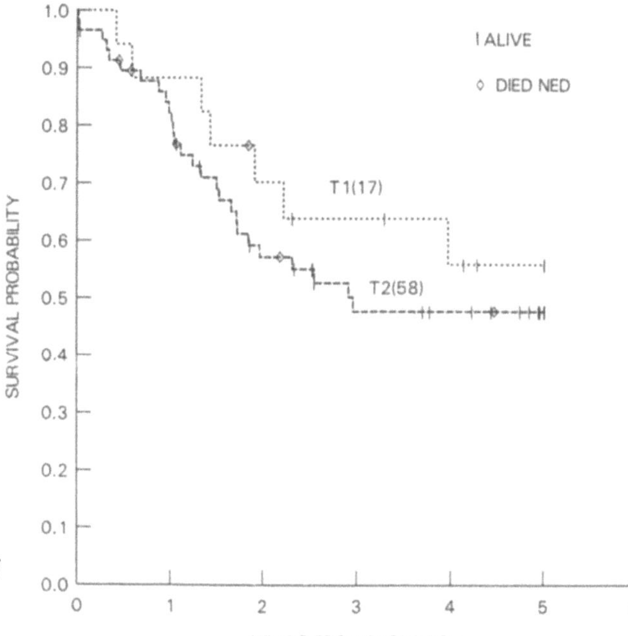

Fig. 4. Actuarial survival of resected T1 N1 and T2 N1, non-small cell carcinoma of the lung

quently distant in adenocarcinomas, with only one patient demonstrating locoregional recurrence. The most common site of distant metastasis was the brain. In epidermoid carcinomas, however, one-half of the patients who failed therapy demonstrated local or regional recurrence and the other half had distant metastases. Perhaps in this group of patients, radiation therapy to further sterilize the mediastinum may contribute to better control of the regional disease.

Most investigators believe that the incidence of stage I or II carcinoma presenting for treatment in various institutions is low and ranges from 10% to 15% of all lung cancers seen. We have observed in our tertiary cancer institute that one-third of our total lung cancer accrual is in the stage I or II disease state (Fig. 5 [2]. This may be due to our particular referral pattern or to a more diligent use of a routine chest roentgenogram on all patients.

In general we and most other investigators consider lobectomy, bilobectomy, or pneumonectomy with mediastinal node dissection as optimum primary therapy for clinically operable patients with stage I or II non-small cell lung carcinoma [14]. By definition this includes patients with localized disease of one hemithorax completely confined by unaffected perietal pleura without extension to carina nor metastases to mediastinal lymphatics. Lobectomy is the procedure of choice when disease is limited to a lobe or lobar bronchus. With tumor present within the right bronchus intermedius, bilobectomy should be performed. When the tumor is in a main bronchus, at the pulmonary hilum, or across a lobar fissure, pneumonectomy, or occasionally bilobectomy for right-sided lesions, is necessary in order to en-

117

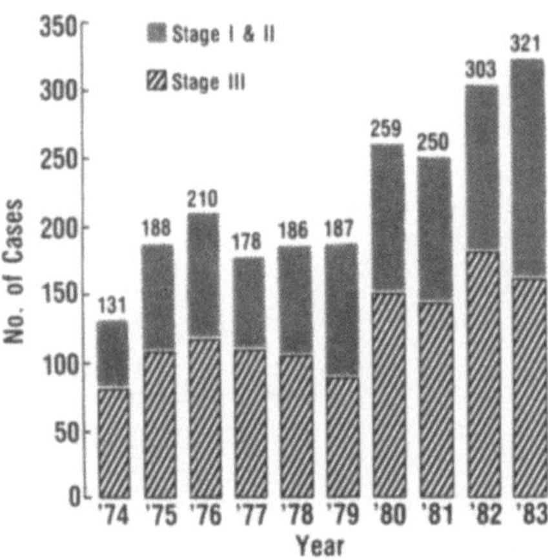

Fig. 5. Yearly accrual of non-small cell carcinoma of the lung at Memorial Sloan-Kettering Cancer Center by clinical stage

compass all disease and obtain clear margins of resection. Technically we prefer stapled closure for all bronchial stumps in these cases.

For tumors protruding from a lobar orifice into the main bronchus, particularly in patients with limited pulmonary reserve, sleeve lobectomy, consisting of resection of the involved lobe and a segment of the main bronchus with reanastomosis of distal and main bronchial margins, may be considered. This procedure serves to conserve pulmonary parenchyma and offers lower morbidity and mortality rates than radical pneumonectomy but comparable curability when complete resection is possible. We consider bronchoscopy performed by the operating surgeon to be an essential part of every pulmonary resection for cure in order to assure both proper clinical staging of disease and proper choice of curative procedure.

Although advocated by others, we do not recommend elective segmentectomy or wedge resections as adequate operative therapy for non-small cell lung carcinoma. We limit such procedures only to select, physiologically compromised, usually elderly patients with limited cardiopulmonary reserve who would be left with an FEV1 of less than 0.8 litres were they to undergo major lobectomy or pneumonectomy, as estimated by quantitative pulmonary function testing. Our results with 53 of such lesser resections for stage I disease (43 T1 N0 and 10 T2 N0) demonstrated a 5-year actuarial survival of 50% and a local recurrence rate of 19% [10]. In confirmation, a much larger series of 259 patients reported by Jensik to have undergone curative segmentectomy demonstrated a 5-year survival of 53% [15]. In contrast, 128 consecutive patients treated by lobectomy or pneumonectomy with mediastinal node dissection yielded a 72% 5-year survival for stage I disease without nodal involvement. Moreover, there was no local pulmonary recurrence in any patient and only three regional recurrences to mediastinal lymph nodes have been observed. A similar favorable surgical experience in stage I non-small cell lung cancer corroborating our findings has been published by the Mayo Clinic group [16].

118

Surgery in Patients with Advanced Disease

Unfortunately, the majority of lung carcinomas presenting for clinical management are advanced tumors and are currently classified as stage III by the American Joint Committee on Cancer. These patients represent two-thirds of our clinical case material of primary lung cancer at Memorial Sloan-Kettering Cancer Center [2]. The factors that limit curability in lung cancer include mediastinal lymph node involvement, extension of the primary tumor to chest wall, mediastinum, diaphragm, trachea, or opposite main bronchus, development of a pleural effusion with or without positive cytology, and the development of distant metastases.

In the absence of distant metastases or M1 disease, many of the advanced non-small cell lung carcinomas are also amenable to surgical treatment, with prolonged survival benefit in many and potential cure in some. From 1968 to 1972, we treated 654 patients with non-small cell carcinoma of the lung [17]. All categories of patients whose tumors could be completely resected exhibited favorable survival statistics. However, there were no 5-year survivors among patients who had inoperable stage III disease without distant metastases (M0) at the time of diagnosis, despite their receiving chemotherapy or radiotherapy.

We also recently looked at the prognostic indicators of long-term survival in 118 patients with carcinoma of the lung who were treated at our institution and were alive at 10 years from their initial diagnosis and treatment [18]. Although the majority had stage I cancers, a third had stage II or III disease. Of 118 patients, 115 had surgery and 3 received radiation therapy only. None of the 10-year survivors had distant metastases at presentation.

In the group of potentially curable stage III disease are three major categories: (1) tumors invading the chest wall, (2) tumors with mediastinal lymph node metastases (N2), and (3) central tumors with extension to within 2 cm of the carina.

Tumors Invading Chest Wall (T3)

In patients with tumors involving the chest wall, resection of the tumor with all involved tissues is still the most effective form of treatment provided the resection can encompass all disease. Many of these peripheral tumors extending into the chest wall present without lymphatic metastases and are amenable to effective pulmonary and chest wall resection. The prognosis for patients with carcinoma of the lung invading chest wall is influenced principally by three factors: (1) resectability, (2) mediastinal lymph node status, and (3) depth of penetration of the tumor into the chest wall proper. We recently reviewed our experience with 111 patients with non-oat cell carcinoma of the lung invading chest wall that were treated surgically [19]. Seventy-seven patients, or two-thirds of this group, underwent a complete resection of the primary tumor and the adjoining affected chest wall, and a complete mediastinal lymph node dissection. The 5-year survival of this group of patients was 40% (Fig. 6). The remainder were either found unresectable or underwent in-

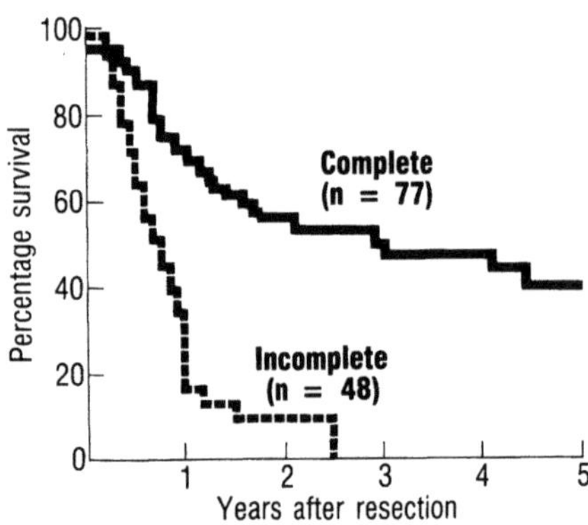

Fig. 6. Actuarial survival of all operated patients with primary chest wall invasion by non-small cell lung carcinoma

complete resection. In this group with incomplete resection were a few patients who had only microscopic residual disease at the margins of resection. Although these patients received a postoperative course of radiation therapy, none survived beyond 2½ years from treatment. It is essential therefore that when resection is done in this group of patients a complete resection of all involved tissue with clearance of all margins microscopically be obtained if prolonged survival is to be attained.

The depth of penetration of the tumor within the chest wall also affects survival. In patients where the tumor extended to the parietal pleura, but did not penetrate beyond the parietal pleura into the soft tissues of the chest wall and the ribs, the 5-year survival following complete resection was better than in patients with deeper involvement of the chest wall (48% vs. 16% respectively for all patients, and 62% vs. 35% for those patients without lymphatic metastases) [19].

The extent of resection is determined by the nature of the chest wall invasion, the site and size of the primary tumor, the ability to resect all tumor, and the medical condition of the patient. In 66 patients extrapleural mobilization of the tumor in the region of its chest wall attachment facilitated the resection. However, 45 patients required en bloc resection of lung and segments of ribs and intercostal muscles because of tumor extension beyond the parietal pleura. Segments of from 1 to 5 ribs were removed and the skeletal defect was reconstructed in 30 patients. Marlex mesh was used alone in 26 patients and Marlex combined with methyl methacrylate in 4 patients. Skeletal reconstruction was not performed in those patients with small chest wall defects or in those with posterosuperior defects lying under cover of the scapula [19].

The extent of surgical resection necessary for peripheral carcinomas of the lung found at thoracotomy to have a parietal attachment remains controversial. Some have advocated that all patients with involvement of the parietal pleura should undergo en bloc resection of lung and chest wall rather than an extrapleural dissection [20, 21]. Our approach has been different. When faced with parietal attachment, we attempt an extrapleural dissection if there is no evidence of extension of disease beyond the parietal pleura. If during the extrapleural approach any resistance to dissection is encountered, dissection is ceased and en bloc resection of chest wall and lung carried out. Employing this technique, more than 88% of

120

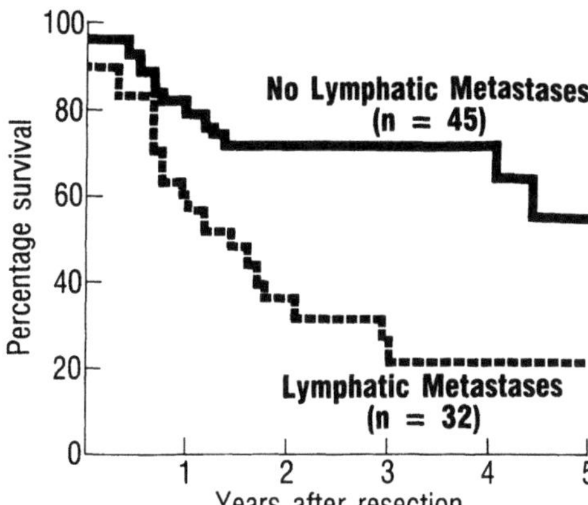

Fig. 7. Actuarial survival for completely resected carcinoma of the lung with chest wall invasion by pathologic nodal involvement

tumors invading only parietal pleura could be resected in this manner. It was necessary in only six patients, found subsequently at pathological examination to have only involvement of the parietal pleura, to perform en bloc resection of chest wall with lung [19]. The pattern of survival in these patients was not different to those undergoing an extrapleural resection. While we recommend an initial attempt at extrapleural dissection we do not hesitate to proceed with chest wall resection when we suspect or find tumor extending beyond the parietal pleura. If extrapleural dissection reveals gross or microscopic evidence by frozen section of deeper chest wall invasion, a *post facto* discontinuous chest wall resection of involved rib and muscle should then be performed. In our experience we have found no survival compromise with this discontinuous technique of chest wall resection compared with en bloc resection with pulmonary parenchyma, provided all resection margins are free of tumor. This observation has also been supported by the Toronto group [22].

We favor chest wall reconstruction with a Marlex mesh/methylmethacrylate sandwich technique whenever there is suspicion of chest wall instability, but rarely find this necessary with resection of fewer than three contiguous rib segments. For such smaller defects Marlex mesh patch closure will ensure acceptable cosmetic results. In either case, we use a double-thickness patch fashioned from a single-folded sheet of Marlex mesh which is tautly and securely fixed to the margins of the chest wall defect with interrupted, nonabsorbable monofilament suture. In the sandwich technique for larger defects methylmethacrylate resin is first moulded to match the defect between the leaves of the Marlex mesh and then allowed to harden and cool prior to implantation of the composite patch [23].

The prognosis in patients who underwent complete resection and were found to have no lymphatic metastases was better than in those who were found to have metastases to the regional lymph nodes. The 5-year survival following resection in the absence of lymphatic metastases was 56% at 5 years compared with 21% in patients with positive local or regional lymph node involvement [19]. It is important to note, despite the presence of positive hilar or mediastinal lymph node metastases and chest wall invasion, that 33 patients treated by complete resection have demonstrated a 5-year survival of 20% (Fig. 7). There was no survival advantage noted between patients with adenocarcinomas or epidermoid carcinomas when evaluated stage by stage and related to the extent of resection and lymph node involvement. We continue to recommend surgical resection whenever possible for all patients with tumors extending to the chest wall. We do not recommend postoperative radiation therapy or chemotherapy if the resection is complete. We have continued to recommend postoperative external radiation therapy to those patients with unresectable tumors, or to those with residual disease following resection.

Superior Sulcus Tumors

Within the subset of T3 lesions invading the chest wall are the superior sulcus tumors. These are apical lung tumors that invade early on, ribs, superior cervical ganglion, brachial plexus, and vertebrae and are often referred to as Pancoast tumors. For this group of patients, the treatment of choice is combined preoperative radiation therapy and resection of all residual disease. Any visible tumor that is not resected is treated by intraoperative implantation of radioisotopes when possible. In this group of patients, treatment by radiation therapy alone is insufficient, resulting in a 5-year survival of less than 10%. Treatment by surgery alone improves survival somewhat, but better survival is noted when preoperative radiation therapy is combined with surgery. These patients are generally symptomatic at presentation, with shoulder pain extending to the arm. Patients generally report to their physicians early and it is rare to note patient delay in seeking management. The usual delay in diagnosis and treatment is physician's delay. Often superior sulcus tumors are mistakenly diagnosed as shoulder bursitis and treated by instillation of steroids into the shoulder joint. Some patients are referred for neurologic evaluation, assumed to have cervical arthritis, and are treated with cervical collars and, occasionally, cervical traction. In general, there is a 6- to 8-month delay from the time of the patient's symptoms to the time of the suspicion of a superior sulcus tumor in this group of patients. Unfortunately many present at the time of their diagnosis with palpable cervical lymph nodes or advanced carcinomas beyond the expectations of control by combined radiation and surgery [24].

Most superior sulcus tumors are initially diagnosed histologically or cytologically by a transcutaneous needle biopsy performed under fluoroscopic or CT guidance. Diagnostic bronchoscopy is less helpful in establishing a tissue diagnosis in this group of patients because of the peripheral position of the lesion. The vast majority of Pancoast tumors are squamous cell carcinomas or adenocarcinomas, but 3%–5% are small cell or oat cell carcinomas with vastly different therapeutic implications, hence the importance of a tissue diagnosis before treatment. It is not acceptable to proceed with treatment in Pancoast disease without a histologic diagnosis [25].

Treatment of superior sulcus tumors begins by a preoperative course of external radiation therapy to a biologic dose of 4000 rad to the tumor [25]. This can be given in 300-rad fractions over 2 weeks or in increments of 1000 rad/week for a period of 4 weeks. The radiation portal includes the primary tumor, adjacent mediastinum, and ipsilateral supraclavicular area. Following a rest period of 1 month, these patients are assessed for surgical treatment. If no distant disease is evident, these patients are offered surgical exploration for removal of the residual tumor. The presence of a Horner's syndrome or ipsilateral supraclavicular node involvement is not a contraindication for combined preoperative radiation and surgery. Of the patients considered for this therapeutic approach, 25%–40% have Horner's syndrome and 20% present with supraclavicular lymph nodes. Paulson first advocated the combined use of preoperative radiation and resection and demonstrated a 31% 5-year survival [26]. He also noted that in a small percentage of these patients mediastinal lymph node metastases (N2) may coexist and that very few of this group survive longer than 1 year. Mediastinoscopy has consequently been recommended in the evaluation of these patients to rule out the presence of N2 disease. We have not undertaken a routine mediastinoscopy in these patients, but have encompassed the mediastinal lymph nodes in our resection whenever feasible at the time of the surgical exploration and have supplemented postoperatively a course of external radiation therapy to the mediastinum. Paulson has reported that in most patients who present with localized disease amenable to surgical consideration in Pancoast tumors, preoperative radiation followed by surgical exploration can result in complete resection of all disease at the time of surgical exploration. The standard resection described by Paulson encompasses en bloc removal of affected lobe and chest wall including the entire first rib and posterior segments of ribs 2, 3, and often 4, transverse processes of contiguous thoracic vertebrae, nerve roots C8 and T1–3, the lower trunk of the brachial plexus, and the dorsal sympathetic chain with mediastinal node dissection. His series suggests that nearly 90% of the patients explored have undergone complete resection [26]. At Memorial Sloan-Kettering, we have also combined preoperative radiation therapy with surgical management but have observed that only 21% of all patients surgically explored after irradiation had a complete resection of their tumor [25]. Reviewing our 40-year experience through 1978 of 170 patients treated for superior sulcus tumors, of which 127 were operated, we have found that preoperative irradiation roughly doubles resectability while nearly halving the postoperative complication rate to 8%. Total operative mortality was 3%, all in the nonirradiated group. Locoregional failure rate was 29% in preoperatively irradiated patients compared with 48% in those operated without external radiation. Distant failure rates were equivalent at 56%–58% [25].

The determinants of unresectability have generally been widespread invasion of the major divisions of the brachial plexus, the subclavian artery, and the vertebral body with or without cord compression. In the vast majority of patients where the tumor was incompletely resected or found unresectable, interstitial implantation of radioiostopes has been used to increase the radiation dose to unresectable disease. The 5-year survival results obtained by us following resection are similar to that reported by Paulson. Overall survival for 66 preoperatively irradiated patients was 19% [25]. Of these, 43 had localized disease pathologically staged as T3 N0 M0, with a cumulative 5-year survival of 26% compared with only 8.4% in 23 patients with regional mediastinal or supraclavicular nodal metastases. In those with localized disease, 9 of 43 were completely resected, with an observed 5-year survival of 55%. Long-term survival in the remaining unresectable subgroup, all treated with interstitial implantation and postoperative external radiation, ranged from 15% to 25%.

We have recently been attempting to evaluate the merits of extended radical resection without preoperative radiation therapy by the combined efforts of neurosurgical and thoracic surgical teams in removing all diseased tissue extending to rib, brachial plexus, and spine with reconstruction of the vertebral bodies when indicated with orthopedic endoprostheses and methylmethacrylate. Preliminary results suggest that patients treated in this manner derive survival benefit from this approach, provided radiation therapy is appended either intraoperatively or postoperatively to treat any residual tumor and so enhance locoregional disease control. A more recent approach under evaluation is the use of preoperative chemotherapy to reduce tumor burden and enhance resectability This is a pilot study and no conclusions can as yet be drawn.

Treatment of N2 M0 Tumors

Metastasis to mediastinal lymph nodes (N2 disease) is probably the most frequent deterrent to cancer cure despite a localized presentation. This is noted in 45% of patients with non-small cell lung carcinoma. It is this large group of patients that is viewed by many to have incurable disease despite the best efforts of surgery and radiation therapy. Mediastinoscopy is thus used extensively in many centers for all patients presenting with operable carcinoma of the lung, to detect and identify all sites of mediastinal lymph node metastases in order to exclude these patients from effective locoregional management by combined surgery and radiation therapy, A few centers utilize mediastinoscopy to select those patients with N2 disease that should be treated surgically [27, 28].

It has been our firm belief that the factors that affect outcome in lung cancer patients with mediastinal lymph node metastases are site of the involved nodes, number of the involved nodes, extent of tumor involvement within the nodes, and histologic cell type. We seriously believe that many patients with ipsilateral N2 disease can benefit from effective management by combined surgery and radiation therapy. It is generally agreed that patients with N2 disease in contralateral hilar or mediastinal nodes, patients who present with distant metastases, and patients with small cell or oat cell carcinomas are clearly not candidates for management by surgery or radiation. However, all other patients presenting with N2 disease require serious consideration for surgical treatment. In an attempt to clarify this issue, we undertook a prospective study in 1974 at Memorial Sloan-Kettering Cancer Center [29]. From 1974 to 1978, 445 patients with N2 disease were seen and treated at our institution. Nearly one-half of these patients also manifested distant metastases, malignant pleural effusion, or superior vena caval syndrome, or had small cell carcinomas and were clearly not candidates for surgical management. The remaining, 217 patients, were surgically explored to assess disease extent, to identify and label the site and number of involved nodes, and at the same time to attempt to resect the primary tumor and all involved nodes or treat unresected disease by interstitial implantation of radioisotopes. In this group of surgically explored patients, 80 patients had a curative resection despite the presence of positive mediastinal lymph nodes.

Curative resection was defined as removal of the primary tumor by lobectomy or pneumonectomy as indicated, with a complete systematic mediastinal lymph node dissection of all N2 disease. For right-sided tumors we perform a thorough resection which entails removal of lymph node levels 1 through 4, and 7 through 9 (Fig. 3). We expose the superior mediastinal lymph node compartment by incising the mediastinal pleura longitudinally between the subclavian artery and azygos vein. The pleura is reflected and the fat pad with all included nodes is dissected away from the vena cava, trachea, and underlying ascending arch of the aorta. The vagus nerve, including its recurrent branch, and the azygos vein are spared. The mediastinal contents anterior to the superior vena cava are not routinely included unless palable nodes are present. We expose subcarinal, paraesophageal, and inferior pulmonary lymph nodes by incising the posterior mediastinal pleura from the level of the main stem bronchus to the inferior pulmonary ligament. Under direct visualization with lateral retraction of the esophagus, we are able to clear the subcarinal space to the deep boundaries of contralateral main stem bronchus and pericardium.

For left-sided tumors we routinely remove nodal levels 5 and 6, clearing all fatty tissue between the left pulmonary artery and the aortic arch from the recurrent laryngeal to the phrenic nerves. We dissect the supraaortic compartment between the phrenic and vagus nerves only when nodes are palpable or apparent. We complete all left-sided dissections including nodal levels 7 through 9 as described for right-sided lesions.

In our study, all margins of resection were negative in those patients in whom potentially curative resection had been undertaken. These 80 patients were subsequently evaluated for histology and survival; 44 of these were adenocarcinomas, 25 were epidermoid cancers, and 11 were various other histologic types including 3 with small cell carcinoma. In this prospective study, the 3-year survival in the 80 patients who underwent complete resection was 49% [29]. It has since been followed to 5 years with an observed survival of 29% (Fig. 8). By histology, there was no evidence of survival advantage in this group of patients between the epidermoid carcinomas and adenocarcinomas. These patients were clinically staged before treatment without the benefit of mediastinoscopy, and 57% of 116 patients with no clinical evidence of N2 disease preoperatively on chest roentgenograms and bronchoscopy were completely resectable. Overall it was evident that 80 of 445 patients with N2 disease had potentially curative resections despite the presence of mediastinal involvement, representing 20% of all N2 patients [29].

From 1974 to 1981 a total of 1598 consecutive patients underwent treatment for non-oat cell carcinoma of the lung at Memorial Sloan-Kettering Cancer Center. Of these, 706 patients, or 44%, were found to have N2 nodes, and 151 of these patients, or 9.4% of all patients presenting with non-small cell lung carcinoma, had N2 disease that was completely resected at thoracotomy [30]. Analysis of this latter group was performed to assess postoperative survival. Histology in the 151 resected N2 patients was adenocarcinoma in 94 or 62%, epidermoid carcinoma in

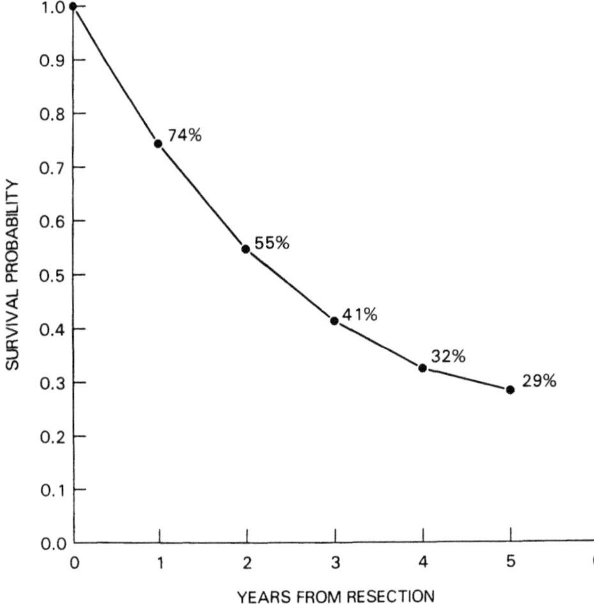

Fig. 8. Overall actuarial survival for completely resected non-small cell lung cancer metastatic to mediastinal lymph nodes

46 or 30%, and large cell carcinoma in 11 or 7%. Though the vast majority underwent a lobectomy with mediastinal lymph node dissection, 26 patients or 1 out of 6 underwent a pneumonectomy with complete resection of the tumor and the mediastinal lymph nodes. The overall 5-year survival of this group of patients was again 29% and there was no observed survival advantage between patients with adenocarcinoma and epidermoid cancers (32% vs. 30% respectively) [30].

Treatment results of specific sites of N2 nodal involvement were assessed in these 151 resected lung carcinomas [31]. The majority of the N2 nodes were located in the right lower paratracheal area, an incidence of 80% in those undergoing right-sided operations. The second most frequent site was the aorticopulmonary window, which was positive in 81% of patients with tumors in the left lung. The third most frequent site was the subcarinal region in both right- and left-sides lesions. Despite the opinion of many that the presence of upper paratracheal lymph nodes precludes curability by surgery, 37 patients in this series had upper paratracheal nodes at levels 1 and 2, completely resected at the time of the thoracotomy. The survival in this group of patients was compared with patients with N2 disease at other sites and there was clearly no survival advantage in either category. Patients with N2 disease in the subcarinal region had a 5-year survival of 18% as compared with 37% in patients with N2 disease in other sites of the mediastinum. Subcarinal metastases suggest a more serious extension of the disease but are still amenable to surgical excision with a resultant 5-year survival of 18% [31]. The majority of these patients again were clinically staged without the benefit of mediastinoscopy, and, in general, consisted of patients with peripheral tumors of T1 or

126

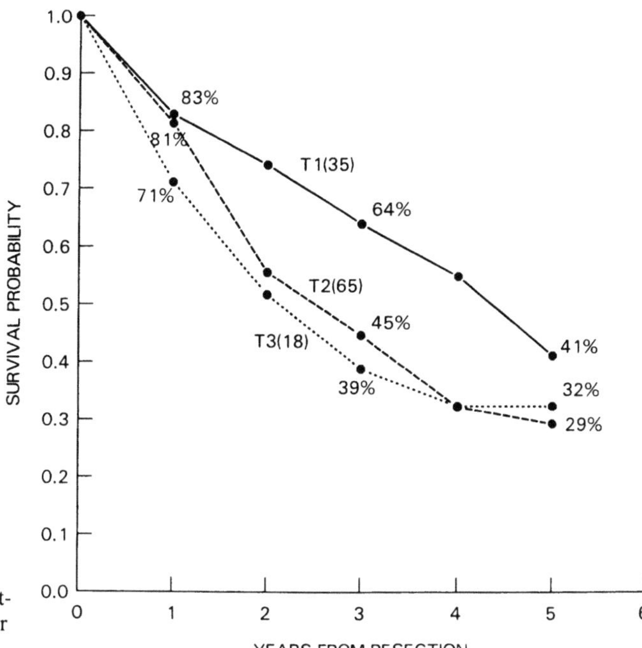

Fig. 9. Survival from resected N2 lung cancer by tumor size

T2 size with absent evidence of mediastinal involvement on routine chest roentgenograms and on bronchoscopy. There were a total of 24 patients who were classified clinically to have T1N0 or T1N1 disease. All 24 were surgically explored and a complete resection was possible in 23 of 24 patients (96%). It is clearly evident that patients with small peripheral tumors without apparent mediastinal involvement on routine chest roentgenogram have nodal metastases of sufficiently small burden as to permit their resection with the primary tumor despite their involvement. It is in this group of patients that a mediastinoscopy, though helpful in identifying metastases in these regions, should not preclude such patients from surgical management. Similarly 55 patients presented with T2, N0 or N1 disease clinically were evaluated without mediastinoscopy. All were surgically explored and 62% or approximately two out of three of these patients had a complete resection of their primary tumor and all involved mediastinal nodes. Again this group of patients clearly benefits from surgical consideration since two-thirds of these patients can have completely resectable tumors despite the involvement of N2 lymph nodes (Fig. 9). However, those who present clinically with more advanced tumors with central T3 or gross N2 involvement demonstrated by routine chest roentgenograms or by invasion of trachea or carina on bronchoscopy clearly have a poorer prognosis. One hundred and ninety-six patients were classified to have had gross N2 disease manifest on routine chest roentgenograms and only half of these patients underwent surgical exploration, of which 14, or 7% of all N2 patients noted clinically, had resectable lesions. There were 33 patients who underwent surgically complete resection of their primary tumor and their mediastinal nodes despite clinically noted N2 disease on routine chest roentgenograms. The 3-year survival in this group of patients was only 9%, representing less than 2% 3-year survival for all patients presenting with N2 disease that is clinically manifested on routine plain chest roentgenograms or bronchoscopy. This suggests that patients with cancer involvement in lymph nodes, with enlargement extending 1–3 cm in diameter, which may be detected on CT scan but not on plain chest roentgenograms, are patients who have well-encapsulated lymph nodes despite their metastases and whose tumors are amenable to surgical excision. Patients with lymph node involvement and enlargement greater than 3 cm in diameter, generally seen on routine chest roentgenograms as well as on CT scan, and in this group of patients the resectability rate is low, and despite complete resection the survival rate is equally low due to distant failure. It is in this group of patients that new and innovative treatment alternatives are necessary [31].

At MSKCC, patients found to have extensive unresectable disease at thoracotomy and whose tumors are still localized to one hemithorax have been treated by surgical exploration and interstitial implantation of radioiodine seeds to the primary tumor followed by external radiation therapy to the mediastinum. In so doing a 2-year survival of 30% has been obtained in this group of patients, despite their unresectable disease [32]. Although the 5-year survival of these patients is less than 3%, the palliation of survival with locoregional control in 80% of the patients for at least the duration of the survival justifies this surgical alternative. All patients with N2 disease who are surgically explored, whether resected or found unresectable, also receive a course of external radiation therapy to the mediastinum postoperatively to a tumor dose of 4000–4500 rad. Although such adjuvant external radiation therapy decreases regional recurrence rates, it has not been shown to prolong survival. The majority of treatment failures remain due to distant metastases. Adjuvant prospective trails of effective systemic agents are clearly indicated for this group of patients.

More recently, CIS-platinum-based combination regimens of chemotherapy have demonstrated favorable response rates in advanced unresectable non-small cell carcinomas of the lung. At MSKCC, a 43% partial response was noted with the use of CIS-platin combined with vindesine in patients presenting with advanced disease and distant metastases, with a median duration of response of 12 months and a median survival of 20 months [33]. A partial response was defined as greater than 50% reduction in the maximum diameter of all measurable lesions at the time of evaluation. Because of this encouraging approach, a preoperative course of chemotherapy is now considered in patients with advanced mediastinal involvement in the absence of distant metastases. Many of these patients are first offered a chemotherapy regimen consisting of CIS-platin, a vinca alkaloid (vindesine or vinblastine), and mitomycin C. Two cycles of this treatment are given preoperatively. All responders are subsequently offered an exploratory thoracotomy to resect all residual disease or implant unresectable tumors by interstitial implantation of radioisotopes. In this early pilot study, a 50% partial response to chemotherapy has been noted and 4 of 15 patients were found to have totally sterilized tumors at the time of surgical treatment. Despite these encouraging observations it is too early to state whether this would translate into prolonged survival in the more advanced forms of non-small cell carcinomas of the lung.

During the past 3 years we have also been investigating the role of adjuvant postoperative chemotherapy in a prospective randomized trial for all patients found to have non-small cell carcinoma with mediastinal nodal metastases at surgery. This study was motivated out of a desire to improve on the best 5-year salvage rate of approximately 30% for N2 disease achieved by locoregional methods alone, i.e., resection, brachytherapy, and external radiation therapy [30]. Based on the analysis of our present accrual, we cannot as yet endorse the efficacy of adjuvant chemotherapy with CIS-platin/vinca alkaloid-based regimens in prolonging survival or reducing the incidence of distant recurrence in completely resected and postoperatively irradiated patients. At this time we feel there is no role for such adjuvant chemotherapy outside of established controlled investigational trials at clinical centers well versed in the surgical treatment of N2 disease.

Treatment of T3 Lesions Due to Proximity to Carina

An additional subset of stage III carcinomas that benefits from surgical management is patients with central tumors that extend within 2 cm of the carina. In many instances, the carina itself is not involved despite a T3 presentation and in many instances also a surgical extirpation of the tumor is possible. In some, no lymphatic metastases are evident at the time of the resection. In patients in whom resection can be undertaken despite the proximity of the lesion to the carina but without its involvement, the 5-year anticipated survival following resection is currently reported at 36% [34].

The presence of tumor at a major lobar orifice and the need to conserve lung tissue are the main indications for sleeve resection. A pneumonectomy is required to encompass all of a tumor protruding from a lobar orifice into the main bronchus and to provide a clear margin of resection. This may not be possible because of a compromised pulmonary reserve. In such situations a sleeve lobectomy is a worthwhile alternative and has lower morbidity and mortality rates than pneumonectomy. When a complete excision is possible, curability by sleeve lobectomy is comparable to that obtained by pneumonectomy. Faber et al. performed 101 sleeve lobectomies over a 21-year period, with only two postoperative deaths in the entire series [34]. The survival in this group of patients was 30% at 5 years and 22% at 10 years. The benefit derived from preoperative external radiation therapy in this group of patients is controversial.

Primary lesions which extend to and invade carina bear a much poorer prognosis. Some advocate aggressive pneumonectomy with tracheal sleeve resection and direct reanastomosis of trachea to contralateral main stem bronchus in young patients who are good surgical risks. Best results for this procedure approach 20% 5-year survival, but often in the face of 13%–30% operative mortality [35]. We prefer at present to treat most such patients with combined interstitial und external irradiation without resection. Transbronchoscopic laser photodynamic therapy with and without hematoporphyrin derivative may play an important role in the future management of such localized tracheal invasion [9, 36].

Conclusion

It is clearly evident that there are subsets of patients with advanced non-small cell lung carcinoma that benefit from surgery or surgery combined with radiation and/ or chemotherapy. One subset of patients has been identified as tumors extending to chest wall that can be completely resected. It is also noted that nearly 45% of all lung carcinoma presents with mediastinal lymph node metastases and that 20% of this large group of patients is amenable to surgical resection despite the presence of these metastases [30]. This represents a total of nearly 10% of all non-oat cell lung carcinomas presentling to treatment. In patients with stage I lung carcinoma, treatment by resection currently holds an 83% 5-year survival for the small tumors and 65% for the larger ones [10]. Hence stage I carcinoma of lung treated by resection clearly has a very favorable prognosis with two out of three patients anticipated to remain alive and well many years hence. In patients with N1 disease, a 50% 5-year survival is also attainable by surgical resection, but adjuvant therapy needs to be explored in this group of patients to enhance the control both locally and distally in those patients who fail treatment [13].

From 1973 to 1980 a total of 1493 patients were seen at Memorial Sloan-Kettering Cancer Center for management of their lung carcinoma. Thoracotomy for control of their tumor was offered to 961 patients or 64% of the patients; 18% of these were 70 years or older and the male/female ratio was 2 to 1 [37]. Of these nearly 1000 consecutive thoracotomies for primary lung carcinoma, despite the liberal surgical indications presented, only 20 postoperative deaths were noted, an operative mortality of 2%. Proper case selection and careful preoperative and perioperative management are necessary to minimize complications. We have identified high-risk groups to be: (1) patients over 70 years of age in whom a major resection is being considered, (2) patients with cardiovascular disease, and (3) patients with severely restricted pulmonary reserve regardless of their age. To minimize complications a lesser resection may be considered in the elderly and in all physiologically compromised persons who present an increased risk for surgery.

Assuming these precautions, we continue vigorously and confidently to promote operative intervention combined where indicated with appropriate adjuvant therapy as the best means of cure or palliation for non-small cell lung cancer. Indeed, in our retrospective 23-year experience, for those treated patients with primary lung carcinoma who most closely reach an operational definition of cure, i.e., 10-year disease-free survival without death from original disease, less than 3% were treated by means excluding surgery [18]. Thus, to deny thoracotomy to a clinically operable patient with stage I, stage II, or herein specified subsets of localized stage III non-small cell lung carcinoma is in our opinion to capitulate to his disease.

References

1. Silverberg E, Lubera J (1968) Cancer Statistics. CA 36: 9–25
2. Martini N, Beattie EJ Jr (1980) Current views in primary pulmonary cancer. In: International advances in urgical oncology. 3: 275–297. Liss New York
3. Minna JD, Higgins GA, Gladstein EJ (1985) Cancer of the lung. In: DeVita VT, Hellman S, Rosenberg SA (eds), Principles and practice of oncology. 2nd edn. Lippincott Philadelphia pp 509–598.
4. Vincent RG, Pickren JW, Lane WW, et al (1977) The chaning histophathology of lung cancer: a review of 1682 cases. Cancer 39: 1964
5. American Joint Committee on Cancer (1983) Manual for staging of cancer 2nd edn. Lippincott, Philadelphia, pp 99–105
6. Martini N, Melamed MR (1980) Occult carcinomas of the lung. Ann Thorac Surg 30: 215–223
7. Flehinger BJ, Melamed MR, Zaman MB, Heelan RT, Perchick WB, Martini N (1984) Early lung cancer detection, results of the initial (prevalence) radiologic and cytologic screening in the Memorial Sloan-Kettering study. Am Rev Respir Dis 130: 555–560
8. Cortese DA, Kinsey JH, Woolner LB, Sanderson DR, Fontana RS (1982) Hematoporphyrin derivative in the detection and localization of radiographically occult lung cancer. Am Rev Respir Dis 126: 1087–1088
9. Hayata Y, Kato H, Konaka C, Amemiya R, Ono J, Ogawa I, Kinoshita K, Sakai H, Takahashi H (1984) Photoradiation therapy with hematoporphyrin derivative in early and stage I lung cancer. Chest 86: 169–177
10. Martini N, McCaughan BC, McCormack P, Bains MS (1986) Lobectomy for stage I lung cancer. In: Kittle CF (ed) Current controversies in thoracic surgery. Saunders Philadelphia
11. NCI cooperative early lung cancer detection program (1984) Results of initial screen (prevalence) summary and conclusions. Am Rev Res Dis 130: 565–570
12. Melamed MR, Flehinger BJ, Zaman MB, Heewlan RT, Perchick WA, Martini N (1984) Screening for early lung cancer: results of the Memorial Sloan-Kettering Study in New York. Chest 86: 44–53
13. Martini N, Flehinger BJ, Nagasaki F, Hart B (1983) Prognostic significance of N1 disease in carcinoma of the lung. J Thorac Cardiovasc surg 86: 646–652
14. Martini N (1985) Preoperative staging and surgery for non-small cell lung cancer. In: Aisner J (ed) Contemporary issues in clinical oncology, vol 3. Churchill Livingstone, London, pp 101–130
15. Jensik R (1985) Conservative resection for lung cancer. In: Delarue NC and Eschapasse HE (eds) International trends in general thoracic surgery, vol 1. Saunders Philadelphia, pp 100–103
16. Williams DE, Pairolero PC, Davis CS, Bernatz PE, Payne WS, Taylor WF, Uhlenhopp MA, Fontana RS (1981) Survival of patients surgically treated for stage I lung cancer. J Thorac Cardiovasc Surg 82: 70–76
17. Kemeny NM, Block LR, Braun DW Jr, Martini N (1978) Results of surgical treatment of carcinoma of the lung by stage and cell type. Surg Gynecol Obstet 147: 865–871
18. Temeck BK, Flehinger BJ, Martini N (1984) A retrospective analysis of 10 year survivors from carcinoma of the lung. Cancer 53: 1405–1408
19. McCaughan BC, Martini N, Bains MS, McCormack P (1985) Chest wall invasion of carcinoma of the lung: therapeutic and prognostic implications. J Thorac Cardiovasc Surg 89: 836–841
20. Grillo HC, Greenberg JJ, Wilkins EW Jr (1966) Resection of bronchogenic carcinoma involving thoracic wall. J Thorac Cardiovasc Surg 51: 417
21. Piehler JM, Pairolero PC, Weeland LH, Offud KP, Payne WS, Bernatz PE (1982) Bronchogenic carcinoma with chest wall invasion: factors affecting survival following en-bloc resection. Ann Thorac Surg 34: 684–691
22. Patterson GA, Ilves R, Ginsberg RJ, Cooper JD, Todd TRJ, Pearson FG (1982) The value of adjuvant radiotherapy in pulmonary and chest wall resection for bronchogenic carcinoma. Ann Thorac Surg 34: 692–697
23. McCormack PM, Bains MS, Beattie EJ Jr, Martini N (1981) New trends in skeletal reconstruction after resection of chest wall tumors. Ann Thorac Surg 31: 45–52

24. Martini N (1981) When lung cancer masquerades as a shoulder problem. Your patient and cancer 1: (5)25-32
25. Martini N, Hilaris BS (1982) Multimodality therapy of superior sulcus tumors In: Bonica JJ (ed) Adavances in pain research and therapy. vol 4 Raven New York, pp 113-122
26. Paulson DL (1985) The "superior sulcus" lesion. In: Delarue and Eschapasse (eds) International trends in general thoracic surgery vol 1. Saunders Philadelphia, pp 121-133
27. Paulson DL, Urschel HC Jr (1971) Selectivity in the surgical treatment of bronchogenic carcinoma. J Thorac Cardiovasc Surg 62: 554
28. Pearson FG (1985) Mediastinal adenopathy-the N2 lesion. In: Delarue and Eschapasse (eds) International trends in general thoracic surgery vol 1. Saunders Philadelphia, pp 104-107
29. Martini N, Flehinger BJ, Zaman MB, Beattie EJ Jr (1980) Prospective study 445 lung carcinomas with positive mediastinal lymph node metastases. J Thorac Cardiovasc Surg 80: 390-397
30. Martini N, Flehinger BJ, Zaman MB, Beattie EJ Jr (1983) Results of resection in non-oat cell carcinoma of the lung with mediastinal lymph node metastases. Ann Surg 198: 386-397
31. Martini N, Flehinger BJ, Bains MS, McCormack PM (1985) Management of stage III disease: alternate approaches to the management of mediastinal adenopathy. In: Delarue and Eschapasse (eds) International trends in general thoracic surgery vol 1. Saunders Philadelphia, pp 108-120
32. Hilaris N, Nori D, Beattie EJ Jr, Martini N (1983) Value of perioperative brachytherapy in the management of non-oat cell carcinoma of the lung. Int J Radiat Oncol Biol Phys 9: 1161-1166
33. Gralla RJ, Casper ES, Kelsen DP, Braun DW Jr, Dukeman MD, Martini N, Young CW, Golbey RB (1981) CIS-platin and vindesine combination chemotherapy for advanced carcinoma of the lung: a randomized trial investigating two dosage schedules. Ann Intern Med 95: 414-420
34. Faber LP, Jensik RJ and Kittle CF (1984) Results of sleeve lobectomy for bronchogenic carcinoma in 101 patients. Ann Thorac Surg 37: 279-285
35. Deslauriers J (1985) Involvement of the main carina. In: Delarue and Eschapasse (eds) International trends in general thoracic surgery vol 1. Saunders, Philadelphia, pp 139-145
36. Oho K, Ogawa I, Amemiya R, Ohtani T, Yamada R, Taira O and Hayata Y (1983) Indications for endoscopic Nd-YAG laser surgery in the trachea and bronchus. Endoscopy 15: 302-306.
37. Nagasaki F, Flehinger BJ, Martini N (1982) Complications of surgery in the treatment of carcinoma of the lung. Chest: 82: 25-29
38. Martini N (1976) Improved methods of recording data in lung cancer. Clin Bull Memorial Sloan-Kettering Cancer Center 6: 97

12. Treatment at Brompton Hospital and Royal Marsden Hospital

P. Goldstraw, S. G. Spiro, and J. R. Yarnold

Pretreatment Preparation (Treatment at Brompton Hospital)

P. Goldstraw

Whatever treatment is decided upon, it is clearly necessary to get the patient into the best condition prior to commencing therapy.

Any infective focus should be eradicated. As the majority of sufferers from lung cancer are smokers, infection in the tracheobronchial tree is common. These patients may well have had recurrent winter bronchitis over many years, for which the primary physician has used a variety of broad spectrum antibiotics, often without any bacteriological guidance. As a result their airways are often colonized by upper respiratory commensals such as *Haemophilus influenzae* and *Streptococcus pneumoniae,* which may be resistant to first-line antibiotics. There are additional mechanical factors predisposing to chest infection. The mucosal changes associated with cigarette smoking, mucuos gland hyperplasia, and squamous metaplasia, result in excessive sputum production and decreased sputum clearance. The stage is therefore set for serious chest infections should there be any reduction in the patient's immunological competence, as may occur with chemotherapy or radiotherapy, or additional mechanical problems imposed by surgery. After pulmonary resection, lung volume is reduced, often dramatically. There is further trouble with expectoration because of pain, and this may be exacerbated by resection of the recurrent laryngeal nerve, phrenic nerve, or chest wall. Anesthesia and dehydration will adversely affect sputum viscosity, and there will be a further reduction in ciliary clearance. All of these factors make sputum difficulties the commonest postoperative complication following pulmonary resection.

Pretreatment preparation should concentrate on the mechanical factors associated with chest infections. If time permits, the patient should discontinue smoking for 3–4 weeks before treatment. This is a realistic delay if contemplating surgery for a localized squamous carcinoma, but impossible if urgent chemotherapy is needed to relieve superior vena caval obstruction in small cell lung cancer. Much improvement in sputum clearance and airway resistance can be achieved with a few days of in-patient physiotherapy coupled with bronchodilators. The patient will be taught the maneuvres required of him following treatment, and, if there is any reversibility to airway resistance, instructed in the correct use of inhalers and nebulizers. Antibiotics are of little value unless there is an acute infection with an identifiable pathogen. In other circumstances it is exceptionally difficult to obtain a representative specimen of sputum without contamination by the mouth flora.

Any nidus of infection in the upper respiratory tract requires attention. This may lie in the sinuses where, once more, mechanical factors are most important, and decongestant drugs are of more value than antibiotics. In severe dental infection, improvement in oral hygiene is recommended. If treatment is urgent, it may be necessary to delay dental treatment. If there is any intercurrent infection, appropriate cultures should be taken and eradication of infection confirmed prior to commencing treatment.

It is customary to correct anemia before undertaking chemotherapy, radiotherapy, or surgery. It is unlikely that there is any merit in such an approach unless the anemia is substantial (with a hemoglobin of < 10 g%). Less severe anemia has no effect on wound healing, patient stamina, or peripheral oxygen uptake. Should anemia require transfusion, it is best undertaken more than 24 h prior to treatment so that any equilibration of blood volume and acid-base balance may take place.

The patient's nutrition may suffer greatly with treatment due to the catabolic stimulus of trauma, anorexia, and possible vomiting. No advantage has been shown, however, of preoperative dietary supplementation. It is recognized that dietary support via the nasogastric or intravenous routes is necessary if the patient does not commence an adequate oral diet shortly after surgery. Dehydration may result from excessive vomiting, and this should be corrected by intravenous crystalloids.

The endocrine effects of bronchogenic cancer may require treatment. With all such paraneoplastic syndromes the best control comes from effective tumor treatment. Supportive measures are occasionally necessary to put the patient in the best state temporarily, in order to permit definitive tumor treatment. This may prove an impossible goal for some patients.

Attention paid to the social problems which afflict many patients will pay dividends, allowing patient and clinician to devote their attention to the primary treatment freed of the anxiety of outside social pressures.

The aim of pretreatment preparation is to bring the patient speedily to definitive treatment in the best possible condition to minimize the risk of morbidity and mortality. A few days spent achieving this goal may save considerable time dealing with complications after treatment.

Surgery

P. Goldstraw

The role of surgery in lung cancer is to effect cure or greatly extend survival over that achievable by other treatment modalities. Whether this is possible requires an individual cost-benefit analysis for each patient.

The cost of pulmonary resection concerns not only the financial implications of staging and surgery but also of inpatient care, which entails 8–14 days in hospital and the loss of earnings consequent on 4-6 weeks' recovery. It also encompasses the morbidity and mortality after the operation There is a scar, some pain, and several weeks of discomfort. Inevitably pulmonary resection will result in some loss of exercise tolerance. This should be minimal after lobectomy, and the ratio of forced expired volume in 1 s to the forced vital capacity (FEV1.0/FVC%) should return to the preoperative level within 6 weeks of surgery. After pneumonectomy there is usually a noticeable reduction in effort tolerance and for most patients the FEV1.0/FVC% will be reduced by one-third over preoperative figures. The risk of severe limitation of exercise tolerance with respiratory invalidity has been overstated and probably only occurs if there is damage to remaining lung tissue from postoperative complications. The risk of death around the time of surgery will depend upon the patient's age, general health, and respiratory function. In most Western centers lobectomy carries an operative mortality (inpatient death) of 1%-2%, and pneumonectomy of 5%-8%. The question of age is a vexed one, but there is no doubt that biological age is more important than the chronological one. Many patients in their 70s are in better condition than people suffering from arteriopathy in their 50s. One should, however, assess anyone over the age of 70 particularly critically since many will survive but lose their much valued prowess and independence. An assessment of general health should include past medical history and present concurrent diseases such as myocardial ischemia and hypertension, and other smoking-related diseases. Of the many tests of respiratory function used in preoperative assessment, only two have been shown to correlate with postoperative morbidity and mortality. These are the resting $pCO\hat{2}$ and forced expiratory maneuvres such as peak expiratory flow rate (PEFR), forced expired volume in 1 s (FEV1.0), forced vital capacity (FVC), and the FEV1.0/FVC%. The former is self evident; if the patient is in respiratory failure preoperatively, pulmonary resection is contraindicated. It is interesting to speculate as to why relatively crude tests of lung function such as FEV1.0/FVC% have proven of predictive value where more sophisticated tests have not. The answer probably lies in the postoperative problems associated with sputum clearance. Forced expiratory maneuvres simulate coughing and if patients can expectorate forcefully, they will survive the ordeal of surgery and have reasonable postoperative lung function. There can be no arbitrary level of FEV1.0/FVC% which permits safe surgery. Much will depend upon the extent of the proposed resection and the state of the lung to be removed. If the tumor has produced collapse of a lobe or lung prior to surgery, then removal of this lung has no effect on lung function! As a general rule, as preoperative FEV1.0 falls below 1.5 liter and the FEV1.0/FVC% falls below 50%, the risks associated with pneumonectomy rise. It is still feasible to operate on these patients, but greater vigilance and more assistance with sputum removal by bronchoscopy and/or tracheostomy are required. It is rarely possible to undertake pneumonectomy safely if the FEV1.0 is < 1 liter, or the FEV1.0/FVC% ratio is < -40%.

The other side of the surgical equation - benefit - will depend upon the cell type and stage of the tumor. Discussion of the cell type effectively hinges upon the distinction between small cell lung cancer (SCLC) and the other varieties - squamous, adeno, and large cell - collectively termed non-small cell lung cancer (NSCLC). SCLC is rarely localized sufficiently to permit surgery, whereas surgery may be the best form of treatment for up to one-third of patients suffering from NSCLC. Surgery is the only treatment resulting in large numbers of cures, and one should not be too easily deterred by insubstantial results of investigations having a low specificity. The establishment of tissue diagnosis has been considered in another section of this manual. It should be remembered, however, that cytology of the sputum and needle biopsy are frequently misleading, and even histology of fiberoptic bronchoscopic biopsies will not always be representative. Discussion of staging methods has been undertaken elsewhere. The results of surgery in the most favorable categories of squamous carcinoma show an 80% 5-year survival (T1N0 tumors) and up to 60% for all stage I tumors.

If the decision is made that in an individual case the risk of surgery is balanced by a reasonable chance of cure, then this recommendation should be put forcefully to the patient by the surgeon who will undertake the operation. It must be remembered that statistics are confusing to lay people and that cure or death for an individual is 100%.

Prior to thoracotomy the surgeon will wish to make his own assessment of bronchoscopic operability. This can most easily be accomplished under general anesthesia immediately prior to thoracotomy. The rigid bronchoscope has much to commend it in such circumstances. It permits a more accurate measurement of tumor proximity and reveals fixation and compression by extrabronchial extension not appreciated on fiberoptic bronchoscopy. Should there remain any doubt as to cell type, it is a convenient occasion to take a further and larger biopsy.

The final, most critical staging maneuvre – surgical exploration of the mediastinum by cervical mediastinoscopy, supplemented for left upper lobe tumors by left anterior mediastinotomy – will be undertaken by the surgeon. This may be done immediately prior to thoracotomy or several days prior to surgery. The former approach requires rapid frozen section analysis of node biopsies and is somewhat extravagant on theater time since there is a delay while awaiting the results of frozen section, and the surgeon will not know whether to allocate sufficient time for pulmonary resection. The other approach, allowing an interval between mediastinoscopy and thoracotomy, is less attractive to the patient, involving two anesthetics and a longer inpatient stay. If thoracotomy is indicated but delayed more than 1 week after mediastinoscopy, subsequent evaluation of the mediastinum at thoracotomy becomes more difficult. The individual surgeon must make his own decision on the timing of mediastinoscopy based upon local, logistical considerations.

The technique of thoracotomy will be dictated by the surgeon's training. In general, however, lateral thoracotomy provides better access and greater flexibility than the older technique using a posterior approach with the patient face down. With modern anesthesia and wider expertise in the use of endobronchial intubation, the situation which led to the earlier approach is now obsolete.

A description of the techniques of pulmonary resection is beyond the scope of this book. A few basic points will be explained. It is suggested that the surgeon proceed in each case to answer these questions at thoracotomy:

1. Have we established a tissue diagnosis? Here the concern is not so much that cell type be accurately known but rather that extensive and unnecessary resec-

tions are not performed for what is later shown to be a benign disease. Pulmonary resection should not be undertaken on the basis of cytology alone. A histological confirmation of malignancy is required, and if it is not available prior to thoracotomy, then a frozen section analysis of the mass is recommended. The surgeon should be satisfied that such a biopsy is representative of the underlying pathology. Shallow peripheral wedges may not be representative, and a more ominous disease may lurk deeper in the lung substance. If macroscopically involved glands dictate more extensive resection, they may provide a more reliable frozen section histology than the lung mass. Occasionally, the surgeon will decide that representative biopsies of the mass cannot be safely performed and must proceed with resection based on macroscopic appearances. It will be rare for these circumstances to accompany a lesion so extensive as to require pneumonectomy.

2. Was preoperative (cTNM) staging accurate? The local extent of the primary tumor is reassessed with evaluation of invasion of hilar and mediastinal structures and, laterally, visceral pleura or chest wall. Here also macroscopic appearances may be misleading, and inflammatory adhesions distal to a central, obstructing carcinoma provide a common pitfall. If there is serious doubt, and this feature would affect staging and subsequent resection, then frozen section analysis is mandatory. Lymph nodes within the mediastinum, at all points around the hilum, should be excised as a biopsy and labeled separately for pathology using a gland chart such as that of Naruke (see section on staging). Each gland group should be sliced by the surgeon, and if there is doubt on macroscopic appearance, then frozen section histology is necessary. It is unrealistic to attempt this examination on all excised glands, but as a decision frequently hinges on one gland group, a representative biopsy of the most suspicious area of these glands would suffice.

3. Is the lesion operable by pneumonectomy? By the time that sufficient exploration has been done to answer the first two questions, the answer to this third question is usually obvious. No irreversible damage should have occurred up to this point. In the vast majority of cases the surgeon is concerned only with the possibility of complete excision since so-called palliative or incomplete resections have only an adverse influence on survival. Occasionally incomplete resection is justified if the tumor residue is minimal, and it is tagged with metal markers to facilitate postoperative radiotherapy. Pancoast type tumors provide a ready example of such a combined approach, but occasionally invasion of the chest wall in an area not amenable to surgical excision, such as vertebral bodies, may also justify such an approach.

Should the lesion prove irresectable, then the surgeon should pause to consider what other procedure might help the patient before closing the chest. If troublesome hypertrophic osteoarthropathy is present, division of the vagus nerve, high in the mediastinum, has occasionally provided relief. Marking the tumor and involved glands with metallic clips may facilitate later radiotherapy as tumor margins may be obscured by atelectasis or pleural collections.

4. If the lesion is operable, is resection possible by less than pneumonectomy? It is at this stage that the surgeon's attention turns to the pulmonary hilum. There is no advantage in undertaking a resection more extensive than that which will re-

move the primary and its involved lymphatics, producing resection margins clear of tumor. Careful dissection of the pulmonary hilum will show whether the tumor involves structures vital to adjacent lobes, and whether involved glands lie in the resection line of any possible lobectomy. Once again, macroscopic appearances may require histological confirmation by frozen section analysis if the surgeon is in doubt. Lobectomy is always preferable to pneumonectomy if such an operation satisfies these basic tenets of cancer surgery. Bronchoplastic procedures, such as sleeve lobectomy, provide an infrequent but satisfactory way of dealing with tumors that would otherwise prove to be operable by lobectomy except for the involvement of or close proximity to the descending bronchus. The position of segmentectomy is as yet undecided. In this operation the line of resection crosses the first nodal station, that is, in intersegmental glands. The use of this operation should therefore probably be restricted to patients with peripheral tumors, without nodal metastases, in whom poor lung function would make lobectomy more hazardous.

5. If the lesion is operable, should resection be undertaken? The surgeon now has all the information needed to make this final decision before proceeding with resection. Equally, he has not committed himself by damage to any vital structures and can yet retreat. With knowledge of the patient's fitness and lung function, an updated staging (sTNM), and an accurate assessment of the resection necessary to remove the tumor, the surgeon should decide whether to proceed with resection or not. Such decisions should be made with reasonable speed, but unhurriedly. There are difficult situations which require a lifetime of experience, and opinions will change as experience is gained and as information becomes available from other centers. One such taxing problem concerns the discovery at thoractomy of mediastinal gland metastases, which eluded preoperative evaluation. As the surgeon develops proficiency at mediastinoscopy, it will be come uncommon to find gross involvement of high mediastinal glands. Such a situation contraindicates resection. What happens then if there is limited involvement of glands low in the superior mediastinum or beyond the reach of the mediastinoscope? In squamous carcinoma there is some evidence which suggests that if this mediastinal gland involvement is ipsilateral and limited, then complete resection may yield up to 40% 5-year survival. It is such decisions which ensure that pulmonary resection for lung cancer will never become a "standardized" operation.

The complications succeeding pulmonary resection are fully dealt with in standard surgical textbooks and will not be covered here.

Adjuvant Therapy (Treatment at Brompton Hospital)

P. Goldstraw

Radiotherapy

Previous trials using radiotherapy prior to or following surgery in NSCLC have shown no added benefit. Indeed, in most such studies, operative morbidity and mortality are increased. As staging concepts become more widely disseminated, and greater accuracy of pTNM staging becomes available, these attitudes must be reexamined. The situation regarding Pancoast tumors is unique (see above).

Chemotherapy

Currently available chemotherapeutic agents are too ineffective to influence the results of surgery for NSCLC. There may be some value to adjuvant chemotherapy coupled with surgery in stage I SCLC. Although not proven, this approach would seem reasonable with our present knowledge, but controlled clinical trials are still awaited.

Rehabilitation and Follow-Up

On discharge from hospital the patient should be encouraged to resume full mobility and to exercise daily so that mobility is back to normal within 1 month. Following pneumonectomy there undoubtedly will be a reduction in the patient's exercise tolerance, but he should still be encouraged to exercise as much as possible each day.

Follow-up should take place after 1 month and then every 3 months for 1 year, every 6 months for 1 year, and subsequently annually. There is no need for any sophisticated tests other than physical examination, chest X-ray, and investigation of any specific complaints by the patient. Regular sputum cytology, CT scanning, or any other investigation not directed by specific symptoms is not indicated since at relapse, cure is impossible.

Role of Radiotherapy
(Treatment at Brompton Hospital and Royal Marsden Hospital)

J. R. Yarnold

Treatment Selection

Non-Small Cell Lung Cancer

Curative Radiotherapy

Patients with early stage disease confined to the primary site with or without hilar lymph node involvement (T1-2 NO 1MO) are best considered for surgical resection. Patients with resectable disease who are inoperable for medical reasons, such as ischemic heart disease or chronic obstructive airways disease, may be fit enough for high-dose radiotherapy with curative intent. Patients with central tumors encroaching on the carina are unresectable but may also be suitable for curative radiotherapy if nodal disease is confined to the ipsilateral hilum.

Most patients with non-small cell lung cancer are inoperable by virtue of mediastinal disease and they are often unsuitable for curative radiotherapy. The following criteria exclude a patient from curative therapy:

1. Pathologically enlarged supraclavicular lymph nodes
2. Bulky mediastinal adenopathy causing:
   - Signs of superior vena cava obstruction
   - Hoarseness due to recurrent laryngeal palsy
   - Paralysis of hemidiaphragm
   - Horner's syndrome
   - Dysphagia due to extrinsic compression of the esophagus
3. Malignant pleural or pericardial effusion
4. Involvement of chest wall (with the possible exception of superior sulcus tumors)

Relative contraindications include old age and infirmity, both associated with poor tolerance to high-dose radiotherapy. Greater than 10% weight loss due to dis-

Table 1. Unresectable non-small cell lung cancer: local failure by tumor size after randomization to different levels of total dose. (Perez et al. 1982)

Tumor size (cm)	Local failure after primary irradiation (No. of patients)			Level of significance
	4000 rad	5000 rad	6000 rad	
1-3	(19)58%	(13)46%	(10) 0%	$P=0.003$
4-6	(61)57%	(21)29%	(17)35%	$P=0.023$
>6	(29)45%	(7)43%	(11)46%	NS
Nonmeasurable	(92)48%	(51)47%	(47)40%	NS

ease is also a relative contraindication for curative radiotherapy, being associated with a high incidence of occult metastases.

Opinions vary regarding the eligibility for curative radiotherapy of patients with obvious mediastinal adenopathy unassociated with the clinical syndromes listed above. In Europe, patients with macroscopic mediastinal involvement are regarded as having such poor prognoses as to seldom, if ever, justify curative treatment. There are two reasons for this: firstly, these patients have a very high probability of metastatic disease and, secondly, these patients often have bulky primary and nodal disease which is difficult to eradicate. In the United States, however, many of these patients are treated with curative intent for the sake of a very small proportion of long-term survivors.

A reasonable therapeutic strategy is to exclude patients from curative treatment if the mediastinal adenopathy can be seen on a good-quality chest radiograph. Disease of this size is rarely radiocurable even if it is truly limited in extent to the thorax. Even if the mediastinum is normal on the chest radiograph, mediastinal involvement is present in approximately half the patients. Identation of the esophagus on a barium swallow or widening of the carina seen at bronchoscopy is additional indirect evidence of bulky mediastinal involvement precluding curative radiotherapy.

If facilities for CT scanning exist, a normal mediastinal scan is a good basis on which to consider curative radiotherapy. If enlarged lymph nodes are seen it should be borne in mind that enlargement > 1.5 cm may be associated with reactive changes only. Thus, positive tomography may be an indication for direct assessment by mediastinoscopy or mediastinotomy.

Considering the difficulties of accurate staging by noninvasive means, many radiotherapists forgo detailed mediastinal examinations in favor of patient selection for curative treatment on the basis of good general condition, less than 10% weight loss, and no evidence of mediastinal adenopathy or distant metastases on physical examination, chest X-ray, barium swallow, blood count, or biochemical screen. The best chances of cure are seen in fit patients with N0–N1 disease and primary tumors < 4 cm in diameter.

Surgery and Curative Radiotherapy

Combined radiotherapy and surgery has a limited role in the curative treatment of patients with non-small cell lung cancer. Randomized trials have failed to demonstrate a survival advantage for combined modalities in operable patients irradiated prior to surgery. Randomized studies have also failed to demonstrate a survival advantage for postoperative radiotherapy in patients undergoing curative resections for tumors unassociated with regional lymph node involvement. On the other hand there is a strong suggestion from several retrospective studies that patients with hilar or mediastinal lymph node involvement undergoing complete resection of all visible disease are benefitted in terms of local-regional control and long-term survival by postoperative radiotherapy to the mediastinum and tumor bed. There appears to be no curative role for postoperative radiotherapy if macroscopic residual disease remains after surgery. The other situation where combined radiotherapy and surgery might offer an advantage is in patients with T3N0 superior sulcus tumors of squamous cell subtype. Retrospective studies suggest that high-dose radiotherapy confined to the tumor bed following surgical resection of the primary disease, with or without adjacent chest wall structures, improves the prospects of long-term survival and even cure.

Palliative Radiotherapy of Intrathoracic Disease

The majority of patients with inoperable non-small cell lung cancer are not eligible for treatment with curative intent and require palliative radiotherapy for the relief of troublesome symptoms such as cough, dyspnea, hemoptysis, or intrathoracic pain. Other indications for palliative radiotherapy include superior vena caval obstruction and other clinical evidence of mediastinal node involvement such as dysphagia. Tumor encroaching on a main bronchus or trachea is a further indication for palliative radiotherapy regardless of symptoms because of the high risk of developing stridor if left untreated.

A minority of patients with incurable non-small cell lung cancer present without significant symptoms arising from their local-regional disease. Depending on the exact location of their local-ragional disease and follow-up facilities, it is reasonable to adopt a watch policy in these patients because a proportion will succumb to metastatic disease without ever requiring thoracic irradiation. So far, attempts to start a randomized comparison of the benifits of a "watch policy" versus immediate radiotherapy in terms of quality and duration of survival in this category of patients have been unsuccessful. This is mainly due to the difficulties in obtaining informed consent from patients in a trial setting.

Palliative Radiotherapy of Metastases

Palliative courses of radiotherapy induce tumor shrinkage with partial or symptom relief in patients with metastases in many solid organs, most commonly the bones and brain. Painful liver metastases unresponsive to high-dose steroids may also respond well to radiotherapy. The treatment prescription is discussed in a separate section.

Small Cell Lung Cancer

The optimal treatment for patients with small cell lung cancer is controversial but includes combination chemotherapy. Despite good initial response rates, local-regional progression occurs in the majority of patients. In randomized clinical studies thoracic irradiation delivered during or after chemotherapy reduces the rate of local-regional relapse but has no advantage for median survival. However, data are now becoming available suggesting that most survivors who are disease free at 2 or more years after completion of chemotherapy had radiotherapy to the mediastinum. However, the numbers of these long-term survivors are too small as yet to permit statistical comparison. Until a clearer picture emerges from trials currently underway it is justified to confine radiotherapy to those patients with the best prospects of permanent cure, that is those limited disease patients who achieve a complete radiological response of their intrathoracic disease following induction chemotherapy.

In parts of the world where facilities for giving effective chemotherapy are limited but where radiotherapy is available, it is reasonable to select fit patients with no signs of extrathoracic disease for high-dose thoracic irradiation. Unfortunately, the majority of patients will be suitable for palliative treatment only.

Radiotherapy Treatment Planning

Non-Small Cell Lung Cancer

Curative Radiotherapy

It is advisable to plan the treatment in two phases, the first encompassing the primary tumor and most of the mediastinum via anteroposteriorly opposed fields, and the second phase to a reduced volume confined to visible disease at the time of commencing this second phase.

Planning of the First Phase

The patient lies supine with the arms by the sides. The margins around visible disease should not be less than 2 cm especially if cobalt gamma rays are used.

Superior border – 2 cm above the sternal notch (higher for tumors in the apical segment of the upper lobe).

Inferior border – 5 cm below the carina (lower for tumors in the basal segments of the lower lobe).

Ipsilateral border – leave 2-cm margins around the primary tumor and regional adenopathy.

Contralateral border – 1 cm lateral to the vertebral bodies (note this does not completely encompass the contralateral hilum).

If a simulator is not available remember that in the treatment position the carina lies at the level of the manubrium sterni, which is easily palpated. It should be kept in mind that the position of the thoracic viscera as seen on a PA chest radiograph differs from that with the patient lying in the treatment position, and that the primary tumor can move several centimeters during deep inspiration/expiration.

Planning of the Second Phase

The patient position is supine with the arms raised above the head to allow the entry of posterior oblique fields if these are used. The length of the treatment volume is reduced to encompass all known disease at the time of treatment with 2-cm margins above and below. A transverse contour of the patient is taken halfway between the upper and lower borders. AP and lateral chest radiographs are taken at the appropriate source-skin distance for the treatment machine, using opaque centimeter markers on the anterior and posterior skin surfaces to allow calculations of magnification. The lateral, anterior, and posterior extents of the treatment volume are marked on the radiotherapy check films. Making allowances for film magnifi-

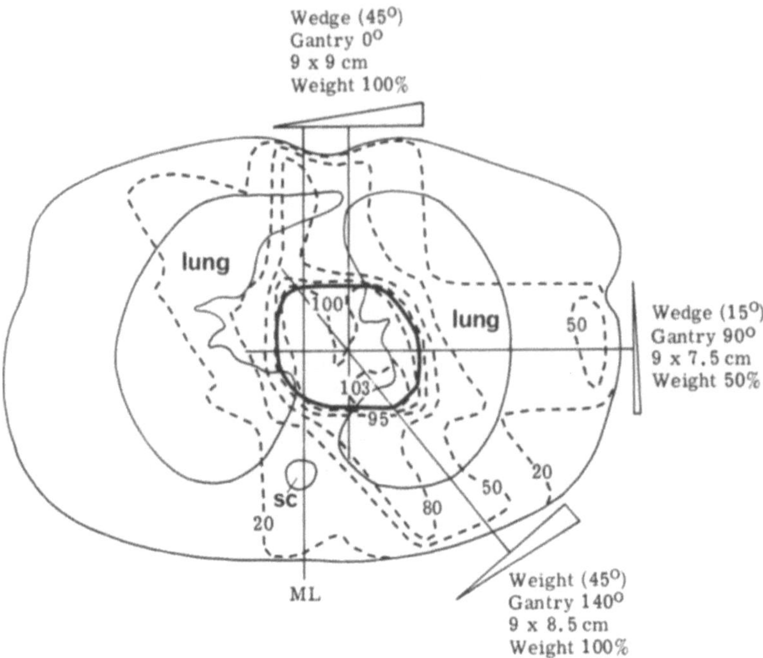

Fig. 1. Three fields encompassing residual disease at the hilum during a second phase of radiotherapy. The tumor dose is supplemented by a lateral field from the same side (with a 50% weighting) rather than by a contralateral posterior oblique field which would pass through the spinal cord

cation, these points are transferred to the transverse mid-plane contour and the marks joined in a continuous line to demarcate the treatment volume. Likewise, the position of the spinal cord is transferred to the patient contour. Using the appropriate isodose curves the treatment volume is encompassed with three fields or oblique opposed fields (Fig. 1, 2). For dosimetric purposes reduced lung attenuation is corrected for by subtracting 2.5% from the applied dose for every centimeter of lung traversed by the beam. Alternatively, cross-sectional CT data linked to a computerized planning system are used to localize the treatment volume and calculate the dosimetry.

Note that no spinal shielding should be used during the first phase of treatment but that the spinal cord should be excluded from the high-dose volume during the second phase. In practice, the spinal cord is usually on the fringe of the high-dose zone during the second phase. Spinal cord tolerance depends on the length of cord in the high-dose zone, the fractionation schedule, the age of the patient, and preexisting disease such as diabetes or hypertension. Attempts should be made not to exceed a cord dose of 45 Gy in fractions of 2 Gy, whenever possible. Doses in excess are associated with a rising risk of myelopathy, particularly over 50 Gy.

144

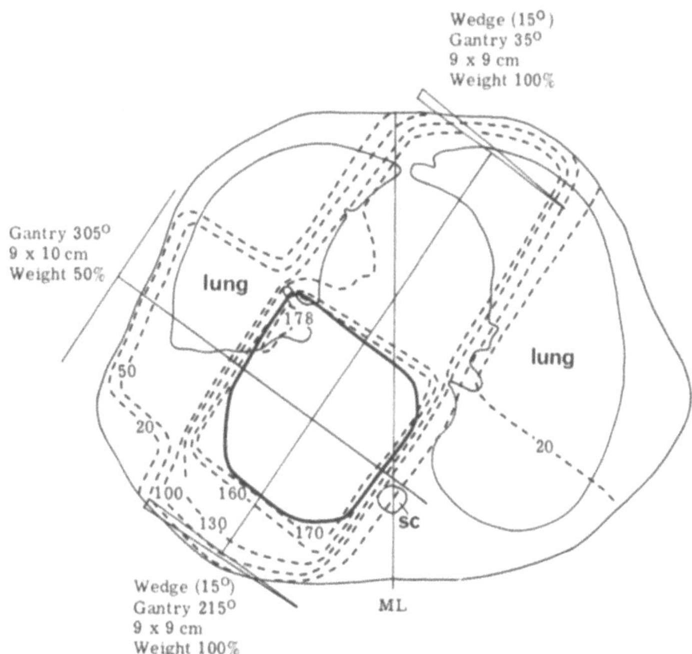

Fig. 2. Oblique opposed fields encompassing a bulky tumor at the hilum during a second phase of radiotherapy. The tumor dose is supplemented by a lateral field with a weighting of 50%; this may not be essential in a small patient

Palliative Radiotherapy to the Chest

It is usually sufficient to confine the high-dose volume to the primary tumor and hilar lymph nodes including the carina with 2-cm margins all around, thereby avoiding large portions of the mediastinum and healthy lung. This reduces the morbidity of treatment in terms of fatigue, nausea, esophagitis, and pneumonitis. Note that for the treatment of the superior vena cava obstruction the whole mediastinum should be treated from 2 cm above the sternal notch to 5 cm below the level of the carina. Anteroposterior opposed fields are used.

Palliative Radiotherapy to Metastases

Whole brain irradiation is best given via opposed lateral fields using cobalt-60 gamma rays or megavoltage X-rays, with the patient lying supine. The surface markings of the base of skull coincide with a line drawn between the superior tragus of the ear and a point 1 cm superior to the outer canthus of the eye. Simulator or treatment machine check films should be taken to confirm proper localization. Most radiotherapists administer a dose of 30 Gy in 10 fractions. An alternative would be 20 Gy in 5 fractions – but the former regime is the commonest. In the case of an isolated deposit the dose to the tumor area itself can be given a dose of 10 Gy in 5 fractions after completion of the whole brain irradiation.

Single appositional fields are often adequate for painful bone metastases but opposed fields are preferable in the pelvis and for pathological fractures of long bones.

Small Cell Lung Cancer

If thoracic irradiation is confined to limited disease patients who respond completely to induction chemotherapy, the radiotherapy portals should include the whole mediastinum plus the visible extent of disease at diagnosis with 2-cm margins during the first phase. During the second phase attempts should be made to reduce the volume to the regions of residual visible disease after chemotherapy with 1-cm margins via a three-field technique which avoids the spinal cord.

Radiotherapy Treatment Prescription

Curative Radiotherapy to Local-Regional Disease

Continuous daily schedules and split-course regimes are both widely used. A 60 Gy tumor dose in 30 fractions over 6–7 weeks is delivered as a continuous regime in two phases, with 40 Gy delivered in 4–5 weeks via large opposed fields and a second phase delivering 20 Gy in 10 fractions to a reduced volume. Local boosts to 65 Gy in 7 weeks are occasionally possible to small peripheral tumors. One of the commonest split-course regimes delivers a 30 Gy tumor dose in 10 fractions over 2 weeks followed after a 3-week rest by a second phase of a 25- to 30-Gy tumors dose in 10 fractions to a reduced volume over a total treatment time of 7 weeks.

The advantages of split-course therapy are chiefly those of convenience to the patient and institution, involving fewer visits to hospital and fewer setups on the machine. Potential biological advantages include tumor shrinkage and reoxygenation between split courses but there is no clinical evidence that this can be exploited. In a multicenter randomized trial of the Radiation Therapy Oncology Group (RTOG), patients randomized to a 40-Gy tumor dose as a split course over 4 weeks faired less well in terms of initial tumor response rate and 2-year survival rate, compared with 50 or 60 Gy in 25 or 30 fractions delivered daily (Perez et al. 1982). Other small randomized studies have failed to demonstrate significant differences between split course and continuous regimes.

In the absence of clear evidence for superior tumor response rates with split-course therapy, and evidence from one large randomized study that they might be worse, the treatment of choice is to use daily fractions of 2 Gy, to a total of 60 Gy using shrinking field techniques, thereby minimizing the late damage to critical normal tissues, such as the lungs, esophagus, and spinal cord.

Nevertheless in terms of palliation there are practical advantages to split-course radiotherapy. The initial course can be quite intensive, giving the irradiation to a dose of, for example, 20 Gy in 5 days, which is more rapid than for a single-treatment course. The patient is then allowed to recover and when the second part of the course is due, if there has been no response to initial irradiation, one could consider withholding further treatment as the tumor is unlikely to undergo a useful reduction in size. This approach allows the responsiveness of a tumor to radiotherapy to be tested and it may be wise to limit the treatment and prevent possible toxicity in the nonresponders.

Palliative Radiotherapy to Intrathoracic Disease

The aim of palliative treatment is the lifelong relief of distressing symptoms achieved in the shortest possible treatment time and with the minimum side effects in terms of fatigue, nausea, esophagitis, and pneumonitis. Palliation is thus concerned with the quality as well as the duration of survival; yet, several studies addressing the optimal dose of palliative radiotherapy use duration of survival as the only measure of palliative effect. This is not surprising in view of the lack of quantitative end points available for scoring symptoms and side effects of treatment.

A common policy is to give a 30-Gy tumor dose in 10 daily fractions, a dose sufficient to relieve respiratory symptoms and pain partially or completely in the majority of patients. One course of treatment is enough for patients with distant metastases or in poor general condition who have a very poor prognosis. In these patients a second phase of treatment involves pointless extra visits to hospital and extra toxicity, especially esophagitis. The second phase should be held in reserve if symptoms recur.

Nausea accompanying radiotherapy should be treated by metoclopramide 10 mg by mouth three times daily. Other antiemetics such as prochlorperazine may also be used.

Patients may develop a persistent cough with or without dyspnea and the expectoration of small amounts of frothy mucoid sputum due to radiation pneumonitis 3–11 months or more after high-dose radiotherapy. The syndrome lasts several weeks to a few months and may respond to short-term steroid therapy, e.g., prednisolone 10 mg three times daily. Simple linctus, codeine, or methadone linctus may be necessary to relieve exhausting cough in severely affected patients. Steroids to not affect the incidence or severity of pulmonary fibrosis which supercedes the pneumonitis in a proportion of patients. In patients with poor cardiac or respiratory reserve, inappropriately prescribed high-dose radiotherapy can induce pulmonary fibrosis severe enough to prevent even mild exertion.

Other serious late sequelae of high-dose radiation include esophageal stenosis, myelopathy, and pericardial fibrosis, all of which are rare when the correct techniques are used.

Further Reading

Kjaer M (1982) Radiotherapy or squamous, adeno- and large cell carcinoma of the lung. Cancer Treat Rev 9: 1–20
Perez CA, Stanley K, Grundy G et al (1982) Impact of irradiation technique and tumour extent in tumour control and survival of patients with unresectable non-oat cell carcinoma of the lung. Cancer 50: 1091–1099
Salazar OM, Creech RH (1980) "The state of the art" toward defining the role of radiation therapy in the management of small cell bronchogenic carcinoma. Int J Radiat Oncol Biol Phys

Chemotherapy (Treatment at Brompton Hospital)

S. G. Spiro

Chemotherapy for Inoperable Non-Small Cell Lung Cancer

Over 50% of patients with lung cancer present with evidence of metastatic disease and metastases will appear in many others following failure of initial treatment to control the disease. There have been more than 200 studies of chemotherapy for inoperable non-small cell lung cancer, but evidence for a worthwhile prolongation of survival is lacking. Single agents produce a response rate (at least a 50% reduction in tumor diameter) in the region of 10%, and combinations of cytotoxic drugs may result in a larger percentage of "responders." However, a response to chemotherapy does not equate simply to a prolongation of survival. The majority of reported studies do not contain a randomized prospective control group and either compare their data with retrospective control subjects or compare responders with nonresponders. The latter is open to strong criticism as nonresponder cases often have more advanced disease or poorer general health, or lower performance status. As yet the case for cytotoxic chemotherapy in non-small cell lung cancer is not made and should be considered a subject for careful future clinical studies.

At present no specific recommendations can be made for any single agent or combination of chemotherapeutic agents for the treatment of non-small cell lung cancer. Reviews of recent additions to the cytotoxic range have included examination of drugs such as vindesine, mitomycin C, epipodophyllotoxin, ifosfamide, and *cis*-platinum. As yet these drugs, whether alone or in combination, are little better than the older studies on single agents such as nitrogen mustard, methotrexate, adriamycin, the nitrosoureas, and vincristine. The tendency has always been to try drugs in combination in the hope that some form of synergy will develop. However, the response rates with combination chemotherapy even with the newer agents are no better than for single agents. Most studies that have given promising results have included too small a group of patients and have provided only a

148

rough guide to response. When subdivided into histological subtypes there are many studies in which fewer than ten patients have been treated. A single response will then distort the results. Usually large studies have failed to confirm any promise shown by small studies.

Until studies of potentially effective drugs are compared with untreated control closely matched populations it is not possible to make any statement about the effectiveness of new agents. This report therefore is not making any recommendations for any particular cytotoxic drug or combination of cytotoxic drugs for the treatment of inoperable advanced non-small cell lung cancer.

It should be borne in mind that the toxicity of many of the regimens that have been examined has been considerable as has been the expense. Toxicity may shorten patients' lives. The toxicity is the usual predictable type with myelosuppression, alopecia, nausea, and vomiting.

Other Methods of Treatment – Adjuvant Therapy with Surgery

The poor overall results of surgery have led to many studies of adjuvant therapy including chemotherapy, radiotherapy, and, more recently, immunotherapy. Many studies published to date have not given adequate details of staging and this has made interpretation of results extremely difficult. Adjuvant therapy must be safe and toxicity acceptably low as some patients, especially those with stage 1 tumors, may already have been cured by their operation.

Immunotherapy

During the past 6 years many studies have investigated an immunological approach to surgical adjuvant therapy. This follows the observation that patients developing postoperative empyema had lower relapse rates than those with an uncomplicated postoperative course, and the study by McKneally et al. [1] using intrapleural instillation of Tice BCG. At a follow-up of 2 years McKneally et al. found that the immunotherapy-treated group with stage I disease had 93% of cases disease free, compared with 67% of controls. There was no benefit in patients with stage II or III disease. Other methods of administering BCG – subdermal, scarification, or interdermal – have failed to show any benefit in preventing relapse. To date McKneally's results have not been reproduced and results in a recent study at Brompton Hospital have shown no improvement in survival at 1 year in stage I patients using an identical protocol to McKneally et al. with matched controls, and there was a disturbing incidence of local side effects [2].

Levamisole, an anthelminthic drug, alters T-cell function and has been given orally as an immunostimulant. There has been no evidence of clear efficacy, and shorter survival in the treated patients with an excess of deaths due to cardiorespiratory causes, tentatively related to the drug, has been reported [3].

Another agent, *Corynebacterium parvum,* was claimed to give encouraging results when given intravenously [4]. However, many subsequent studies have proven disappointing and the injection of the organism, particularly by the intravenous route, is associated with a high incidence of side effects including fever, pain, and malaise for several hours.

It would appear that the likelihood of immunotherapy fulfilling its earlier promise is small, but the slight possibility remains that benefit may accrue for stage I tumors, and this is likely to be answered by the large studies currently in progress evaluating intrapleural BCG.

Radiotherapy

Several studies of preoperative radiotherapy have failed to prolong survival [5, 6]. Preoperative radiotherapy is, however, still advocated for superiorsulcus tumors provided the mediastinal structures are not involved [7], although a 40% 5-year survival is possible by surgery alone [8].

Surprisingly the role of postoperative radiotherapy is still not clear. This is due to inadequate information on staging and whether resections were considered "curative" or not. Two recent studies advocating postoperative radiotherapy for patients with mediastinal and hilar node involvement are uncontrolled [9, 10]. In the study of Kirsch et al. [10] the 5-year survival of patients with squamous cell cancer undergoing radiotherapy with mediastinal metastases was 34% compared with 53% 5-year survival for NOMO disease. With adenocarcinoma none of the patients with hilar nodal involvement who received radiotherapy survived 5 years, but 12% of those with mediastinal nodal involvement were disease free at 5 years. Controlled studies are important in this area to confirm the tendency (not statistically significant in *any* study) that postoperative irradiation to the mediastinum in patients with either residual macroscopic disease or resected involved mediastinal lymph nodes confers any survival benefit.

Chemotherapy of Small Cell Lung Cancer

Recently the natural history of SCLC has been considerably modified by combination chemotherapy [11–13]. Several cytotoxic agents are active in this condition, producing a response rate far higher than for other lung cancers: methotrexate (30%), cyclophosphamide (40%), vincristine (33%), doxorubicin (25%), epipodophyllotoxin (45%), and lomustine (CCNU) (18%). However, these encouraging single-agent responses failed to prolong median survival any further than local radiotherapy – another treatment to which small cell carcinoma of the lung is highly sensitive (Table 2). Combining three or four drugs resulted in marked improvement in median survival (Table 2). The most frequent combinations include methotrexate, cyclophosphamide, adriamycin, vincristine, or epipodophyllotoxin; and a median survival in limited disease of 15 months and in extensive disease of 9 months is now relatively common. A vital factor in improving survival is the attainment of a complete response, i.e., a clinical, radiological, and bronchoscopic

Table 2. Incidence of complete responses and overall survival in small cell carcinoma of the lung. (Adapted from Greco et al. 1978 [12])

Therapy	Complete responses (%)	Median survival of all patients (months)	1 year (survival %)
Placebo	0	2.5	5
Radiotherapy	<20	6.0	20
Cyclophosphamide	1	5.0	18
Eight other active single drugs	3	5.5	15
Combination chemotherapy (two, three, and four drugs)	15	8.5	25
Combination chemotherapy (three and four drugs)	23	9.0	40
Combination chemotherapy plus radiotherapy	31	11.0	47

clearing of visible tumor (Fig. 3). Although this is not equivalent to eradication of the tumor, it seems the most important prognostic factor as well as a yardstick of treatment efficacy. Limited disease patients treated by one of several available regimens attained a complete response rate of about 60% as compared with 20% with extensive disease patients [12], although most studies have reported lower percentages using the same drugs. A minority of patients have remained in complete remission for longer than 2 years, a duration perhaps close to cure in this very rapidly growing tumor. Of 225 limited disease patients compiled from 10 institutions and treated with effective chemotherapy alone or in combination with radiotherapy, 72% had complete responses and 42 of these 184 patients (23%) were free of detectable disease 2 years or more after starting treatment [14]. These results have yet to be equaled or bettered.

All the effective regimens are associated with some toxicity, the severity of which is a function of the dose of drugs, the number and type of drugs, the frequency of administration, stage of the disease, and the patient's performance status. As so many of the patients are symptomatic at presentation and as up to 90% of patients show at least a partial response to chemotherapy, there can be a gratifying improvement in symptom control, albeit often for only a few months. Personal experience of four courses of chemotherapy in 100 patients with small cell carcinoma of the lung caused an improvement in cough and dyspnea in 65% of sufferers (Fig. 4), hemoptysis in 77% (Fig. 5), malaise and weakness in 63%, pain relief in 60% (Fig. 6), and relief of dysphagia and/or superior vena cava obstruction in 80% (Fig. 7). The cytotoxic agents used in this study were adriamycin 50 mg/m^2 and vincristine 1.4 mg/m^2 alternating every 3 weeks with cyclophosphamide 1 g/m^2 and methotrexate 50 mg/m^2. Most regimens are associated with transient granulocytopenia and infection is a major risk. Approximately 5%–10% of patients will require admission to hospital with a presumed infection and occasionally an established septicemia. The risk of a lethal infection is 1%–4% [14].

It would appear that in its current form and using conventional dose schedules combination chemotherapy is unlikely to extend significantly the median survival

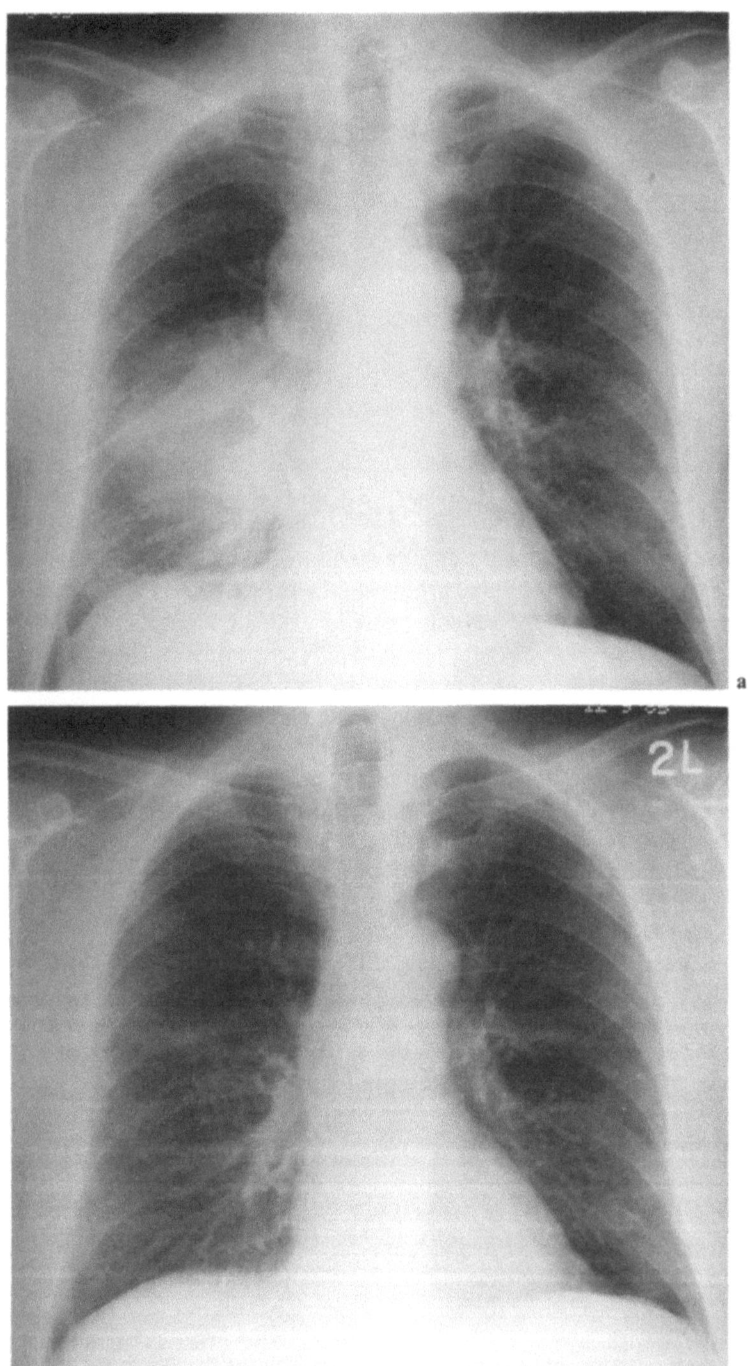

Fig. 3. **a** Pretreatment chest radiograph of patient with SCLC. **b** After completion of 6 months chemotherapy. Patient is now asymptomatic

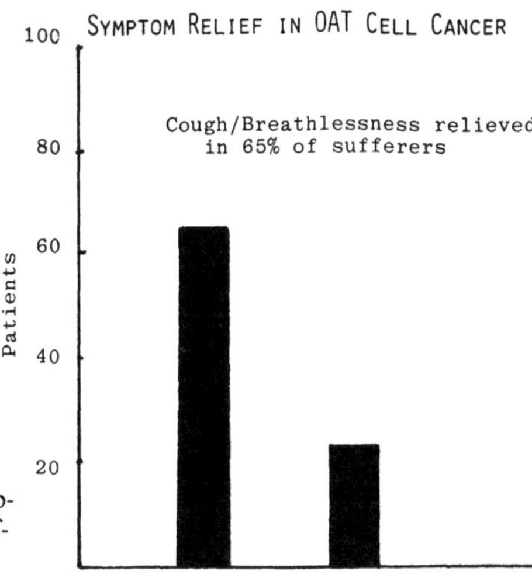

Fig. 4. The effect of 3 months (4 courses) of chemotherapy on the symptoms of cough and dyspnea. The number of sufferers of these symptoms *(left)* from 100 patients, and the number after treatment *(right)* who still had these complaints

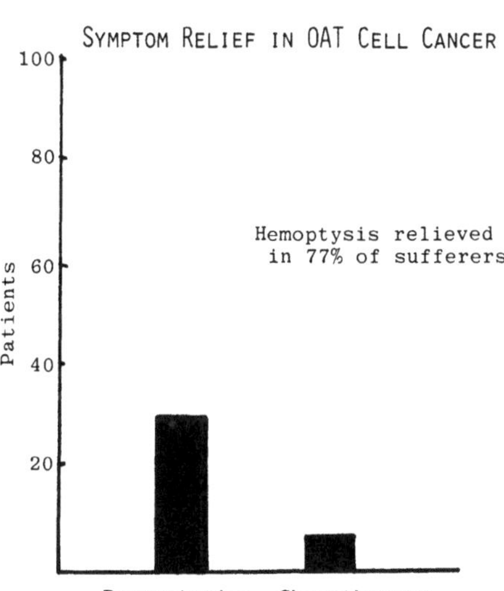

Fig. 5. Similar effects for hemoptysis

from that currently reported. There are, however, several possibilities for the future: newer drugs such as *cis*platin and ifosfamide are yet to be assessed in detail. *Cis*platin as a single agent has been disappointing, with a response rate of $< 20\%$. It is also nephrotoxic and has a high incidence of nausea and vomiting. It is particularly poorly tolerated by the elderly (i.e., patients with lung cancer). New, less toxic analogues are becoming available for clinical trials. The possible use of existing drugs at a much higher dosage to achieve greater tumor-killing potential with autologous bone marrow support, and the question of maintenance chemotherapy after intensive cyclical chemotherapy, which however is only tolerated by most for up to 9-12 months, is under study.

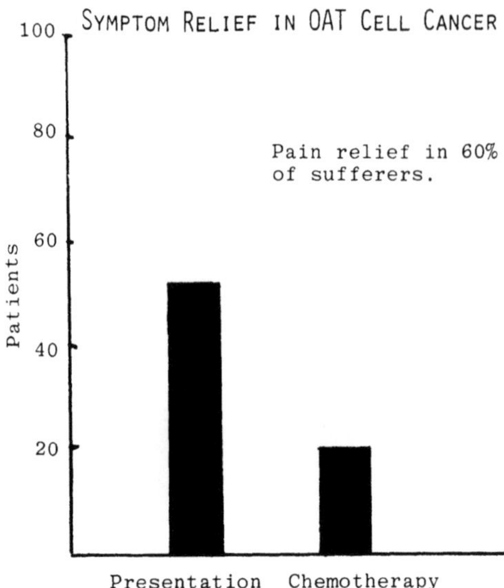

Fig. 6. Similar effects for pain

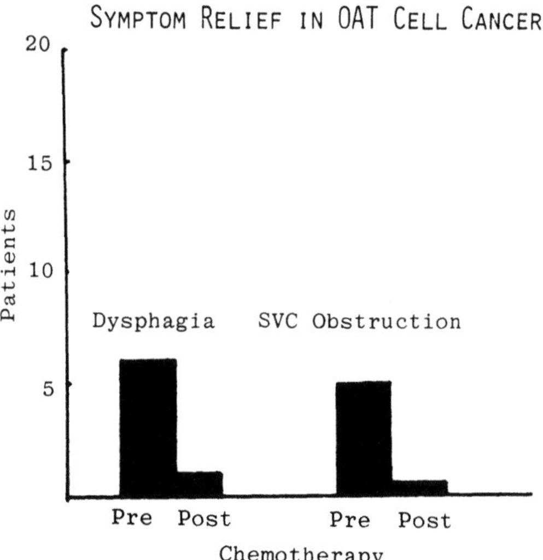

Fig. 7. Similar effects for dysphagia and superior vena caval obstruction

At present the minimum duration of treatment compatible with a worthwhile survival in small cell lung cancer is not established. Many centers treat patients until they relapse, or for 1 year or more once a complete response is established. It is our recommendation that patients considered for treatment should be treated while they respond for a maximum of 8 courses of cyclical chemotherapy – each treatment being given every 3 weeks. Possible combinations of chemotherapy are shown in Table 3. It is very likely that elderly patients (above the age of 70) will tolerate chemotherapy poorly. Similarly patients with a poor performance status and extensive disease with metastases in two or more sites with a history of weight

Table 3. Suggested cytotoxic regimens for small cell lung cancer[a]

1.	Cyclophosphamide	1 g/m^2 i.v.	
	Vincristine	2 mg i.v.	q 3/52
	Epipodophyllotoxin	100 mg p.o. 8 hrly × 9 doses	
2.	Cyclophosphamide	1 g/m^2 i.v.	
	Adriamycin	40 mg/m^2 i.v.	q 3/52
	Vincristine	2 mg i.v.	
3.	Cyclophosphamide	1 g/m^2 i.v.	
	Adriamycin	40 mg/m^2 i.v.	
	Vincristine	2 mg/m^2 i.v.	q 3/52
	Epipodophyllotoxin	100 mg p.o. 8 hrly × 9 doses	
4.	Cyclophosphamide	1 g/m^2 i.v.	
	Methotrexate	50 mg/m^2 i.v.	q 3/52
	Vincristine	2 mg i.v.	
5.	Epipodophyllotoxin[b]	200 mg p.o. stat, then 100 mg 8 hrly × 8 doses q 3/52	

[a] Before administration of any cycle of chemotherapy the total WBC ≥ 3500 *and* platelets > 100000. If not, withhold chemotherapy and repeat blood count weekly until satisfactory. If Hb < 10 g transfuse

[b] For elderly or poor performance status patients

The optimal duration for treatment is not known. Most suggest six to eight cycles provided the patient continues to respond

loss are likely also to do poorly. Patients with extensive disease with a reasonable or good performance status and metastases in only one site may do well. Patients with limited disease also are in the best prognostic category for doing well.

In deciding whether to treat patients the following staging investigations should be done:

1. Evaluation of performance status.
2. Posteroanterior chest X-ray.
3. Bronchoscopy (the most probable way of making a diagnosis), together with sputum cytology, liver function tests, urea and electrolytes, and full blood count.
4. If possible, bone marrow aspiration should be carried out as this yields a surprisingly high positive rate. Marrow trephine is often necessary for a positive result.
5. Brain, bone, and liver scans should only be done if clinical indications are present or in the case of the liver if liver function tests are abnormal.

In patients who respond to treatment there is an advantage in giving prophylactic cerebral irradiation. We recommend the dose of 2000 rad (20 Gy given in 5 doses over 7 days). Only patients who show a good response (partial response or complete response) to chemotherapy after four courses should receive prophylactic cerebral irradiation. It will reduce the incidence of cerebral metastatses and therefore reduce significant patient morbidity. Other regimes of 3000–4000 rad (30–40 Gy) over 3–4 weeks neither prolong survival nor do they appear to reduce the incidence of metastases any further than does 2000 rad (20 Gy). The five-fraction treatment over 7 days has been used extensively by our group with excellent tolerance and acceptable typical results of the incidence in prevention of the emergence of clinical disease.

Superior vena caval obstruction (SVCO) – a presentation in approximately 10% of patients with small cell carcinoma – will respond as effectively to cytotoxic chemotherapy as it will to radiotherapy. Since radiotherapy centers are scattered and cytotoxic agents are usually available to most hospitals, it is our recommendation that cytotoxic chemotherapy is commenced in patients in whom a diagnosis of small cell carcinoma is made who have superior vena caval obstruction. The survival in patients with small cell carcinoma who present with SVCO is identical to any other presentation of this disease. To reduce edema, dexamethasone, 4 mg orally 6 hourly, should be commenced with cytotoxic chemotherapy and continued for 4 days and then reduced by 50% of the dose every 3 days.

References

1. McKneally MF, Maver CM, Kausel HW (1976) Intrapleural BCG immunostimulation in lung cancer. Lancet 1: 377–379
2. Law MR, Spiro SG, Geddes DM, Hodson ME (1981) Side effects of intrapleural BCG. Thorax 36: 236
3. Anthony HM, Mearns AJ, Mason MK, Scott DG, Moghissi K, Deverall PB, Rozycki ZJ, Watson DA (1979) Levamisole and surgery in bronchial carcinoma patients: increase in deaths from cardiorespiratory failure. Thorax 34: 4–12
4. Israel L, Edelstein R, Depierre A, Dimitrov H (1975) Brief communication: daily intravenous infusion of *Corynebacterium parvum* in twenty patients with disseminated cancer. J Natl Cancer Inst 55: 29–33
5. Shields TW, Higgins GA, Lawton R, Keilbrunn A, Kreehn RJ (1970) Preoperative x-ray therapy as an adjuvant in the treatment of bronchogenic carcinoma. J Thorac Cardiovasc Surg 59: 49–61
6. Warram J (1975) Preoperative irradiation of cancer of the lung: final report of a therapeutic trial. Cancer 36: 914–920
7. Paulson DL (1966) The survival rate in superior sulcus tumours treated by presurgical irradiation. JAMA 196: 342
8. Miller JI, Mansour KA, Hatcher CRJ (1979) Carcinoma of the superior pulmonary sulcus. Am Thorax Surg 28: 44–47
9. Green H, Kurohara SS, George FW, Creuss PG (1975) Post-resection irradiation for lung cancer. Radiology 116: 405–407
10. Kirsch M, Rotman H (1976) Carcinoma of the lung: results of treatment over ten years. Ann Thorac Surg 21: 371–377
11. Bunn PA, Cohen MH, Ihde DC, Fossieck BE, Matthews MJ, Minna JD (1977) Advances in small cell bronchogenic carcinoma. Cancer Treat Rep 61: 333–342
12. Greco FA, Einhorn LH, Richardson RL, Oldham RK (1978) Small cell lung cancer: progress and perspectives. Semin Oncol 5: 323–335
13. Weiss RB (1978) Small cell carcinoma of the lung: therapeutic management. Ann Intern Med 88: 552–531
14. Greco FA, Oldham RK (1979) Current concepts in cancer: small cell lung cancer. N Engl J Med 301: 355–357

Specific Problems in Inoperable Patients and Terminal Care
(Treatment at Brompton Hospital)

S. G. Spiro

The most important part of the follow-up of the patient is to define responsibility
for continuing care. This is either undertaken by the cardiothoracic center at
which the patient was initially diagnosed and treated or at the local referring hospital. The general practitioner or referring physician should also participate in the
patients' continuing care especially if the patient's condition relapses and terminal
care is required.

Treatment of Specific Problems

Ectopic Hormone Production (Nonmetastatic or Paraneoplastic Syndromes)

Hypercalcemia

Hypercalcemia may be caused by generalized bony metastases or by ectopic secretion of parathormone from the primary tumor in squamous cell carcinomas.

The patient may develop symptoms of confusion, dehydration, constipation,
and polyuria with no bony symptoms. A bone scan is often negative in the case of
ectopic hormone secretion. The primary tumor can be treated by radiotherapy,
which will reduce the hypercalcemia. As a first aid measure steroids, e.g., prednisolone 40 mg/day and diuretics can be given together with intravenous fluid rehy-
dration. If the patient is too unwell to undergo radiotherapy because of prostra-
tion, confusion, or lack of ability to cooperate then cytotoxic chemotherapy with
mithromycin 10–20 mcg/kg can be given intravenously daily for 3 days. Alternatively calcitonin 200 u/day may be helpful but may take several days to achieve
the desired effect. It can, however, be totally ineffective even in massive doses. A
daily dose of 200 units is usually as effective as a larger dose.

Syndrome of Inappropriate Antidiuretic Hormone (SIADH)

The blood electrolytes will be clearly and characteristically abnormal in approximately 10% of all cases of small cell lung cancer. The serum sodium is usually <
120 mmol/liter and the urea < 2 mmol/liter. The plasma osmolality will be
250 mosmol/liter or less with a corresponding urinary osmolality of >
700 mosmol/liter. Treatment should comprise cytotoxic chemotherapy to control
the tumor mass. Democlocycline hydrochloride (ledermycin) 600 mg or 1200 mg
daily acts by competing with the ADH-binding sites at the renal tubules and can
by itself be rapidly effective in reversing the effects of the syndrome. There is no
need to restrict fluid intake if the patient is put on democlocycline.

Hypertrophic Pulmonary Osteoarthropathy

This painful periostitis of the lower tibia and fibula and radius and ulna is usually associated with squamous cell carcinoma and finger clubbing. Characteristically the skin above the ankles and wrists is red and edematous and very tender to touch. Treatment with nonsteroidal antiinflammatory drugs is most helpful. Removal of the primary tumor by surgery will very rapidly relieve the symptoms. Radiotherapy is almost as effective. Chemotherapy is usually not successful as it is an inactive treatment for squamous cell lung cancers.

Syndrome of Ectopic ACTH Secretion

This occurs almost exclusively in SCLC. However, due to the short natural history from diagnosis to death the effects of excessive ACTH (Cushing's syndrome) hardly ever fully manifest themselves. However, some patients develop a Cushingoid appearance with proximal myopathy and perhaps diabetes. Diagnosis is by elevated 9 a.m. and 12 midnight plasma cortisols and disappearance of the diurnal rhythm. Direct estimations of plasma ACTH will be elevated. Therapy is aimed at control of the tumor itself often with dramatic, although usually transient, benefit. Hypokalemia may be severe enough to require replacement therapy and the diabetes occasionally requires insulin. These sufferers rarely respond well to chemotherapy and their overall prognosis is far worse than with SCLC patients without ectopic hormone production.

Superior Vena Caval Obstruction

If possible a specific diagnosis should be made including the cell type of the neoplasm. Although in most cases the diagnosis obviously is carcinoma of the bronchus, the histological cell type is important as small cell carcinoma is best treated with chemotherapy while non-small cell carcinoma is best treated by radiotherapy. Fiberoptic bronchoscopy with brush cytology or careful biopsy should be carried out if there are no lymph nodes accessible to biopsy. Mediastinoscopy in the presence of superior vena caval obstruction is not contraindicated and usually glands high in the paratracheal region are pathological and therefore very accessible to biopsy.

Treatment should commence with diuretics and oral dexamethasone 4 mg 6 hourly. Chemotherapy or radiotherapy should then be given according to cell type. In most cases there is relief within 3–5 days of commencing therapy.

Hoarseness

This is due usually to the recurrent laryngeal nerve being involved by tumor in the subaortic fossa. Specific treatment aimed at the tumor mass causing the hoarseness is unlikely to be helpful. For example, radiotherapy very rarely relieves this symptom. If the patient's general condition is good and there is no adequate compensatory adduction of the other vocal cord, then Teflon paste can be injected into the paralyzed cord to bring it to the midline and improve the voice and minimize aspiration.

Pleural Effusion

Large pleural effusions can develop rapidly in lung cancers of all cell types, but are commonest with adenocarcinoma. They can cause profound dyspnea. As detailed in the section on surgical staging a pleural effusion should always be diagnosed to be malignant by pleural fluid cytological examination or pleural biopsy (repeated if initially negative). Clearly heavily blood stained effusions in patients known to have advanced lung cancer are almost inevitably malignant, but clear straw-colored effusions should be examined critically and if necessary repeatedly, especially in new cases who present with an effusion as part of their disease.

Initially the effusion should be only in part aspirated with samples sent for cytology, microbiology, and biochemistry (including pleural and *serum* glucose estimation). A pleural biopsy should be taken at this time. The effusion should not be aspirated to dryness in case the diagnosis is not established and further samples are required.

Once the diagnosis is made (or at least other possible diagnoses such as tuberculosis and empyema are excluded) the effusion should be aspirated to dryness. However, no more than 1 liter should be removed at any single aspiration in order to minimize the possibility of rapid reexpansion of the lung with cough, shortness of breath, pain, and rarely acute pulmonary edema. Several aspirations may be required over a few days.

It will become clear within a few days or weeks whether the effusion is returning. If so a chemical pleurodesis should be attempted. This should always be carried out by initially inserting a large intercostal drain (22°–26° F) and taking off the effusion slowly using a clamp to control the rate of flow over, say, 12 h using a conventional underwater seal technique.

There is no one especially effective agent for producing the pleuritis necessary for adherence of the two pleural surfaces. Tetracycline injectable powder (1 g), bleomycin (about 100 mg), or *Corynebacterium parvum* (7 mg vial) are equally effective, with tetracycline being much the cheapest. The effectiveness depends on the technique used. It is the author's strong belief that success depends on:

1. Complete drainage of the hemithorax.
2. The insertion of the chosen irritant (in the case of tetracycline with the addition of 100 mg 1% lidocaine) and then, after clamping the intercostal drain, the bed is raised to the head-down position and the patient turned by 90° every 10 min – i.e., a complete rotation of the patient to "spread" the irritant over the pleural surface over a period of 40 min.
3. The bed is returned to the normal position and the tube remains clamped for a further 90 min.
4. The tube is unclamped and the distal end of the tubing connected to a high-volume low-pressure pump and vigorous pressure applied (about 20 cm water) continuously for 48 h.
5. After 48 h the intercostal drain is removed. Effective pleurodesis occurs in 80% of cases.

If Corynebacterium *parvum* is used it is not necessary to insert an intercostal drain, but to inject 7 mg (1 ampoule) into the pleural cavity when a residuum of fluid remains. The patient is rotated as described above. This procedure can be repeated several times if not successful. The patient may develop a pyrexia and rigors. Soluble aspirin 600 mg 6 hourly should be prescribed. Most patients undergoing a clinical pleurodesis can expect pleuritic pain, which should be treated with papaverine or morphine as required.

If pleurodesis is unsuccessful and the symptoms recur, a surgical pleurectomy can be attempted, provided the general condition of the patient justifies this. Colloidal gold, inserted following needle aspiration, is often most effective but the patient has to be isolated while radioactive and it is difficult to obtain colloidal gold. The initial chemical pleurodesis procedure described above could also be repeated.

Cerebral Metastases

The treatment of choice is radiotherapy as described previously. An initial decision has to be made whether the general condition of the patient is sufficiently good to justify radiotherapy. Clearly if the patient is hemiplegic or confused or comatosed it may be wisest not to consider radiotherapy. An initial response to dexamethasone 4 mg orally, intramuscularly, or intravenously 6 hourly for 48 h may aid this decision. If there is a substantial improvement with steroids then much of the disability was caused by the edema secondary to the tumor. If improvement with steroids is considered worthwhile we suggest that these patients should now receive radiotherapy rather than merely continue with high-dose dexamethasone. Some patients can rapidly develop myopathies on steroids and this will often become as gross a handicap as the original cerebral disease. Radiotherapy often allows withdrawal of steroids once treatment is completed and also may cause useful prolongation of life.

Bone Metastases

If isolated and localizable then radiotherapy is the treatment of choice as detailed previously on pp. 140 ff. Any analgesic should contain aspirin or other non-steroidal antiinflammatory medication as these potentiate the effects of analgesics.

Analgesia

The commonest cause of pain in lung cancer is due to bony metastases. Initially analgesics containing codeine should be tried. Dihydrocodeine tartrate or dextropropoxyphene hydrochloride are effective. Aspirin should be added with the codeine medication as aspirin has a beneficial effect in controlling bone pain.

If the codeine containing medications is not adequate then combined tablets of papaverine (Papaveretum 10 mg) and aspirin 500 mg can be tried.

For severe pain morphine salts should be introduced relatively early. Morphine can be given as morphine sulfate (MST) continuous tablets b.d. beginning at 10–20 mg b.d. MST is a particularly useful preparation of 10-mg, 30-mg, and 60-mg tablets, often very effective on twice daily dosage. This allows the patients to return home and to be freed from regular injections. Similarly morphine sulfate elixir 5–10 mg in 5 ml together with prochlorperazine 5 mg/dose is also extremely effective. Many patients tolerate morphine elixir very well and continue pain free with a reasonable quality of life for a considerable time.

Whenever using codeine or morphine medication, laxatives should also be given in order to ensure constipation does not occur. Constipation can become the overriding complaint and obsession of patients with opiates and should be anticipated rather than merely allowed to develop and become a major problem.

General Matters

Anorexia becomes an increasing problem as the patient's condition deteriorates. Care should be given to give light foods and to give build-up preparations such as Complan in order to maintain as nutritious a diet as possible. Corticosteroids such as prednisone 15–20 mg/day often have a nonspecific beneficial effect.

In many cases patients can continue to live at home on morphine elixir, appropriate laxatives, prednisolone, a light diet, and home nursing care from the Community Nursing Service. If possible such patients should be seen once a week at the hospital or should be in contact with the hospital once a week so that the optimal pain control, etc. can be continued.

13. Prognosis and End Results

S. G. Spiro

Non-Small Cell Lung Cancer

As detailed previously surgery offers the only major prospect of cure in non-small cell lung cancer. Of all patients presenting with this disease only 25% undergo thoracotomy following staging and, on average, about 5% of these subjects will still be unresectable despite a negative mediastinoscopy. This is almost always due to nodal involvement beyond the range of the mediastinoscope or tumor invading vital structures in the mediastinum. Thus about 20% of all patients will undergo a curative resection of which 4%–5% will be alive and tumor free at 5 years - a 25% 5-year survival rate overall for this selected group of resected patients (Fig. 1). The other 15% of patients will die of local or distant recurrence within 5 years. The overall 5-year survival figure of 20%–30% and 10-year survival of 16%–18% (there is a significant falloff between 5 and 10 years due to metastatic spread from slowly growing lung cancers) has not changed during the last 30 years. These figures can,

SELECTION FOR SURGERY IN NON-SMALL CELL LUNG CANCER

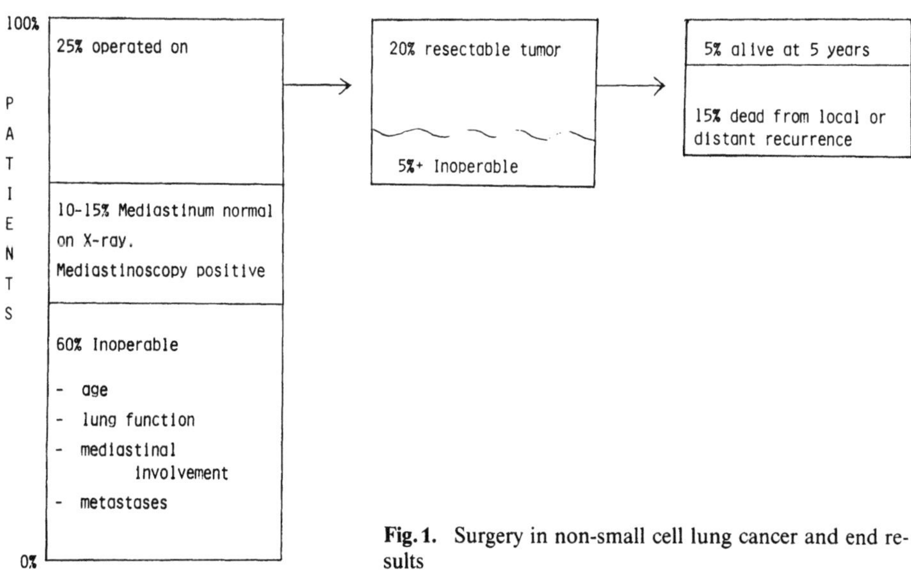

Fig. 1. Surgery in non-small cell lung cancer and end results

Table 1. Main staging categories of lung cancer with survival at 2 years (%). (Adapted from Mountain et al. 1974)

		Squamous	Adeno	Large cell	Small cell
Stage 1	T1 NO MO				
	T1 N MO	47	46	43	6
	T2 NO MO				
Stage 2	T2 N1 MO	40	14	13	5
Stage 3	T3 any N or M				
	N2 any T or M	11	8	13	3
	N1 any T or N				

Table 2. Survival in lung cancer (all cases). (Huhti et al. 1981)

Survival (%)	Squamous	Small cell	Adeno	Large cell
3 months	87	68	68	62
6 months	70	46	46	48
9 months	52	26	40	33
1 year	39	17	34	29
3 years	12	3	10	10

however, be somewhat misleading as they include 40%–50% of patients with stage I disease. In stage I disease the 2-year survival when staging was originally looked at by Mountain et al. in 1974 was 47% for squamous cell carcinoma (see Table 1).

Recent results have been much more encouraging for stage I disease, particularly for squamous cell carcinoma, and this is the result of more accurate staging and the exclusion of inoperable patients preoperatively. The 3-year natural history for survival in lung cancer is shown in Table 2. It is clear therefore that for stage I and II disease surgery confers a survival advantage, particularly for squamous cell carcinoma but perhaps only in stage I disease for adenocarcinoma. However, surgery is still recommended for stage II adenocarcinomas as these tumors are chemo- and radioinsensitive.

Natural History of Inoperable Disease

As previously discussed there is no convincing evidence that the decision to give radiotherapy to patients found to be inoperable with disease confined to the thorax confers any survival benefit upon them. Clearly if patients have symptoms which would be palliated by radiotherapy it should be given. As stated previously, there is no good evidence that postoperative radiotherapy confers survival advantage. It is of course often given in a fit patient, as one feels "one must do everything one can". However, the logic remains unproven (Table 3).

Table 3. Radiotherapy compared with "no treatment" (inoperable disease limited to one hemithorax). (Roswitt et al. 1968)

Cell type	Twelve-month survival			
	Radiotherapy		No treatment	
	No. assessed	% Surviving[a]	No. assessed	% Surviving
All	236	18	210	13
Epidermoid	98	23	76	13
Small cell	53	7	31	7
Adeno	25	18	31	10
Large cell	60	20	72	11

[a] There was no significant advantage for any of the cell types treated with radiotherapy

Table 4. Natural history of untreated small cell lung cancer. (Hyde et al. 1965)

	Survival in months from time of first symptoms	Survival in months from time of diagnosis
No. of cases	76	72
Mean	7.2	4.0
Median	6.0	2.8
% surviving at end of:		
3rd month	74%	39%
6th month	41%	10%
9th month	19%	4%
12th month	9%	4%
24th month	0%	0%

Chemotherapy has never convincingly been shown to add any survival benefit to patients with inoperable advanced non-small cell lung cancer. Of the many studies performed there are occasional patients who do surprisingly well on chemotherapy having obtained a good response but most of these studies are uncontrolled and therefore the natural growth rate of the responding tumor is not compared with that in an untreated patient.

We do not recommend cytotoxic chemotherapy for the prolongation of survival in non-small cell lung cancer. We do recommend that further controlled trials are carried out.

Small Cell Lung Cancer

The natural history of small cell lung cancer is extremely poor, with only 4% of patients surviving for 12 months from the time of diagnosis (Table 4). With effective chemotherapy, and where indicated additional radiotherapy, this percentage has risen to 40%–50%.

Further Reading

Huhti E, Sutinen S, Saloheimo M (1981) Survival among patients with lung cancer: an epidemiological study. Am Rev Respir Dis 124: 13-16
Hyde L, Yee J, Wilson R, Patno ME (1965) Cell type and the natural history of lung cancer. JAMA 193: 52
Martini N, Beatie EJ (1977) Results of surgical treatment in stage I lung cancer. J Thorac Cardiovasc Surg 74: 499-507
Mountain CR (1977) Assessment of the role of surgery for control of lung cancer. Am Thorax Surg 24: 365-373
Mountain CF, Carr DT, Anderson WAD (1974) A system for the clinical staging of lung cancer. Am J Roentgenol Radium Ther Nucl Med 120: 130-138
Roswitt B, Patno ME, Rapp R, Veinburgs A, Feder B, Stuhlbarg J, Reid CB (1968) The survival of patients with inoperable lung cancer: a large scale randomized study of radiation therapy versus placebo. Radiology 90: 688-697

Part II

Tumors of the Mediastinum,
Pleura, and Chest Wall

14. Pathology of Mediastinal Tumors

B. J. Addis

Precise localization of a mediastinal tumor often helps to narrow the differential diagnosis (Table 1, Fig. 1) and modern imaging techniques can provide much information regarding its likely nature. However, treatment and prognosis depend on an exact histological diagnosis and this is greatly facilitated by correct handling of adequate tissue samples.

Since the widespread adoption of immunohistochemistry routine fixation in formalin-based fixtures is no longer ideal. The intact, unfixed specimen should be delivered to the laboratory without delay and with accurate clinical information.

Table 1. The usual location of mediastinal tumors

Superior Mediastinum

    Thyroid and parathyroid tumors and hyperplasias

Anterior Mediastinum

    Thymic cysts and tumors
        Thymoma
        Thymic carcinoma
        Carcinoid
        Germ cell tumors
        Lymphomas
        Thymolipoma
        Sarcoma

Middle Mediastinum

    Bronchogenic and pericardial cysts

Posterior Mediastinum

    Neurogenic tumors
        Neurofibroma
        Schwannoma
        Malignant nerve sheath tumor
        Neuroblastoma
        Ganglioneuroblastoma
        Ganglioneuroma
        Paraganglioma

Middle, Anterior or Superior Mediastinum

    Lymphadenopathy
    Mediastinal fibrosis
    Sarcomas

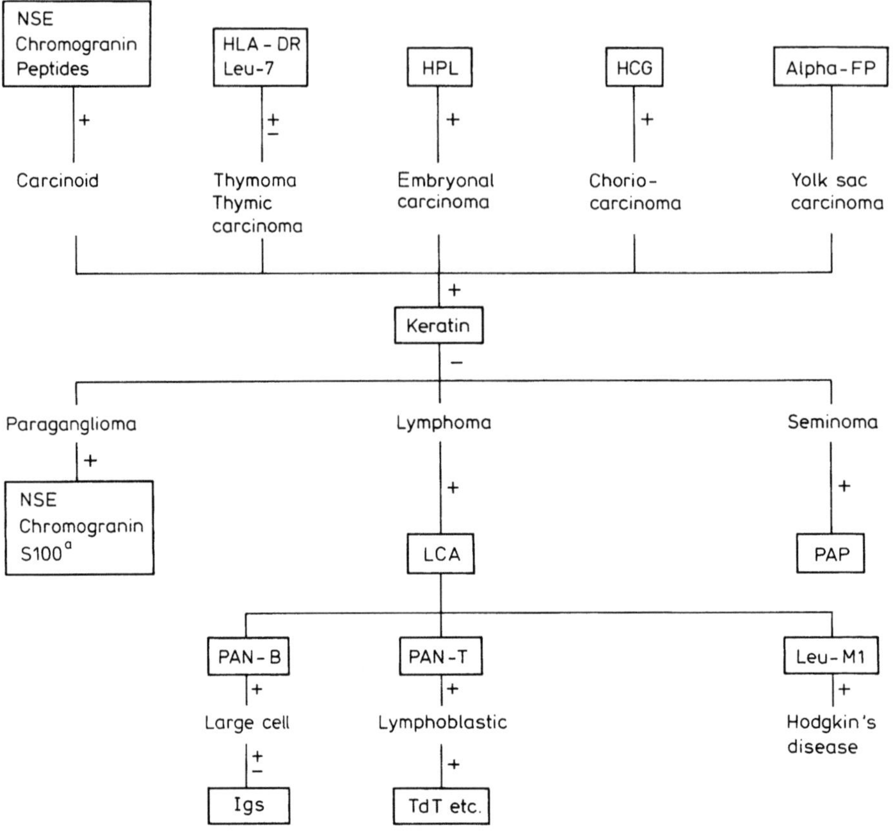

ᵃ supporting cells only

Fig. 1. A guide to the immunohistochemical diagnosis of anterior mediastinal tumors. *NSE*, neuron-specific enolase; *HPL*, human placental lactogen; *HCG*, beta subunit of human chorionic gonadotropin; *Alpha-FP*, alpha-fetoprotein; *PAP*, placental alkaline phosphatase; *TdT*, terminal deoxynucleotidyl transferase; *Igs*, immunoglobulins; *LCA*, leucocyte common antigen

This enables the pathologist to make imprints from the cut surface of the fresh tissue for cytological examination and to snap-freeze suitable blocks for immunohistochemistry and, in the case of lymphomas, gene rearrangement studies. Small representative samples, 1–2 mm in diameter, should be fixed immediately in glutaraldehyde or some other suitable fixative for electron microscopy. The remaining tissue can then be fixed for routine microscopy. Cytological diagnosis of mediastinal tumors, from material obtained by fine-needle aspiration, is not widely practised, although good results are reported from some centers [1].

Endocrine Tumors and Hyperplasias

Thyroid

Abnormalities in development and descent of the thyroid gland may lead to thyroid tissue that is either partially or completely intrathoracic. Usually it lies in the anterior or superior mediastinum, although other sites may be involved, and the appearances are usually those of nodular hyperplasia. The encapsulated mass consists of multiple nodules, of varying sizes, with a vascular, reddish-brown surface. The cut surface usually reveals areas of cyst formation or hemorrhage into nodules as well as solid, pinkish-brown, granular, gelatinous areas. Dense fibrosis and calcification are often present. Microscopically the nodules consist of colloid-filled acini, varying greatly in size and lined by cuboidal or flattened thyroid epithelium. Rarely, the appearances are those of primary thyrotoxicosis. Thyroiditis and tumors, both adenomas and carcinomas, have been described in intrathoracic thyroid tissue [2].

Parathyroid

The thymus and lower parathyroids have a common origin from the third pharyngeal pouch and it is not unusual to find parathyroid tissue associated with the thymus. Enlarged glands may migrate to the posterior mediastinum or hilar region [3]. Functioning intrathoracic parathyroid adenomas, or much less commonly carcinomas, are more likely to present as hyperparathyroidism than as a detectable mediastinal mass [3, 4]. An intrathoracic parathyroid may be involved in cases of hyperparathyroidism due to hyperplasia of all four glands.

Tumors of the Thymus

Thymic Hyperplasia

True Hyperplasia. In childhood a histologically normal, but abnormally large, thymus can simulate a mediastinal tumor. Massive thymic hyperplasia is rare and occasionally associated with peripheral lymphocytosis [5]. "Rebound" hyperplasia may follow cardiac surgery, burns, or malignant disease treated by radiotherapy or chemotherapy [6, 7]. This follows cessation of therapy and occurs during remission of the disease. A trial of steroids will cause shrinkage of the gland and help make the distinction from recurrent malignancy [6]. Retention of the normal lobular architecture, the clear division between cortex and medulla, and the presence of Hassall's corpuscles in the medulla are helpful features in making the important distinction between benign hyperplasia and thymoma, which has a poor prognosis in children.

Lymphoid Hyperplasia. Follicular hyperplasia of thymic lymphoid tissue is occasionally present in normal people but is more often associated with myasthenia gravis, the collagen-vascular diseases, or endocrine disorders, such as thyrotoxicosis. The thymus is rarely sufficiently enlarged to simulate a neoplasm but in patients with myasthenia there may be an associated thymoma. Hyperplastic follicles, with large germinal centers, are usually confined to the medulla with compression of normal medullary structures and a clearly defined cortex. They may arise in an extraparenchymal perivascular compartment [8].

Very rarely a diffuse type of B-lymphoid hyperplasia may produce a mediastinal mass. Germinal centers are less clearly defined than in follicular hyperplasia and the lymphoid infiltrate extends throughout cortex and medulla obscuring the normal architecture and leaving islands of epithelium with Hassall's corpuscles. The distinction from thymoma may be very difficult: the thymus is diffusely enlarged with preservation of Hassall's corpuscles and the B-cell nature of the infiltrate is a usual feature [9].

Cysts of the Thymus

Thymic cysts account for about 1% of all mediastinal masses and may be congenital, degenerative, or neoplastic in origin. Multiple small cysts – Dubois abscesses – were described in children with congenital syphilis but these are now extremely unusual. Degeneration and cystic change in Hassall's corpuscles is occasionally seen and cystic change may occur in thymomas and thymic Hodgkin's disease.

Most thymic cysts are of congenital or development origin, probably originating in third pharyngeal pouch remnants. The majority occur in the anterior or superior mediastinum but they may also arise in the neck along the line of descent of the thymus. They appear as smooth, round, or oval, thin-walled, multiloculated lesions, containing clear fluid or altered blood. The lining epithelium may be stratified squamous, cuboidal, or ciliated columnar in type. Focal calcification may be present and the origin of the cyst is indicated by the presence of islands of thymic tissue in the wall. In contrast to thymomas, this shows normal cortex and medulla with Hassall's corpuscles. Secondary changes may produce thickening and irregularity of the wall with increased fibrosis and cholesterol granulomas.

Thymoma

By current convention the term thymoma is restricted to tumors of thymic epithelium [8, 10]. Like the normal thymus, most tumors also contain a population of lymphocytes. These vary greatly in number and distribution and, although they contribute to tumor mass, are considered to be nonneoplastic.

Thymomas are the most frequent tumors of the anterior mediastinum, with an equal sex incidence. They increase in frequency with increasing age, being most common in the 5th and 6th decades with a mean age of 50 years, and are rare in children [11]. Occasional familial cases are recorded [12].

172

Sites. Most thymomas occur in the anterior and superior mediastinum but they may present in any site where normal thymic tissue is found, such as the neck [13], middle and posterior mediastinum, and lung parenchyma [14].

Gross Appearance. The majority of thymomas, about 75%, are well-circumscribed, encapsulated tumors. The cut surface typically shows irregular pinkish-tan colored nodules separated by white septa continuous with the capsule and which may be calcified. Compressed residual thymic tissue can sometimes be recognized outside the tumor capsule and cysts may develop in both tumor and residual thymus. Invasion of adjacent structures is associated with loss of encapsulation and a more uniform cut surface.

Microscopic Appearances. Most thymomas consist of a mixture of epithelial cells and lymphocytes, with the ratio of the two cell types varying between different tumors and between different areas of the same tumor (Figs. 2, 3). Epithelial cell nuclei have a diameter between two and four times that of a lymphocyte. They are oval and pale staining with small, eosinophilic nucleoli. The cytoplasm is pale and cell borders are often indistinct, particularly when large numbers of lymphocytes are present. Some variation in nuclear size is frequent and occasional mitoses may be seen. Cells may be dispersed, with lymphocytes filling intercellular spaces, or aggregated, with separate clusters of lymphocytes. Their morphology is often seen most clearly around vessels or along septa. Fully formed Hassall's corpuscles are rarely seen but ill-defined cellular whorls with evidence of keratinization are more often present. These may be related to areas of so-called medullary differentiation, which are paler staining due to fewer lymphocytes [10].

Epithelial cells may assume a spindle-cell morphology. This is frequently focal and associated with relative paucity of the lymphocyte population. Pure spindle-

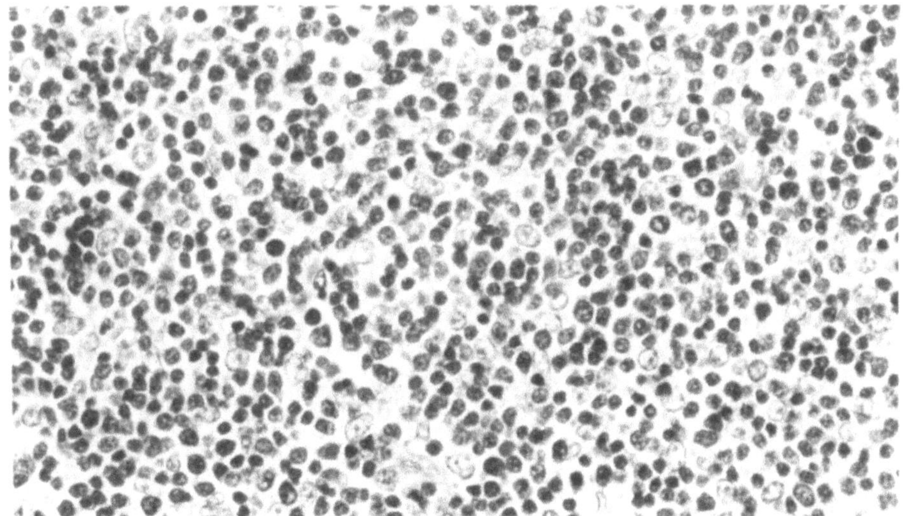

Fig. 2. Thymoma – two cell populations are present. Large numbers of lymphocytes surround thymic epithelial cells, which have larger, paler-staining nuclei

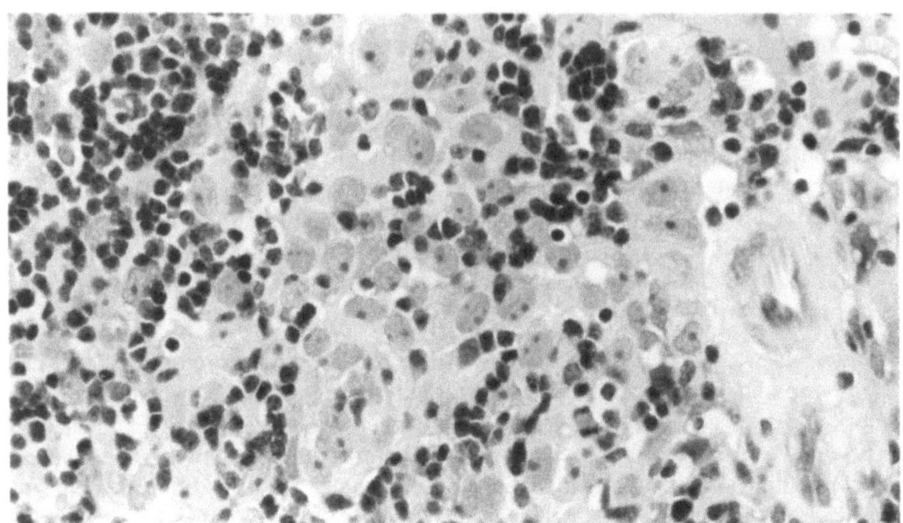

Fig.3. Thymoma – with fewer lymphocytes. Epithelial cells can be more clearly seen

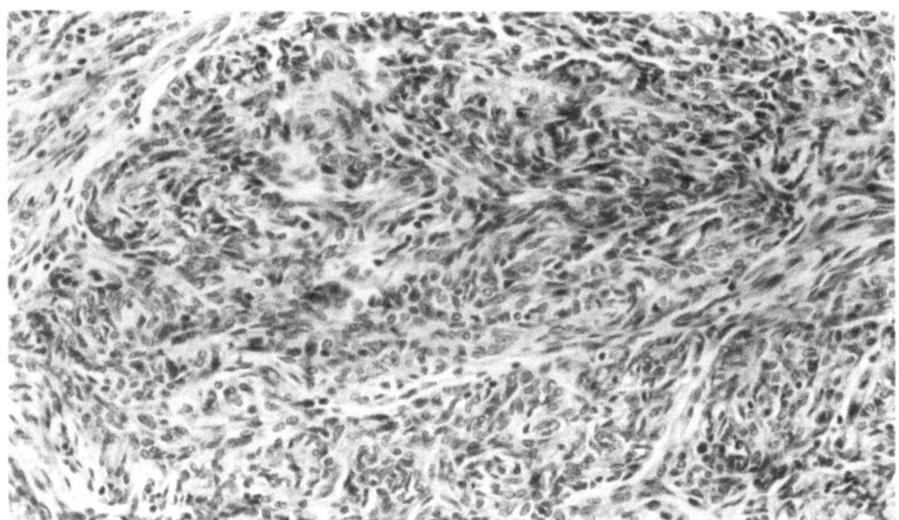

Fig.4. Spindle-cell thymoma – in spindle cell tumors lymphocytes are usually sparse

cell thymomas form a distinctive variant (Fig.4). A variety of other patterns may be seen, including rosette formation, papillary structures, and an appearance resembling hemangiopericytoma. Occasionally true glandular structures, lined by mucus-secreting or ciliated epithelium, are present and myoid cells have been described.

A very characteristic histological feature of thymomas is the presence of perivascular spaces, an exaggeration of those seen in the normal thymus. These are

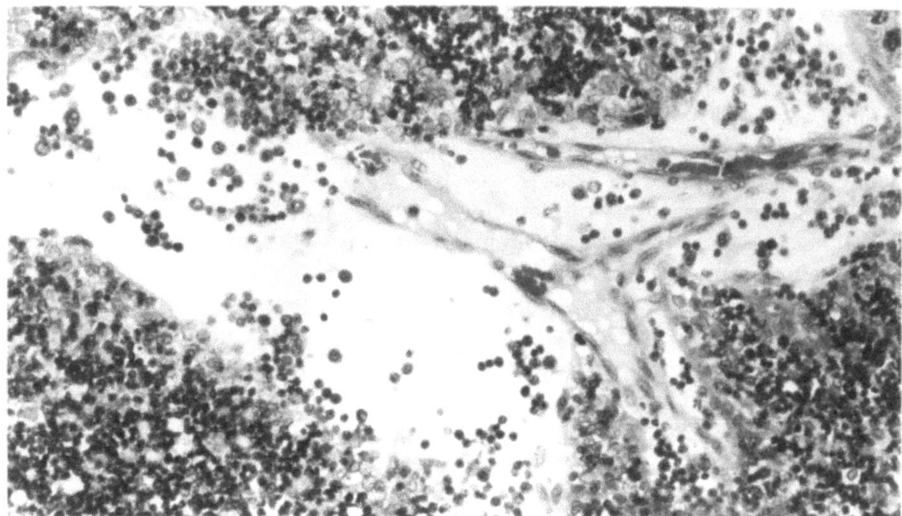

Fig. 5. Thymoma – perivascular space

formed between capillary basement membrane and epithelial basement membrane and contain scattered lymphocytes, plasma cells, and mast cells (Fig. 5). They may be obliterated by hyaline material or dilate to form cysts. Cysts can also result from hemorrhage or degeneration in a thymoma, when the contents may include cholesterol crystals and macrophages and a foreign body giant cell response may be present in the wall. Microscopic, epithelial-lined cysts, ducts, or tubules are a feature of some tumors, often related to the fibrous septa.

Most lymphoid cells in thymomas have the morphology of small lymphocytes but variation in size is common and mitoses are frequent. Benign histiocytes may be scattered throughout the tumor and the presence of phagocytized nuclear debris indicates a high turnover of thymocytes. Germinal centers are an unusual finding.

Ultrastructural Appearances. Electron microscopy shows a relationship between epithelial cells, lymphocytes, and vessels similar to that in the normal thymus. Lymphocytes lie between interdigitating cytoplasmic processes from epithelial cells. Frequent desmosomal attachments are present between processes, and variable numbers of cytoplasmic filaments form bundles near cell junctions. Epithelial cells are separated from perivascular spaces by a basal lamina [15].

Immunohistochemical Features. HLA-DR antigens, normally present on the majority of thymic reticular epithelial cells, are either undetectable or much reduced in thymomas [16, 17] (Fig. 1). Normal thymic epithelial cells also share the antigen p19 with the human T-cell leukemia virus. It is not detectable in invasive thymomas whereas in benign encapsulated tumors variable numbers of cells may express the antigen [17]. The Leu 7 (HNK-1) antigen is present on normal thymic epithelium and has a very variable expression in tumors [16]. Thymomas have a lymphoid population similar to that of the normal thymus [18, 19]. The majority of cells have the phenotype of cortical thymocytes: medullary thymocytes are reduced in number and the corticomedullary ratio is increased [19]. No preferential localization of different T-cell populations in different areas of tumors has been found.

Malignancy in Thymomas. There is no general agreement about the use of the term malignant thymoma. If tumors showing unequivocal histological evidence of malignancy are placed into the separate group of thymic carcinoma, the assessment of malignancy in the majority of thymomas is largely based on behavior. Malignant thymomas are those that spread within the thoracic cavity (invasive thymomas) or give rise to distant metastases.

The incidence of invasive thymoma varies greatly between different series [10, 20, 21]. Macroscopic evidence of invasion of mediastinal structures, pericardium, or lung parenchyma can be confirmed histologically, when intravascular invasion may also be seen. Dissemination may occur by implantation on pleural or pericardial surfaces, leading to recurrence some distance from the primary site. Distant metastases are rare and may occur by lymphatic or hematogenous routes. Sites include lymph nodes, liver, bone, kidney, spleen, central nervous system, and peripheral nerves.

Most authors conclude that the expected indicators of malignancy in thymomas correlate poorly with behavior but in some large series a high ratio of epithelial cells to lymphocytes is associated with invasiveness and a poor prognosis [20, 21].

Associated Diseases [22]. Thymomas may be associated with major abnormalities of the immune system, such as defective cell-mediated immunity with mucocutaneous candiasis, as well as a number of diseases, many of which have an immune basis. Two of the best-known associations are myasthenia gravis and pure red cell aplasia:

Myasthenia Gravis. Between 10% and 15% of patients with myasthenia gravis, particularly those in the older age group, have thymomas . Morphologically these do not differ from tumors in nonmyasthenic patients but, in contrast to patients with pure red cell aplasia, spindle-cell tumors are exceptional.

Pure Red Cell Aplasia (PRCA). Between 3% and 10% of patients with thymoma have PRCA and 30%–50% of patients with PRCA have a thymoma. These are usually of spindle-cell type, except when PRCA and myasthenia gravis coexist.

Thymic Carcinoma [23, 24]

Thymic carcinomas form a heterogeneous group of rare tumors. They are clearly malignant on cytological and histological grounds as distinct from thymomas, which are designated malignant according to their ability to invade or metastasize. Variants include:

Squamous Cell Carcinoma [25]

1. Keratinizing squamous cell carcinomas are similar to other squamous cell carcinomas and, in the better differentiated examples, keratin pearls may resemble

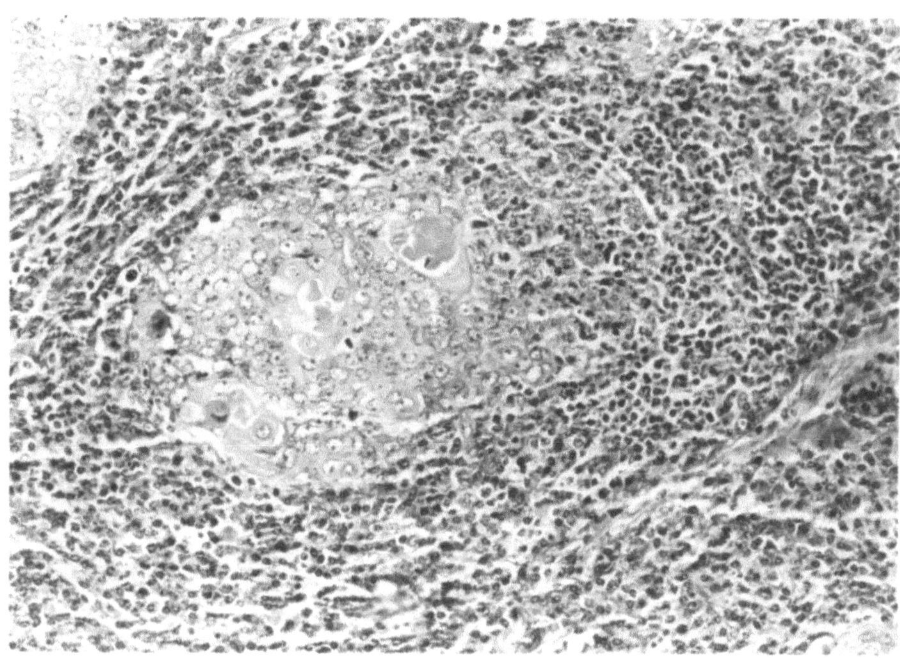

Fig. 6. Thymic carcinoma, squamous cell type – dense chronic inflammatory infiltrate surrounds islands of malignant cells, with foci of keratinization resembling Hassall's corpuscles

Hassall's corpuscles (Fig. 6). Some may be partially cystic and one example apparently originated in a benign cyst. Local invasion may be extensive.

2. Lymphoepithelioma-like poorly differentiated squamous cell carcinoma resembles poorly differentiated nasopharyngeal carcinomas and a link with Epstein-Barr Virus infection has been suggested [26]. Tumor cells have large nuclei and indistinct cytoplasmic borders with no evidence of keratinization. Mitoses are numerous and foci of necrosis are usually present. The variable lymphocytic infiltrate may make the distinction from malignant lymphoma and seminoma difficult.

3. Spindle-cell carcinoma is equivalent to similar tumors in the skin, lung, and elsewhere and results from a tendency shown by pleomorphic squamous cell carcinomas to assume a spindle-cell morphology. The appearance may be uniform throughout the tumor or focal (Fig. 7).

Sarcomatoid Carcinoma

In these tumors spindle or strap-like cells, with large bizarre hyperchromatic nuclei and abundant mitoses, form interlacing fascicles. Some probably represent a further degree of the spindle-cell change described above. Others are described in which malignant fusiform epithelial cells are combined with cells showing myoid differentiation [27, 28]. This may indicate a common origin for epithelial and myoid cells in the thymus.

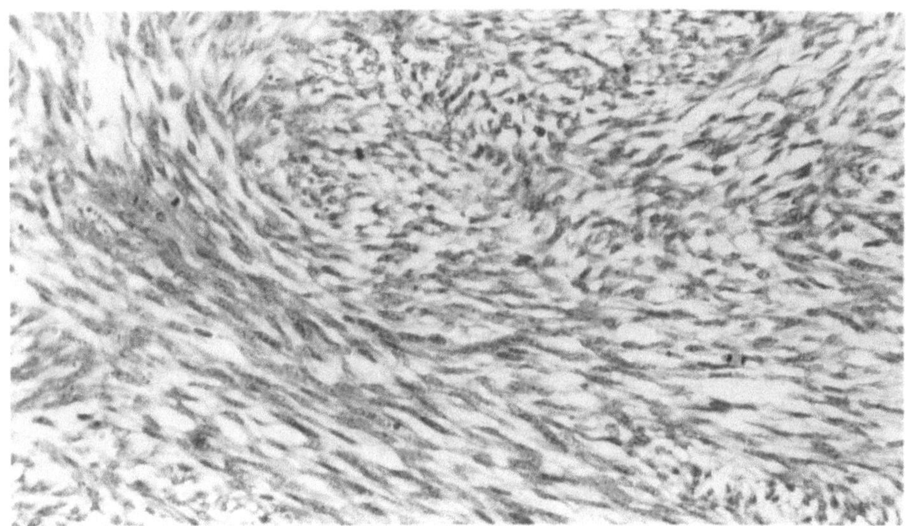

Fig. 7. Thymic carcinoma, spindle-cell type – other areas of the tumor were more clearly epithelial

Basaloid Carcinoma

The three published examples of this tumor were partially cystic, well-circumscribed, and covered by benign squamous epithelium, suggesting an origin in a preexisting thymic cyst. Histologically they resembled basaloid or basal cell tumors elsewhere, with well-defined islands of small uniform polygonal cells and peripheral palisading.

Clear Cell Carcinoma

Abundant clear cytoplasm with large quantities of glycogen give this tumor a distinctive histological appearance but whether it forms a separate entity or is a morphological variant of squamous cell carcinoma is uncertain.

Small Cell Undifferentiated Carcinoma [29, 30]

This may occur as a primary tumor of the thymus, either as a monomorphic tumor or combined with a carcinoid tumor or squamous cell carcinoma. Electron microscopy reveals small numbers of dense core neurosecretory granules.

Mucoepidermoid Carcinoma and Adenoid Cystic Carcinoma

One example of each of these tumors has been described. The morphology is identical to tumors of salivary gland or bronchial gland origin and they may arise in the glandular epithelium occasionally seen in the normal thymus.

Problems in the Diagnosis of Thymic Carcinoma

None of the histological variants of thymic carcinoma is peculiar to the thymus and the possibility that the mediastinal tumor is metastatic must be excluded. The presence of a well-circumscribed mediastinal mass and the absence of detectable tumor elsewhere are clearly important. Useful histological features include the presence of normal thymus around the tumor, coexistent typical thymoma, fibrous septa, a lymphoid infiltrate, and perivascular spaces.

Carcinoid Tumors [29, 31, 32]

Carcinoid tumors are neoplasms of the diffuse endocrine system. In the normal human thymus cells of this system are difficult to demonstrate, but they are present in the thymus of birds and animals and have staining properties similar to those shown by endocrine cells in the respiratory and gastrointestinal tracts.

Thymic carcinoids occur most frequently during middle age and show a strong male predominance. They may be clinically silent or compress mediastinal structures. Ectopic production of ACTH may lead to Cushing's syndrome [33] and thymic carcinoids occasionally form part of the type 1 multiple endocrine adenoma syndrome, associated with pancreatic and parathyroid tumors and hypercalcemia.

Although they appear well circumscribed, thymic carcinoids lack a capsule and infiltration of surrounding structures often makes surgical removal difficult. The cut surface is uniformly pinkish-tan colored with small foci of necrosis, calcification, and hemorrhage.

The histological features are similar to carcinoid tumors elsewhere. In typical areas, cells are of uniform size with moderate granular eosinophilic cytoplasm, finely dispersed nuclear chromatin, and small inconspicuous nucleoli. They form cellular nests, ribbons, and cords with a delicate richly vascular stroma. Rosette formation or a cribriform pattern may be present and some tumors are composed of spindle cells [24]. Rarely the stroma may be more abundant with separation of cell groups by fibrous tissue. Pigmentation may be due to the presence of lipofuscin or melanin [34]. In contrast to lung carcinoids, the majority of thymic tumors have atypical features, such as significant numbers of mitoses, nuclear pleomorphism, and areas of necrosis, which may calcify (Fig. 8). These features correlate with clinical behavior: local recurrence is common and metastases develop in the majority of patients. Mediastinal node involvement may be followed by widespread distant metastases, including sclerotic bone deposits.

The distinction between carcinoid tumors and thymic epithelial tumors may be difficult, particularly if the pattern is unusual, as in spindle-cell variants, or the biopsy is small and crushed. The argentaffin reaction, regarded as being specific for amines such as 5-hydroxytryptamine (serotonin), is insensitive and invariably negative in thymic carcinoid. The chemical basis of arygrophil staining is poorly understood but it provides useful empirical confirmation of the endocrine nature of typical tumors and most thymic carcinoids contain positive cells. Electron microscopy confirms the presence of numerous dense-core neurosecretory granules.

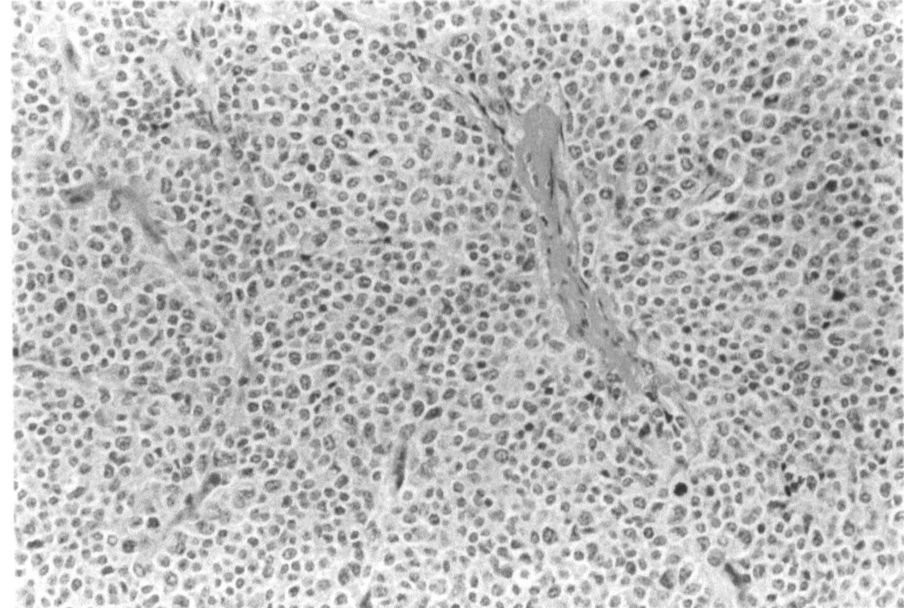

Fig. 8. Thymic carcinoid tumor – cells show atypical features with mitoses and nuclear pleomorphism

Immunohistochemistry may be used to show the endocrine nature of the tumor and to identify amines and peptide hormones. Antibodies to neuron-specific enolase (NSE), PGP 9.5 and chromogranin, a component of the protein matrix of the secretory granules, are valuable in recognizing endocrine tumors (Fig. 1). Hormones identified in thymic carcinoids include ACTH and somatostatin.

Germ Cell Tumors [35, 36]

The occurrence of extragonadal germ cell tumors in the mediastinum and other midline sites such as the pineal region, retroperitoneum, and sacrococcygeal region, is usually explained by misplacement of totipotential cells during the very early stages of embryogenesis or incomplete or misdirected migration of germ cells in the embryo. Between 1% and 5% of all germ cell malignancies occur in the mediastinum, where they constitute 2%–3% of tumors. They arise within, or in close proximity to, the thymus and thymic tissue is frequently intermixed. The possibility of metastasis from a testicular lesion must be excluded but, provided the testes are clinically normal and retroperitoneal nodes are uninvolved, this is unlikely. An association between malignant germ cell tumors of the mediastinum and acute leukemia has been established [37].

The range of tumors is similar to that seen in the gonads:

180

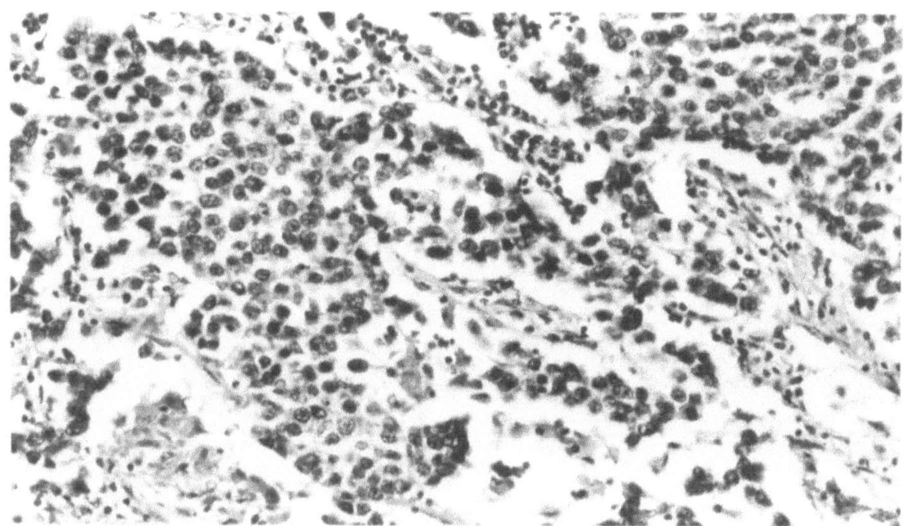

Fig. 9. Seminoma – groups of tumor cells are separated by stroma with a variable infiltrate of lymphocytes and plasma cells

Seminoma [38]

These constitute about 50% of mediastinal germ cell tumors and occur almost exclusively in males with a mean age of 30 years. They are soft, tan-colored tumors with histological appearances identical to the corresponding tumors of the testis and ovary (dysgerminoma). The large cells have uniform, oval, irregular nuclei, prominent nucleoli, and moderate amounts of clear cytoplasm, which contains glycogen. Groups of tumor cells are separated by bands of stromal connective tissue with a variable lymphocyte and plasma cell infiltrate (Fig. 9). Epithelioid granulomata are frequently seen and have no prognostic value but, if present in large numbers, may suggest sarcoidosis. Anaplastic variants are described.

Nonseminomatous Malignant Germ Cell Tumors

These occur exclusively in young males with an average age of 24–26 years. Pure tumors are embryonal carcinoma, yolk sac carcinoma, or choriocarcinoma but these elements are frequently mixed, with each other, with seminoma, or with benign elements (teratocarcinoma). Adequate sampling of a tumor is therefore of great importance.

1. Embryonal carcinoma consists of large, polygonal, pleomorphic cells with vesicular nuclei, prominent nucleoli, and frequent, often atypical, mitoses. Cells may form sheets or tubulopapillary epithelial structures. Extensive necrosis is often present.

2. Yolk sac carcinoma (endodermal sinus tumor) shows a variety of histological patterns. Typically, vacuolated cells form a loose microcystic or glandular pattern with papillary structures (Fig. 10). Mucin production is variable. Two useful features are the formation of cellular rosettes around small vessels, the so-called

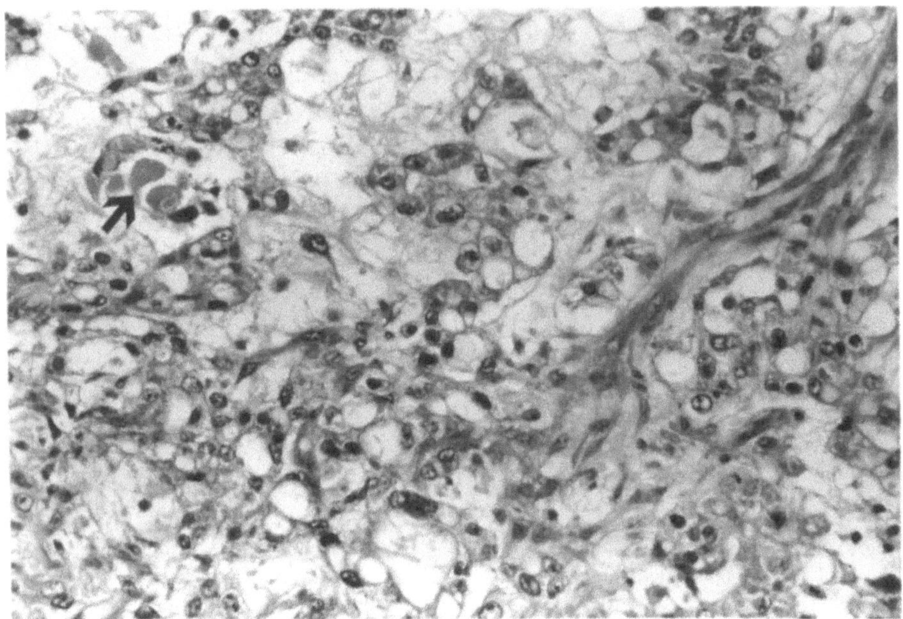

Fig. 10. Yolk sac carcinoma – cells form a delicate lace-like glandular pattern with deposits of eosinophilic material *(arrow)*

Schiller-Duval bodies, and deposition of extracellular eosinophilic material as spherical bodies. Yolk-sac differentiation is associated with the production of alpha-fetoprotein, demonstrable in the tumor by immunohistochemical methods or detectable in the serum.

3. Choriocarcinoma [39] – Pure choriocarcinomas are usually extensively hemorrhagic with only small areas of viable tumor. Both syncytiotrophoblast and cytotrophoblast should be identifiable and in the former the beta subunit of human chorionic gonadotrophin (beta-HCG) can be demonstrated. Serum levels of beta-HCG may be elevated and 50% of patients develop gynecomestia.

Immature Teratoma [40]

Tumors consisting of immature elements from all three germinal layers may contain embryonic mesenchyme, neuroectoderm, and blastema (Fig. 11). In children these behave in a benign fashion but in older patients similar tumors are likely to contain frankly malignant elements.

Immunohistochemical techniques are invaluable in the investigation of germ cell tumors (Fig. 1). Small foci of yolk sac carcinoma or choriocarcinoma, not recognizable by conventional staining techniques, may be identified with antibodies to alpha-fetoprotein and beta-HCG respectively. Single multinucleate cells staining for beta-HCG may be identified in otherwise typical seminomas and these do not significantly alter the prognosis. Embryonal carcinoma, yolk sac carcinoma, and syncytiotrophoblast all express keratin intermediate filaments. Seminoma

182

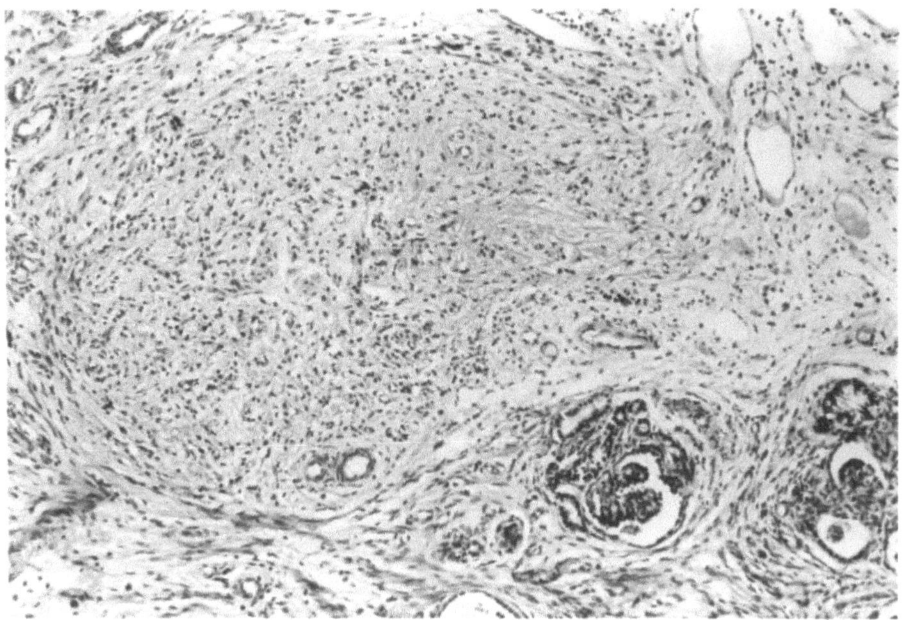

Fig. 11. Immature mediastinal teratoma – this tumor included immature renal tissue with glomeruli and neuroectodermal tissue

cells show variable staining for placental alkaline phosphatase and human placental lactogen is often present in embryonal carcinoma.

Benign Mature Mediastinal Teratoma ("Dermoid Cyst") [36]

Unlike malignant germ cell tumors, benign teratomas in the mediastinum show an equal sex incidence. They may be seen at any age but the majority occur between 10 and 40 years.

Pressure on adjacent structures may lead to wheezing or dysphagia and involvement of the pericardium may be fatal, but most are asymptomatic and the presence of calcification or bone aids their detection on chest X-ray. They are usually multicystic and encapsulated and the cysts contain thin fluid, mucus, or sebaceous material and hair. Skin and skin appendages are invariably prominent histologically and bronchial components, including mucosa, mucous glands, smooth muscle, and cartilage, are frequently present (Fig. 12). Eosinophils and mast cells may be seen in the bronchial mucosa. Bone may be formed in the connective tissue and glandular spaces may be lined by simple intestinal epithelium. Less frequently, neural tissue, including ependyma and ganglia, is seen. Teeth and thyroid tissue, often prominent in ovarian teratomas, are unusual. Pancreatic tissue is frequently present with islets of fetal type, containing relatively large numbers of somatostatin-producing D cells [41].

Infection of the cyst contents may occur, either by blood-borne organisms or due to communication with an airway. Leakage of cyst contents, which may in-

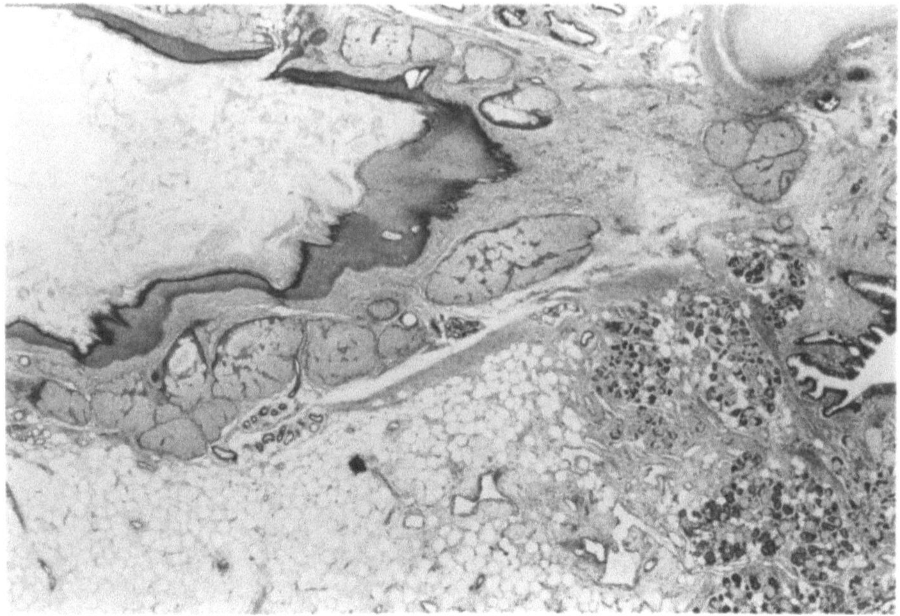

Fig. 12. Mature teratoma – *on the left* skin and skin appendages, including sebaceous glands, surround a lumen. *On the right* bronchial epithelium, glands, and cartilage are seen

clude digestive enzymes from exocrine pancreas, results in inflammation and necrosis of adjacent structures and fistula formation. Rare cases of intrapulmonary teratoma containing normal thymic tissue suggest an origin in aberrant thymus [42].

Thymolipoma

Thymolipomas are rare, benign lesions that account for 2%–9% of all thymic tumors. They may occur at any age but are most frequent in young adults with a mean age of 22 years. Many attain large size, occasionally up to several kilograms, without causing symptoms, but others compress mediastinal structures. Associated diseases include myasthenia gravis [43], thyrotoxicosis, aplastic anemia, and Hodgkin's disease [44].

The thymus is diffusely enlarged with preservation of its original bilobed shape and thin capsule. The tumors are soft in consistency and resemble normal adipose tissue with barely discernible strands of white tissue. Microscopically, normal thymic tissue, with preservation of cortex, medulla, and Hassall's corpuscles, is dispersed in mature adipose tissue (Fig. 13).

Although it constitutes only 5%–10% of the tumor bulk, thymic parenchyma is significantly increased in mass and these tumors are unlikely to represent simply thymic involvement by a benign lipoma. Other explanations include massive thymic hyperplasia with subsequent involution and a hamartomatous origin.

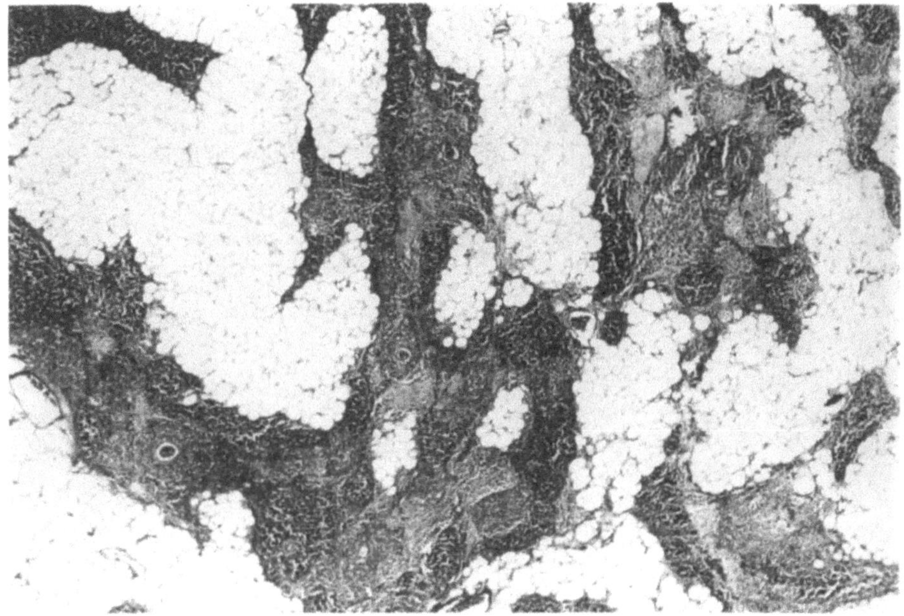

Fig. 13. Thymolipoma – fat separates strands of thymic tissue

Sarcomas of the Thymus

Malignant connective tissue tumors of the thymus are extremely rare and must be distinguished from spindle-cell tumors of thymic epithelium. Both types described have been the subject of single case reports.

Rhabdoid Sarcoma [45]

This tumor, called a malignant histiocytoma by the authors, resembles the rhabdoid sarcoma of the kidney seen in infants but its histogenesis is uncertain. The large polygonal or spindle-shaped tumor cells contain paranuclear, eosinophilic cytoplasmic bodies, consisting ultrastructurally of a meshwork of filaments.

Thymic Liposarcoma [46]

A pleomorphic liposarcoma intimately mixed with histologically normal thymic tissue has been described and may represent a malignant counterpart of benign thymolipoma.

Malignant Lymphomas of the Thymus

Hodgkin's Disease [47, 48]

Hodgkin's disease is limited to the mediastinum in 10% of patients and in half of these it is confined to the thymus. This is more common in young females in the

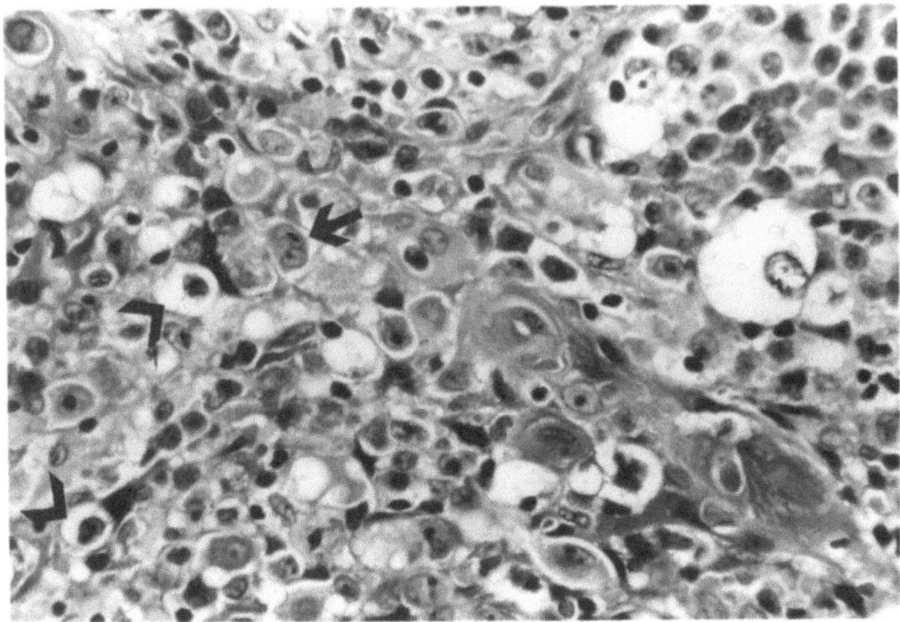

Fig. 14. Thymic Hodgkin's disease – the population of atypical cells includes a Reed-Sternberg cell *(arrow)* and several lacunar cells *(arrowheads)*. A central island of residual thymic epithelium is present

2nd and 3rd decades and is often asymptomatic. Staging procedures usually fail to show evidence of extrathoracic disease. Part of the thymus is replaced by a nodular, well-circumscribed, firm mass and examination of the cut surface shows fibrous septa separating softer nodules. One or more cysts are frequently present, and when a cyst forms the bulk of the lesion careful sampling of the wall may be necessary to determine the underlying pathology. Persistence of the mediastinal mass following therapy may be due to a residual cyst [49].

The microscopic appearances are those of nodular sclerosing Hodgkin's disease, with bands of collagenized connective tissue separating cellular nodules. These contain lymphocytes, histiocytes, plasma cells, neutrophils, eosinophils, and Hodgkin's cells in varying proportions. Lacunar cells are usually prominent but diagnostic Reed-Sternberg cells may be difficult to find. Irregular islands of thymic epithelium are mixed with the Hodgkin's infiltrate (Fig. 14). The cysts may be lined by flattened squamous epithelium or columnar epithelium, which may be ciliated or mucus-secreting. The histological appearances led to the earlier misleading terms "granulomatous thymitis" or "granulomatous thymoma."

Lymphoblastic Lymphoma

Lymphoblastic lymphoma may occur at any age but is commonest in adolescence, accounting for about one-third of cases of childhood non-Hodgkin's lymphoma. About 70% of cases are of T-cell origin (the others being of pre-B-cell type) and are often associated with a thymic mass, the so-called Sternberg sarcoma [50]. In-

186

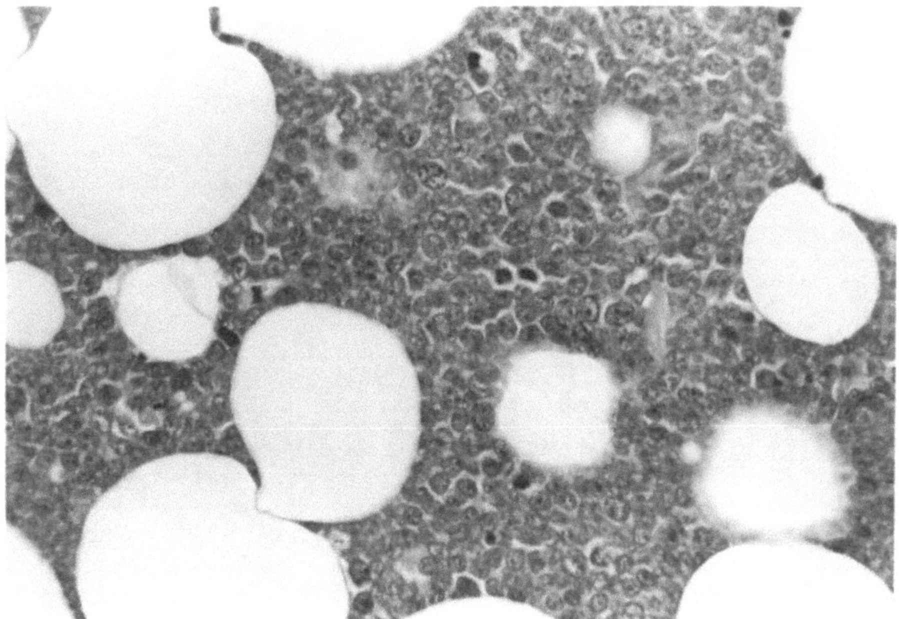

Fig. 15. Lymphoblastic lymphoma – fat is infiltrated by a uniform population of medium-sized lymphoid cells. Nuclear folds are not easily seen in routine sections

volvement of bone marrow and peripheral blood gives rise to a form of acute lymphoblastic leukemia. Lymph nodes may be enlarged due to expansion of the T-cell zone and CSF involvement is frequent.

Tissue from the anterior mediastinal mass is soft and uniformly gray in color. The histological picture is one of sheets of rather uniform, small lymphoid cells with minimal cytoplasm, finely dispersed chromatin, inconspicuous nucleoli, and frequent mitoses (Fig. 15). The presence of scattered benign macrophages gives the so-called "starry-sky" appearance. The cells may show deep nuclear folding giving a convoluted appearance. This is best appreciated on imprint preparations but is not always a feature and the term convoluted T-cell lymphoma may be inappropriate [51]. In the majority of cases the neoplastic cells contain intranuclear terminal deoxynucleotidyl transferase (TdT) but are heterogeneous with regard to cell-surface antigens, sharing markers with cortical thymocytes and reflecting the stages of T-cell intrathymic differentiation [52].

Large Cell Lymphoma with Sclerosis [53, 54, 55]

Another form of non-Hodgkin's lymphoma of probable thymic origin is of large cell type. Patients are usually in their 3rd or 4th decades and there may be some female predominance. Presenting symptoms are due to an anterior mediastinal mass with infiltration of mediastinal structures, lung, and anterior chest wall. Extrathoracic spread is usually to viscera, such as kidney, liver, thyroid, or ovary and involvement of lymph nodes or bone marrow is unusual.

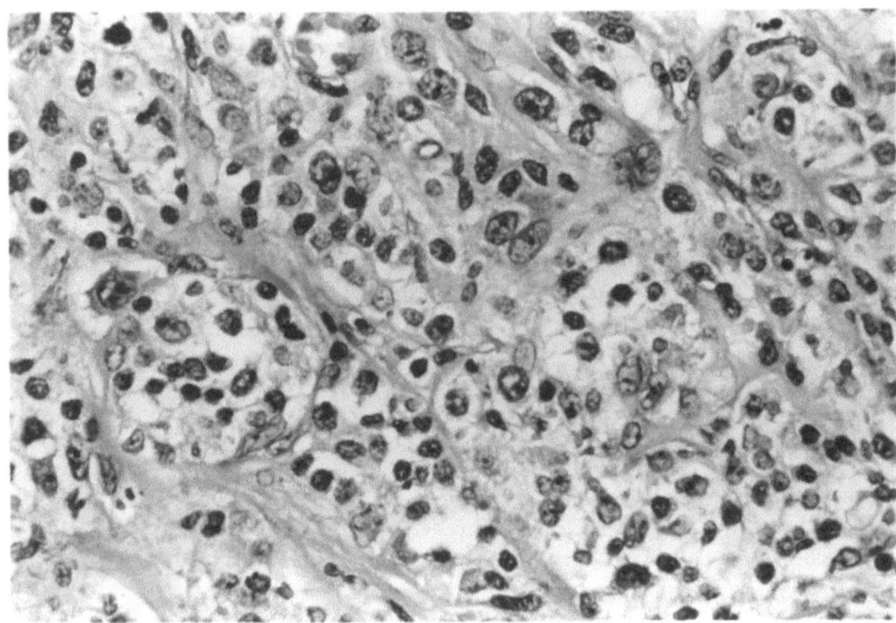

Fig. 16. Large cell lymphoma with sclerosis - groups of tumor cells are segregated by connective tissue

Grossly the tumor is an irregular mass of gray-tan colored tissue, varying in consistency according to the degree of fibrosis. Thymic tissue may be present within or around the tumor. The neoplastic cells have the general morphology of centroblasts or large centrocytes but may show exaggerated nuclear folding or lobation, mimicking Reed-Sternberg cells. Stromal fibrosis, with separation of groups of cells into compartments or cords, is characteristic and may simulate an epithelial malignancy (Fig. 16). Variable numbers of reactive small lymphocytes and eosinophils may be present. Immunohistochemistry demonstrates the B-cell origin of the neoplastic cells in most cases.

Histiocytosis-X of the Thymus [56]

Interdigitating reticulum cells or T-zone histiocytes, sharing the same markers as epidermal Langerhans cells but lacking the characteristic Birbeck granules, are present in the normal thymus. Nevertheless, thymic involvement by histiocytosis X is extremely rare. It is an occasional cause of an anterior mediastinal mass in childhood and the histological features are characteristic with an infiltrate of Langerhans cells, variable numbers of eosinophils, fibrosis, and residual thymic tissue.

Tumors of Neural Origin [57, 58]

Neural tumors in the mediastinum can be divided into tumors of nerve sheath origin, arising from intercostal nerves or occasionally the vagus nerve [59], and tumors of the autonomic nervous system. Multiple peripheral nerve tumors may be accompanied by other features of neurofibromatosis.

Tumors of Nerve Sheath Origin

Benign

These form 75% of tumors of the posterior mediastinum in adults. They are slowly growing tumors that present in the 3rd and 4th decades. Two types are described but a clear distinction is frequently difficult to make:

1. Neurilemomas (Schwannomas) are of Schwann cell origin and occur as round or fusiform swellings located on nerves. The cut surface is white or pale yellow and soft in consistency, often with calcification or cystic change. Nerve fibers are present in the capsule, which is continuous with the epineurium, but not within the tumor. Two types of tissue are described and these are mixed in varying proportions. In the cellular Antoni A areas, spindle cells form closely packed intersecting bundles and their nuclei show a tendency to arrange themselves in parallel rows or palisades to form the so-called Verocay bodies. Antoni B tissue consists of loose, myxoid connective tissue stroma with groups of foamy macrophages and cystic spaces. Degenerate areas in so-called "ancient" Schwannomas may contain large, irregular, hyperchromatic nuclei and thrombosed, thick-walled hyaline vessels (Fig. 17).

2. Neurofibromas arise from perineural and endoneural fibroblasts as well as Schwann cells. When they involve large nerves they are often fusiform and appear encapsulated as the nerve is expanded around them. A true capsule is lacking and the cut surface is more uniform than a Schwannoma, often with a soft mucoid consistency. Neurofibromas are loosely cellular with spindle cells having small elongated wavy nuclei and no particular pattern of organization. Nerve fibers are scattered throughout the stroma and mast cells are present in variable numbers. Glandular epithelial structures are occasionally seen and both neurilemomas and neurofibromas may contain melanin.

Plexiform neurofibromas occur in neurofibromatosis as irregular thickenings of peripheral or autonomic nerves. Nerve fibers are enlarged and separated by a loose stroma containing Schwann cells and fibroblasts.

Malignant

Most malignant nerve sheath tumors (neurofibrosarcomas, malignant Schwannomas) develop in patients with neurofibromatosis. They are commoner in males, with a mean age of 28 years, and some arise in preexisting benign neurofibromas. Malignant change in a neurilemoma is thought to be rare. In patients without neurofibromatosis malignant nerve sheath tumors occur a decade or so later and,

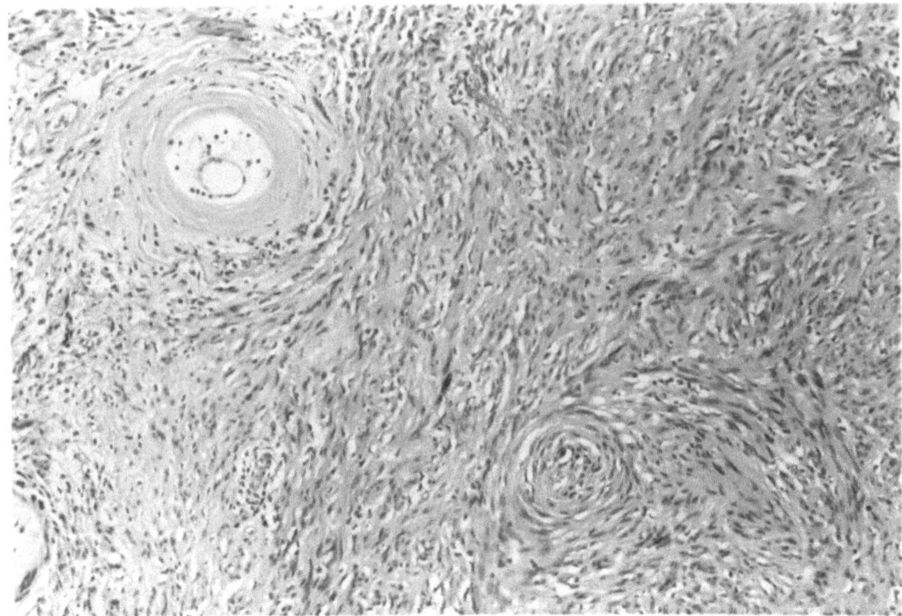

Fig. 17. Schwannoma (neurilemoma) – cellular whorls and a vessel with thick hyaline walls in an Antoni A area

without evidence of a preexisting benign tumor or origin from a peripheral nerve, may be difficult to characterize on histological grounds alone. Like their benign counterparts, they are most frequent in the posterior mediastinum but may also occur in the anterior compartment.

The histological pattern is often indeterminate with interlacing fascicles of malignant spindle cells and variable collagen deposition. A neural origin may be indicated by irregular wavy nuclei, nuclear palisading, and the presence of whorled structures, reminiscent of tactile corpuscles. Heterologous elements such as cartilage and bone are occasionally seen. S-100 protein is a useful marker of Schwann cells in benign and malignant nerve sheath tumors [60].

Tumors of the Autonomic Nervous System

Tumors arising in the posterior mediastinum from autonomic ganglia show a complete spectrum of differentiation from malignant undifferentiated tumors of sympathetic precursor cells (neuroblasts) to benign tumors of fully differentiated ganglion cells.

Neuroblastoma [61]

This is one of the commonest tumors of early childhood. Most occur between birth and 5 years of age and only 10% present after the age of 10 years. Occasional adult cases occur and there is a slight male predominance. The adrenal medulla is the most common site but about 16% occur in the mediastinum.

Symptoms are due to compression of mediastinal structures and occasionally the spinal cord is involved. Hypertension may be present due to catecholamine secretion and metabolites, such as vanillylmandelic acid (VMA) and homovanillic acid (HVA), are excreted in the urine in 80% of patients. Intractable diarrhea may be due to secretion of vasoactive intestinal polypeptide (VIP) by differentiating tumors.

Tumors are usually large and appear encapsulated. The surface is uniformly soft and gray with hemorrhagic areas. Undifferentiated tumors consist of uniform, small cells with scanty cytoplasm. Nuclei are round or oval and hyperchromatic with dispersed granular chromatin and inconspicuous nucleoli. Tumor cells may be aggregated into ill-defined lobules. In better-differentiated tumors rosette formation is seen, with tangled neural processes at the center of small nests of cells, and the stroma contains abundant neurofibrillary material. Glycogen is present in many tumors but this does not generally show the block positivity of Ewing's sarcoma. Staining for neuron-specific enolase is positive [62] and monoclonal antibodies specific for neuroblastoma have been described [63]. Electron microscopy shows dense-core neurosecretory granules and a mesh of interdigitating neural processes. Neuroblastomas metastasize to bone marrow, liver, and lymph nodes but mediastinal tumors may have a better prognosis than adrenal tumors and share a tendency to spontaneous regression or maturation.

Melanin may be present in neuroblastomas and a related but benign tumor of neural crest origin is the melanotic progonoma or pigmented neuroectodermal tumor of infancy, an example of which has been described in the mediastinum [64].

Ganglioneuroblastoma [65]

Maturation of neuroblastoma cells to ganglion cells is indicated by increase in size with more abundant cytoplasm, increased nuclear vesiculation, and prominent nucleoli. If significant numbers of cells show maturation the tumor is known as a ganglioneuroblastoma.

Two patterns are described: the composite type, which is ganglioneuromatous with foci of pure neuroblastoma, and the diffuse type, in which undifferentiated and differentiating neuroblastoma cells are intimately mixed with immature bizarre ganglion cells. The prognosis is most favorable for the diffuse type and for children under the age of 3. Single cases are recorded of anterior mediastinal neuroblastoma and ganglioneuroblastoma, both in adults [66, 67].

Ganglioneuroma

Benign ganglioneuromas occur in older children and young adults and are uncommon under the age of 2. Occasionally they can be shown to result from maturation of a neuroblastoma. They are large, encapsulated tumors with a firm white or pale yellow surface. Calcification is frequent and cystic degeneration may occur. Adjacent structures may be surrounded but without infiltration.

The histological appearances mimic a normal ganglion with bundles of nerve fibers with Schwann cell sheaths and ganglion cells scattered singly or in clusters

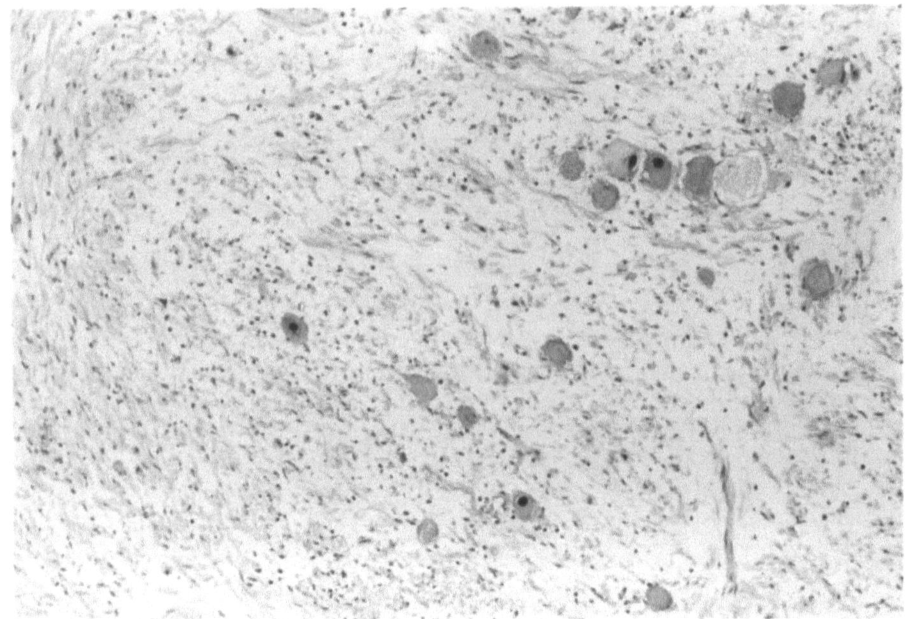

Fig. 18. Ganglioneuroma – ganglion cells are scattered in a loose stroma containing nerve fibers and Schwann cells

(Fig. 18). Satellite cells are usually absent or sparse. Ganglion cells show abnormal variation in size and shape and may contain multiple nuclei. Associated malignant mesenchymal tumors are described and every ganglioneuroma should be thoroughly sampled to exclude foci of neuroblastoma.

Paragangliomas [58]

Paragangliomas may arise in the anterior mediastinum from the parasympathetic aorticopulmonary bodies [68, 69] or in the posterior mediastinum from the sympathetic chain [70].

The aortic or aorticopulmonary bodies have a chemoreceptor function and occur anterolateral to the aortic arch, lateral to the innominate artery in the angle between the ductus arteriosus and descending aorta and on the upper right main pulmonary artery. Tumors have an equal age incidence and occur after the age of 40. They appear as pink, vascular, hemorrhagic lesions with a spongy consistency and consist of nests or balls of cells *(Zellballen)* surrounded by the thin-walled sinusoidal blood vessels of the richly vascular stroma. The chief cells are usually large with round or oval nuclei, inconspicuous nucleoli, and fairly abundant clear or eosinophilic granular cytoplasm. Around the periphery of the cell groups lie inconspicuous spindle cells, the supporting or sustentacular cells (Fig. 19).

The chief cells are argyrophilic and electron microscopy shows dense-core neurosecretory granules. They also stain with antibodies to neuron-specific enolase (NSE) and chromogranin. Antibody to S100-protein stains the supporting

192

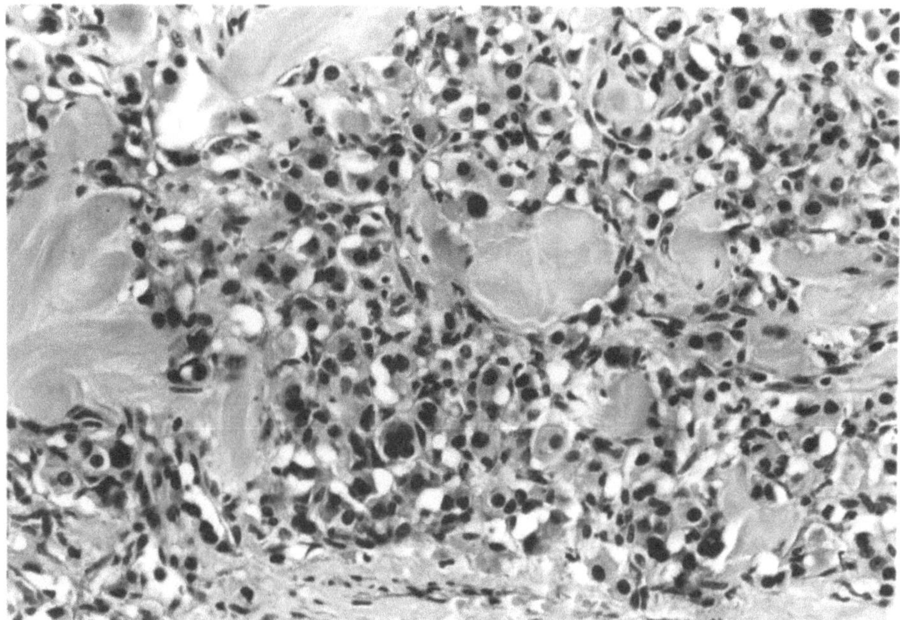

Fig. 19. Paraganglioma – each small nest of chief cells is surrounded by flattened sustentacular cells. A moderate degree of pleomorphism is present

cells, which may be of Schwann cell origin. Unlike thymic carcinoid tumors, keratin intermediate filaments are not expressed by paragangliomas.

Paragangliomas arising in the costovertebral sulcus from residual extraadrenal chromaffin tissue related to the sympathetic chain are far less common and occur in a somewhat younger age group. About half are functional, producing symptoms due to noradrenaline release [71, 72]. The histological features may be identical to other paragangliomas or may closely resemble adrenal pheochromocytomas, with large pleomorphic nuclei, irregular cell outlines, and granular basophilic cytoplasm.

The usual indicators of malignancy, such as nuclear pleomorphism, mitotic rate and even vascular invasion, are considered unreliable in paragangliomas and their behavior is difficult to predict. Although most appear encapsulated, local recurrence is frequent and about 10% metastasize via the bloodstream to lungs and bone.

Mediastinal Lymphadenopathy and Related Disorders

Enlargement of mediastinal lymph nodes may be due to a number of neoplastic or inflammatory conditions. In some, such as infectious mononucleosis or angioimmunoblastic lymphadenopathy, the mediastinal node enlargement forms part of generalized lymphadenopathy. Conditions that may involve mediastinal nodes preferentially are granulomatous inflammation, metastatic carcinoma, malignant lymphoma, and angiofollicular lymph node hyperplasia.

Granulomatous Inflammation

Tuberculosis, fungal infections, and sarcoidosis all commonly involve mediastinal and hilar nodes and granulomas may be found in nodes draining a tumor in the absence of metastases. Granulomas may also be found in association with Hodgkin's disease and non-Hodgkin's lymphomas, both in involved and uninvolved nodes. The appearances closely resemble sarcoidosis and careful examination of residual lymphoid tissue is essential.

Metastatic Carcinoma

This is a common cause of mediastinal lymphadenopathy and superior vena cava compression. The primary tumor is most often in the lung and frequency of spread to mediastinal nodes varies according to tumor type and differentiation. Small cell carcinoma frequently produces early mediastinal involvement. Spread to mediastinal nodes also occurs from carcinoma of the esophagus. Unsuspected primary tumors that may present as mediastinal metastases include breast carcinoma, nasopharyngeal carcinoma, renal carcinoma, and malignant melanoma. Confusion with thymic carcinoma may arise if the primary site cannot be identified.

Malignant Lymphoma

Hodgkin's Disease [47, 48]

The nodular sclerosis variant of Hodgkin's disease shows a particular predilection for the mediastinum, involving either the thymus or lymph nodes or both. Involvement by the other variants usually indicates more widely disseminated disease.

Non-Hodgkin's Lymphoma

Involvement of mediastinal or hilar nodes occurs in 15%–25% of patients with non-Hodgkin's lymphoma, often at a late stage when tumor is widely disseminated and other groups of nodes are also involved. Only 9%–12% of patients present with an enlarging mediastinal mass [72, 73]. Many of these are lymphoblastic or large cell lymphoma originating in the thymus. The remaining tumors are of nodal origin and may be of B-cell type, including plasmacytomas, or of post-thymic T-cell origin. Their histology and classification is identical to nodal lymphomas elsewhere.

194

Angiofollicular Lymph Node Hyperplasia (Castleman's Disease) [74]

Angiofollicular lymph node hyperplasia usually presents as a large, asymptomatic, localized mass in the mediastinum. In most cases the mass appears to involve lymph node groups, particularly at the hilum, and thymic involvement is rare [75]. Lesions have also been reported in the retroperitoneum and superficial lymph node groups as well as in extranodal sites, such as muscle. A multicentric variant involves mainly peripheral nodes [76]. Two histological variants are described. A prominent follicular pattern is common to both and in most cases normal nodal structure is lacking:

Hyaline-Vascular Variant

The follicles are abnormal with a central zone consisting of concentrically layered and flattened follicle center cells and small lymphocytes. Amorphous hyaline material is present between the cells and a thick-walled capillary enters the center of each follicle. The mantle zone is less clearly defined than in a normal reactive follicle. The interfollicular areas are occupied by numerous high-endothelial vessels, which may also show hyaline change (Fig. 20).

Plasma Cell Variant

Follicles are more typically reactive in type than in the hyaline-vascular variant and the interfollicular zone is packed with numerous plasma cells. This variant is

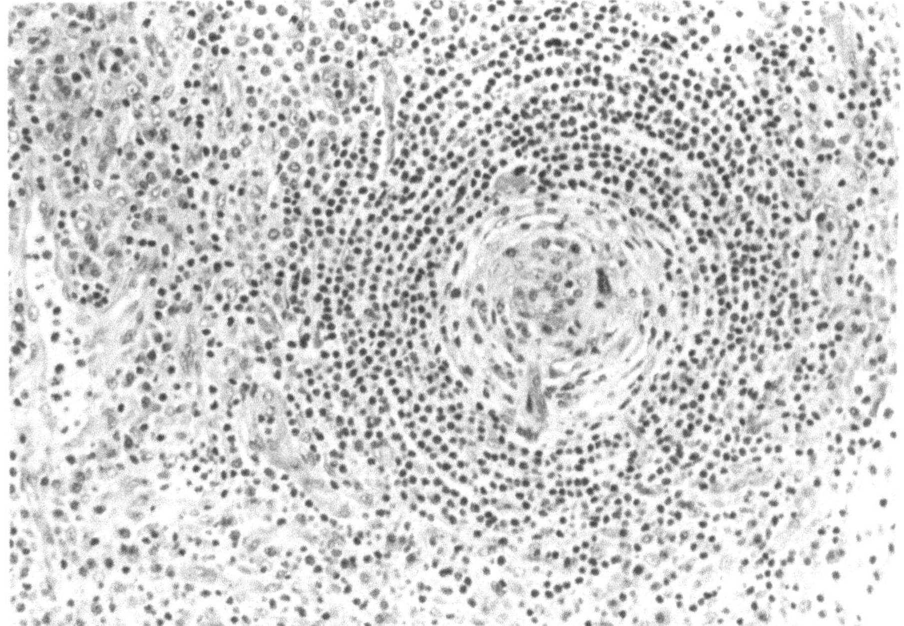

Fig. 20. Angiofollicular lymphoid hyperplasia, hyaline vascular variant – concentric layers of lymphocytes surround the follicle, which is penetrated by a small hyaline vessel

less common and, especially if nodal architecture is preserved, is more likely to be confused with reactive conditions and B-cell neoplasia, such as lymphoplasmacytic lymphoma [77]. Immunohistochemical staining may be necessary to determine the polytypic nature of the infiltrate (Fig. 1).

Systemic effects such as fever, anemia, and hypergammaglobulinemia are particularly likely to occur with the plasma cell variant and associated conditions have included nephrotic syndrome, myasthenia gravis, and peripheral neuropathy. The nature of angiofollicular lymph node hyperplasia is still disputed. Although usually regarded as a form of lymphoid hyperplasia, its occasional association with angiolipomatous elements lends some support to the theory that it is hamartomatous in origin.

Amyloid

Massive enlargement of mediastinal lymph nodes due to deposition of amyloid has been reported in association with multiple myeloma [78] and with primary bronchopulmonary amyloid [79, 80].

Intrathoracic Extramedullary Hemopoiesis [81]

Patients with myeloproliferative disorders or chronic anemia, particularly thalassemia or hereditary spherocytosis, may develop intrathoracic masses of hemopoietic tissue. These may be single or multiple and originate in a paravertebral situation from pleura or extradural space.

Mediastinal Cysts

Classifications of mediastinal cysts based on the type of lining epithelium are unreliable. A more logical approach is to take account of their embryology and anatomical site.

Cysts of Foregut Origin [82, 83]

Bronchogenic Cysts

About half of all congenital mediastinal cysts are of this type. They arise in close association with the main bronchi and are thought to be due to abnormal branching of the bronchial tree. The supernumerary buds are isolated and form cysts either within the lung parenchyma or, more commonly, at the lower end of the trachea or hila. Most do not communicate with the bronchial tree. Many are asymptomatic and are discovered on a routine chest X-ray in the 3rd or 4th decades. Some become infected or produce symptoms due to pressure on adjacent structures. Bronchogenic cysts are spherical or oval with a smooth surface and contain white mucoid material. They may be connected to the bronchial tree by a fibrous band. The wall includes fibrous tissue, smooth muscle, and cartilage and is lined by respiratory epithelium with bronchial glands. Areas of squamous metaplasis are often present.

Intramural Esophageal Cysts

Cysts found in or very close to the wall of the esophagus are regarded as true duplications. The esophageal lumen forms by coalescence of vacuoles, developing in the previously solid tube in the 6-week fetus. Intramural cysts form as a result of isolation of a persistent vacuole. They are usually lined by ciliated columnar epithelium.

Enteric Cysts

Depending on their epithelial lining, enteric cysts have been called by a variety of names, including esophageal, gastric, tracheobronchial, gastroenteric, enterogenous, and tracheoesophageal cysts. They occur in the posterior mediastinum and are often attached posteriorly to vertebral bodies by fibrous tissue. Associated congenital vertebral abnormalities are frequent and the cysts are thought to develop from dorsal displacement of endodermal structures associated with notochordal defects. The epithelium may be esophageal, gastric, intestinal, or respiratory in type, but a muscularis mucosae is usually present together with submucosa and two or three main muscle coats.

Mesothelial Cysts

Depending on their site, mesothelial cysts (spring water cysts or celomic cysts) may be either pericardial or pleural. Although thought to be developmental in origin, they usually present in mid-life. Both pleural and pericardial spaces form by fusion of clefts in embryonic mesenchyme and failure to establish communication results in isolated mesothelial-lined spaces which become cystic. Pericardial cysts usually occur in the right cardiophrenic angle, are unilocular, and contain clear watery fluid. All mesothelial cysts have a thin connective tissue wall lined by flat or cuboidal mesothelial cells.

Thoracic Duct Cysts [84, 85]

Cysts of the thoracic duct are rare and two types are described. Those occurring in elderly patients are usually found incidentally at postmortem and are thought to be degenerative. The wall is fibrotic and calcified atherosclerotic plaques may be present. In younger patients chyle-filled cysts communicating with the thoracic duct are described as lymphangiomatous but they are usually unilocular and may be due to congenital weakness of the duct wall.

Soft Tissue Tumors of the Mediastinum [22, 58]

Mesenchymal tumors of the mediastinum are rare but examples of most types are described. The majority are of adipose tissue or vascular origin.

Tumors of Adipose Tissue [86]

Benign Lipomas

These may be confined to the mediastinum or have an extrathoracic extension, either in the chest wall or base of neck. Intrathoracic tumors are occasionally seen in infants but most occur in adults. They tend to arise in the cardiophrenic angle and may become very large, molding themselves around mediastinal structures without causing symptoms.

Liposarcoma

This is the most frequent malignant soft tissue tumor in the mediastinum [87, 88]. The site varies and tumors often grow to a large size, with infiltration of adjacent structures, before they cause symptoms. Most are low-grade, well-differentiated, or myxoid liposarcomas but tend to recur after excision or radiotherapy. Metastases, usually to lung, pleura, or liver, occur from the more pleomorphic variants.

Tumors of Vascular Origin [89, 90, 91]

Cavernous lymphangiomas usually occur in the neck, where they are thought to arise from sequestered lymphatic tissue. They occur in children and may extend into the mediastinum [92]. Lymphangiomas confined to the mediastinum are usually asymptomatic and discovered in adult life. The majority are located in the anterior mediastinum and are soft cystic or spongy lesions, varying greatly in size. The spaces contain lymph and are lined by endothelial cells with smooth muscle fibers in the walls. Hemorrhage may occur into the lymphatic spaces. Lesions with large cystic spaces are known as cystic hygromas.

Benign hemangiomas also occur in the anterior mediastinum as dark redbrown spongy masses. Histologically they may be cavernous [93], with an appearance similar to lymphangiomas, or of capillary type.

Hemangiopericytomas form a significant group of vascular tumors in the mediastinum. As in other sites, the normal histological criteria of malignancy tend to be unreliable but benign tumors are usually well circumscribed and encapsulated whereas malignant variants may breach the capsule and infiltrate surrounding structures. The diagnosis should be made with caution as some thymomas may mimic the histological pattern of hemangiopericytoma.

Angiosarcoma and the more indolent epithelioid hemangioendothelioma may occur in the mediastinum. Immunohistochemical staining for factor-VIII-related antigen will help to demonstrate an endothelial origin in doubtful cases [94].

198

Tumors of Muscle Origin [86, 95]

Benign leiomyomas are extremely rare in the mediastinum but leiomyosarcomas may originate in the wall of the pulmonary artery, superior vena cava, or even bronchial cysts.

Several cases of mediastinal rhabdomyosarcoma are reported. Benign rhabdomyoma is an extreme rarity, possibly arising from thymic myoid cells [96].

Tumors of Fibrohistiocytic Origin [86]

Both fibrosarcoma and malignant fibrous histiocytoma [97] may occur in the mediastinum. The distinction between sclerosing mediastinitis and a low-grade neoplasm can be difficult but, apart from the presence of histological features of malignancy, the relative absence of inflammatory cells in the latter may be helpful.

Mixed Connective Tissue Tumors [86]

Benign and malignant mesenchymomas have been described in the mediastinum. They are defined as tumors showing differentiation into two or more unrelated types of mesodermal tissue. Most are lipomas, liposarcomas, or rhabdomyosarcomas with focal chondroid or osseous metaplasia, but occasional true mixed tumors occur.

Mediastinal Fibrosis (Sclerosing Mediastinitis) [98, 99]

Mediastinal fibrosis is characterized by compression of mediastinal structures due to proliferation of fibrous connective tissue. In some cases it may represent an exaggerated reaction to infection of mediastinal lymph nodes by mycobacteria, histoplasma [100], or other fungi, but in others no etiology is apparent. In a few instances drugs, such as methysergide, have been implicated.

In the syndrome of multifocal fibrosclerosis, the idiopathic form of mediastinal fibrosis may be associated with a similar pathological process in other sites, such as retroperitoneal fibrosis, Riedel's thyroiditis, sclerosing cholangitis, orbital pseudotumor, and constrictive pericarditis [101, 102]. Very occasionally mediastinal disease is associated with fibrosis in the lungs, producing either a widespread nodular fibrosis or a large fibrous mass [103, 104].

The disease affects all age groups and both sexes but is seen most often in young women and familial cases are described. When fibrosis is maximal in the superior and anterior mediastinum large vessels are surrounded and superior vena caval compression is a frequent feature. Hilar fibrosis, which tends to occur more often in younger patients, leads to involvement of pulmonary vessels and bronchi and may be complicated by infection or pulmonary infarction. Fibrosis around the

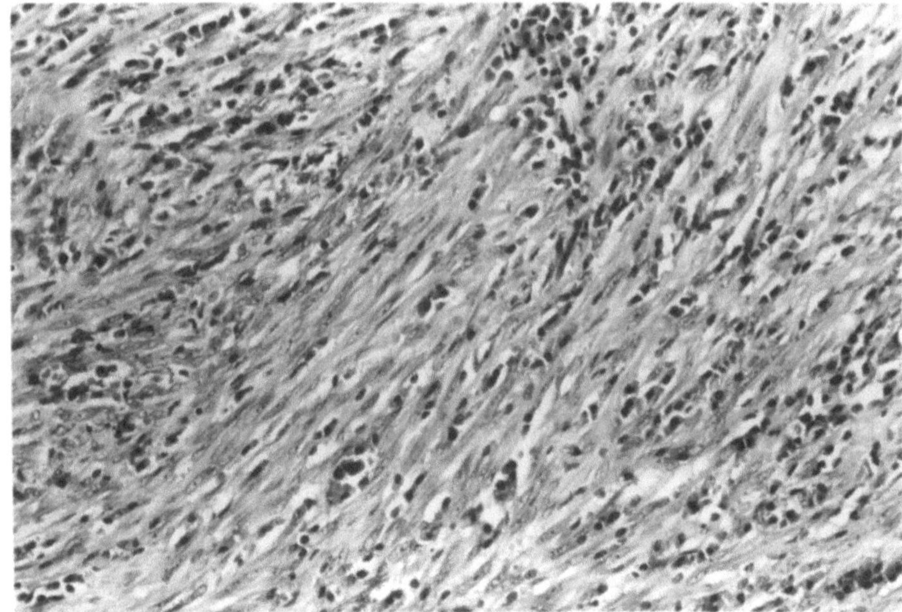

Fig. 21. Sclerosing mediastinitis – a cellular area showing active fibroblast proliferation and numerous inflammatory cells, mainly plasma cells

base of the aorta can involve the coronary arteries. The disease may be self-limiting or pursue an aggressive course.

The microscopic appearances resemble those of retroperitoneal fibrosis. Densely collagenized fibrous tissue merges with more cellular areas of active fibroblast proliferation. Inflammatory cells, including lymphocytes, plasma cells, and histiocytes, are a feature of the active areas, particularly at the periphery (Fig. 21). Eosinophils are occasionally seen and clusters of neutrophils may surround small foci of necrosis. Clear evidence of infection with necrotizing epithelioid and giant cell granulomas is unusual and, if present, staining for mycobacteria or fungi may demonstrate the causative organism.

References

1. Tao L-G, Pearson FG, Cooper JD, Sanders DE, Weisbrod G, Donat EE (1984) Cytopathology of thymoma. Acta Cytol 28: 165–170
2. Fish J, Moore RM (1963) Ectopic thyroid tissue and ectopic thyroid carcinoma: a review of the literature and report of a case. Ann Surg 157: 212–221
3. Nathaniels EK, Nathaniels AM, Wang C-A (1970) Mediastinal parathyroid tumours: a clinical and pathological study of 84 cases. Ann Surg 171: 165–170
4. Massac E Jr, Righini M, Seremetis M (1982) Mediastinal hyperfunctioning parathyroid adenoma. J Natl Med Assoc 74: 385–387
5. Lack EE (1981) Thymic hyperplasia with massive enlargement. Report of two cases with review of diagnostic criteria. J Thorac Cardiovasc Surg 18: 741–746

200

6. Cohen M, Hill CA, Cangir A, Sullivan MP (1980) Thymic rebound after treatment of childhood tumours. AJR 135: 151–156
7. Bell BA, Esseltine DW, Azouz EM (1984) Rebound thymic hyperplasia in a child with cancer. Med Pediatr Oncol 12: 144–147
8. Levine GD, Rosai J (1978) Thymic neoplasia and hyperplasia. Hum Pathol 9: 495–517
9. Addis BJ, Isaacson P. Unpublished observations.
10. Rosai J, Levine GD (1976) Tumours of the thymus. Atlas of tumour pathology. 2nd series. Fascicle 13. Armed Forces Institute of Pathology, Washington DC
11. Deshpande GN, Fisher JE, Jewett TC, Freeman AL (1981) Malignant thymoma in an eight-month old boy. J Surg Oncol 18: 61–66
12. Wick MR, Scheithauer BW, Dines DE (1982) Thymic neoplasia in two male siblings. Mayo Clin Proc 57: 653–656
13. Yamashita H, Murakami N, Noguchi S, Noguchi A, Yokoyama S, Moriuchi A, Nakayama I (1983) Cervical thymoma and the incidence of cervical thymus. Acta Pathol Jpn 33: 189–194
14. Kung ITM, Loke SL, So SY, Lam WK, Mok CK, Khin MA (1985) Intrapulmonary thymoma: report of two cases. Thorax 40: 471–474
15. Pascoe HR, Miner MS (1976) An ultrastructural study of nine thymomas. Cancer 37: 317–326
16. Chan WC, Zaatari GS, Tabei S, Bibb M, Brynes RK (1984) Thymoma: an immunohistochemical study. Am J Clin Pathol 82: 160–166
17. Savino W, Berrih S, Dardenne M (1984) Thymic epithelial antigen, acquired during autogeny and defined by the anti-p19 monoclonal antibody, is lost in thymomas. Lab Invest 51: 292–296
18. Chilosi M, Iannucci AM, Pizzalo G, Menestrina F, Fiore-Donati L, Janossy G (1984) Immunohistochemical analysis of thymoma - evidence for medullary origin of epithelial cells. Am J Surg Pathol 8: 309–318
19. Mokhtar N, Hsu S-M, Lad RP, Haynes BF, Jaffe ES (1984) Thymoma: lymphoid and epithelial components mirror the phenotype of the normal thymus. Hum Pathol 15: 378–384
20. Masaoka A, Mandon Y, Nakahara K, Tanioka T (1981) Follow-up study of thymomas with special reference to their clinical stages. Cancer 48: 2485–2492
21. Verley JM, Hollman KH (1985) Thymoma - a comparative study of clinical stages, histologic features and survival in 200 cases. Cancer 55: 1074–1086
22. Marchevsky AM, Kaneko M (1984) Surgical pathology of the mediastinum. Raven, New York
23. Snover DC, Levine GD, Rosai J (1982) Thymic carcinoma. Five distinctive histological variants. Am J Clin Pathol 6: 451–470
24. Wick MR, Scheithauer BW, Weiland LH, Benatz PE (1982) Primary thymic carcinoma. Am J Surg Pathol 6: 613–630
25. Shimosato Y, Kameya T, Nagai K, Suemasu K (1977) Squamous cell carcinoma of the thymus. An analysis of eight cases. Am J Surg Pathol 1: 109–121
26. Leyvraz S, Henle W, Chahinian AP, Perlmann C, Klein G, Gordon RE, Rosenblum M, Holland JF (1985) Association of Epstein-Barr virus with thymic carcinoma. N Engl J Med 312: 1296–1299
27. Henry K (1972) An unusual thymic tumour with a striated muscle (myoid) component (with a brief review of the literature on myoid cells). Br J Dis Chest 66: 291–299
28. Murakami S, Shamoto M, Miura K, Takeuch J (1984) A thymic tumour with massive proliferation of myoid cells. Acta Pathol Jpn 34: 1375–1383
29. Rosai J, Levine G, Weber R, Higa E (1976) Carcinoid tumours and oat cell carcinomas of the thymus. Pathol Annu 11: 201–226
30. Wick MR (1982) Oat-cell carcinoma of the thymus. Cancer 49: 1645–1647
31. Wick MR, Carney JA, Benatz PE, Brown LR (1982) Primary mediastinal carcinoid tumours. Am J Surg Pathol 6: 195–205
32. Wick MR, Scheithauer BW (1984) Thymic carcinoid: a histologic, immunohistochemical and ultrastructural study of 12 cases. Cancer 53: 475–484
33. Huntrakoon M, Lin F, Heitz PU, Tomita T (1984) Thymic carcinoid tumour with Cushing's syndrome. Arch Pathol Lab Med 108: 551–554

34. Ho FCS, Ho JCI (1977) Pigmented carcinoid tumour of the thymus. Histopathology 1: 363–369
35. Knapp RH, Hurt RD, Payne WS, Farrow MD, Lewis BD, Hahn RG, Muhm JR, Earle JD (1985) Malignant germ cell tumours of the mediastinum. J Thorac Cardiovasc Surg 89: 82–89
36. Lack EE, Wenstein HJ, Welch KJ (1985) Mediastinal germ cell tumours in childhood. J Thorac Cardiovasc Surg 89: 826–835
37. Nichols CR, Hoffman R, Einhorn LH, Williams SD, Wheeler LA, Garnick MB (1985) Hematologic malignancies associated with primary mediastinal germ-cell tumours. Ann Intern Med 102: 603–609
38. Hurt RD, Bruckman JE, Farrow GM, Benatz PE, Hahn RG, Earle JD (1982) Primary anterior mediastinal seminoma. Cancer 49: 1658–1663
39. Knapp RH, Fritz SR, Reiman HM (1982) Primary embryonal carcinoma and choriocarcinoma of the mediastinum. Arch Pathol Lab Med 106: 507–509
40. Carter D, Bibro MC, Touloukian RJ (1982) Benign clinical behaviour of immature mediastinal teratoma in infancy and childhood. Cancer 49: 398–402
41. Dunn PJS (1984) Pancreatic endocrine tissue in benign mediastinal teratoma. J Clin Pathol 37: 1105–1109
42. Holt S, Deverall PB, Boddy JE (1978) A teratoma of the lung containing thymic tissue. J Pathol 126: 85–89
43. Oho HF, Lachenmeyer L, Janzen RWC, Gurtler KF, Fischer K (1982) Thymolipoma in association with myasthenia gravis. Cancer 50: 1623–1628
44. Pillai R, Yeoh N, Addis B, Peckham M, Goldstraw P (1985) Thymolipoma in association with Hodgkin's disease. J Thorac Cardiovasc Surg 90: 306–308
45. Lemos LB, Hamondi AB (1978) Malignant thymic tumour in an infant (malignant histiocytoma). Arch Pathol Lab Med 102: 84–89
46. Havlicek F, Rosai J (1984) A sarcoma of thymic stroma with features of liposarcoma. Am J Clin Pathol 82: 217–224
47. Kaplan HS (1980) Hodgkin's disease. Harvard University Press, Cambridge
48. Keller A, Castleman B (1974) Hodgkin's disease of the thymus gland. Cancer 133: 1615–1623
49. Lindford KK, Meyer JE, Dedrick CG, Hassell LA, Harris NL (1985) Thymic cysts in mediastinal Hodgkin's disease. Radiology 156: 37–44
50. Barcos MP, Lukes RI (1975) Malignant lymphoma of convoluted lymphocytes. A new entity of possible T-cell type. In: Sinks LF, Godden JO (eds) Conflicts in childhood cancer. An evaluation of current management, vol 4, Liss, New York pp. 147–178
51. Nathwani BN, Kim H, Rappaport H (1976) Malignant lymphoma, lymphoblastic. Cancer 38: 964–983
52. Crossman J, Chused TM, Fisher RI, Magrath I, Bollum F, Jaffe ES (1983) Diversity of immunologic phenotypes of lymphoblastic lymphoma. Cancer Res 43: 4486–4490
53. Yousem SA, Weiss LM, Warnke RA (1985) Primary mediastinal non-Hodgkin's lymphomas: a morphologic and immunologic study of 19 cases. Am J Clin Pathol 83: 676–680
54. Waldron JA, Dohring EJ, Farber LR (1985) Primary large cell lymphomas of the mediastinal: an analysis of 20 cases. Semin Diagn Pathol 2: 281–295
55. Addis BJ, Isaacson PG (1985) Large cell lymphoma of the mediastinum: a B-cell tumour of probable thymic origin. Histopathology 10: 379–390
56. Siegal GP, Dehner CP, Rosai J (1985) Histiocytosis X (Langerhans cell granulomatosis) of the thymus. Am J Surg Pathol 9: 117–124
57. Davidson KG, Walbaum PR, McCormack RJM (1978) Intrathoracic neural tumours. Thorax 33: 359–367
58. Enzinger FM, Weiss SW (1983) Soft tissue tumours. Mosby, St. Louis
59. Besznyak I, Toth L, Szende B (1985) Intrathoracic vagus nerve tumours: a report of two cases and review of the literature. J Thorac Cardiovasc Surg 89: 462–465
60. Staffanson K, Wollman R, Jerkovia M (1982) S100 protein in soft tissue tumours derived from Schwann cells and melanocytes. Am J Pathol 106: 261–268
61. Variend S (1985) Small cell tumours in childhood. J Pathol 145: 1–26
62. Dhillon AP, Rhode J, Leathern A (1982) Neurone specific enolase: an aid to the diagnosis of melanoma and neuroblastoma. Histopathology 6: 81–92

63. Kemshead JT, Goldman A, Fritschy J, Malpas JS, Pritchard J (1983) Use of panels of monoclonal antibodies in the differential diagnosis of neuroblastoma. Lancet i: 12–14
64. Misugi K, Okajima H, Newton WA, Kmetz DR, deLorimer AA (1965) Mediastinal origin of a melanotic progonoma or retinal anlage tumor: ultrastructural evidence for neural crest origin. Cancer 18: 477–484
65. Adams A, Hochholzer L (1981) Ganglioneuroblastoma of the posterior mediastinum. A clinicopathologic review of 80 cases. Cancer 47: 373–381
66. Buthker W, Feltkamp-Vroom T, Groen AS, Wieberdink J (1964) Sympathicoblastoma of the anterior mediastinum. Dis Chest 46: 531–536
67. Talerman A, Gratoma S (1983) Primary ganglioneuroblastoma of the anterior mediastinum in a 61-yr-old woman. Histopathology 7: 967–975
68. Olson JL, Salyer WR (1978) Mediastinal paragangliomas (aortic body tumour): a report of four cases and a review of the literature. Cancer 41: 2405–2412
69. Lack EE, Stillinger RA, Colvin DB, Groves RM, Burnette DG (1979) Aortico-pulmonary paraganglioma. Report of a case with ultrastructural study and review of the literature. Cancer 43: 269–278
70. Ogawa J, Inoue H, Koide S, Kawada S, Shotitsu A, Hata J (1982) Functioning paraganglioma in the posterior mediastinum. Ann Thorac Surg 33: 507–510
71. Nigan BK (1981) Intrathoracic chemodectoma with noradrenaline secretion. Thorax 36: 66–68
72. Lichtenstein AK, Levine A, Taylor CR, Boswell B, Rossman S, Feinstein DI, Lukes RJ (1980) Primary mediastinal lymphoma in adults. Am J Med 68: 509–514
73. Levitt LJ, Aisenberg AL, Harris NL, Linggood RM, Poppema S (1982) Primary non-Hodgkin's lymphoma of the mediastinum. Cancer 50: 2486–2492
74. Keller AR, Hochholzer L, Castleman B (1972) Hyaline-vascular and plasma-cell types of giant lymph node hyperplasia of the mediastinum and other locations. Cancer 29: 670–683
75. Karcher DS, Pearson CE, Butler WM, Hurwitz MA, Cassell PF (1982) Giant lymph node hyperplasia involving the thymus with associated nephrotic syndrome and myelofibrosis. Am J Clin Pathol 77: 100–104
76. Weisenberger DD, Nathwani BN, Winberg CD, Rappaport H (1985) Multicentric angiofollicular lymph node hyperplasia. A clinicopathologic study of 16 cases. Hum Pathol 16: 162–172
77. Frizzera G (1985) Castleman's disease: more questions than answers. Hum Pathol 16: 202–205
78. Melato M, Antoniutto G, Falconieri G, Manconi R (1983) Massive enlargement of mediastinal lymph nodes in a patient with multiple myeloma. Thorax 38: 151–152
79. Thompson PJ, Jewkes J, Corrin B, Citron KM (1983) Primary bronchopulmonary amyloid tumour with massive hilar lymphadenopathy. Thorax 38: 152–154
80. Shaw P, Grossman R, Fernandes BJ (1984) Nodular mediastinal amyloidosis. Hum Pathol 15: 1183–1185
81. Verani R, Olson J, Moake JL (1980) Intrathoracic extramedullary hematopoiesis: report of a case in a patient with sickle cell disease – beta-thalassemia. Am J Clin Pathol 73: 133–137
82. Kirwan WO, Walbaum PR, McCormack RJM (1973) Cystic intrathoracic derivatives of the foregut and their complications. Thorax 28: 424–428
83. Salyer DC, Salyer WR, Eggleston JC (1977) Benign developmental cysts of the mediastinum. Arch Pathol Lab Med 101: 136–139
84. Luosto R, Koikkalainen K, Jyrala A, Makinen J (1978) Thoracic duct cyst of the mediastinum. A case report. Scand J Thorac Cardiovasc Surg 12: 261–263
85. Tsuchiya R, Sugiura Y, Ogata T, Suemasu K (1980) Thoracic duct cyst of the mediastinum. J Thorac Cardiovasc Surg 79: 856–859
86. Pachter MR, Lattes R (1963) Mesenchymal tumours of the mediastinum. I Tumours of fibrous tissue, adipose tissue, smooth muscle and striated muscle. Cancer 16: 74–94
87. Schweitzer DL, Aguam AS (1977) Primary liposarcoma of the mediastinum. J Thorac Cardiovasc Surg 74: 83–97
88. Prohn P, Winter J, Ulatowski L (1981) Liposarcoma of the mediastinum – case report and review of the literature. Thorac Cardiovasc Surg 29: 119–121

89. Pachter MR, Lattes R (1963) Mesenchymal tumours of the mediastinum. II Tumours of blood vascular origin. Cancer 16: 95–107
90. Pachter MR, Lattes R (1963) Mesenchymal tumours of the mediastinum. III Tumours of lymph vascular origin. Cancer 16: 108–117
91. Kelley MJ, Mannes EJ, Ravin CE (1978) Mediastinal masses of vascular origin. A review. J Thorac Cardiovasc Surg 76: 559–572
92. Sumner TE, Volberg FM, Kiser PE, Shaffner LD (1981) Mediastinal cystic hygroma in children. Pediatr Radiol 11: 160–162
93. Kissin MW (1977) Mediastinal cavernous hemangioma. Br J Dis Chest 71: 208–210
94. Gibbs AR, Johnson NF, Giddings JC, Powell DEB, Jasani B (1984) Primary angiosarcoma of the mediastinum: light and electron microscopic demonstration of Factor VIII-related antigen in neoplastic cells. Hum Pathol 15: 687–691
95. Rasaretnam R, Panabokke RG (1975) Leiomyosarcoma of the mediastinum. Brit J Dis Chest 69: 63–69
96. Miller R, Kurtz SM, Powers JM (1978) Mediastinal rhabdomyoma. Cancer 42: 1983–1988
97. Chen W, Chan CW (1982) Malignant fibrous histiocytoma of the mediastinum. Cancer 50: 797–800
98. Kittredge RD, Nash AD (1974) The many facets of sclerosing fibrosis. AJR 122: 288–298
99. Light AM (1978) Idiopathic fibrosis of the mediastinum: a discussion of three cases and review of the literature. J Clin Pathol 31: 78–88
100. Weider S, Rabinowitz JG (1977) Fibrous mediastinitis: a late manifestation of mediastinal histoplasmosis. Radiology 125: 305–312
101. Comings DE, Skubi KB, van Eyes J, Motulsky AG (1967) Familial multifocal fibrosclerosis. Ann Intern Med 66: 884–892
102. Hanly PC, Shub C, Lie JT (1984) Constrictive pericarditis associated with combined retroperitoneal and mediastinal fibrosis. Mayo Clin Proc 59: 300–304
103. Engleman P, Liebow AA, Gmelich J, Friedman PJ (1977) Pulmonary hyalinizing granuloma. Am Rev Respir Dis 115: 997–1008
104. Magee JF, Wright JL, Dodek A, Tutassaura H (1984) Mediastinal and retroperitoneal fibrosis with fibrotic pulmonary nodules: a case report. Histopathology 9: 995–999

15. Pathology of Tumors of the Pleura and Chest Wall

B. J. Addis

Pleural Tumors

Malignant Mesothelioma

Etiology

The relationship between asbestos and mesothelioma was first reported by Wagner et al. [1] in 1960. Most cases can be attributed to environmental and occupational exposure to fibrous materials, malignancy being associated with inhalation of straight fibers less than 2 μm in diameter and greater than 8 μm in length. These properties are shared by the amphibole group of asbestos fibers, in particular crocidolite (blue asbestos) and amosite (brown asbestos), and a fibrous zeolite called erionite. Chrysotile (white asbestos), a fibrous form of serpentine, is not clearly associated with mesothelioma. The interval between exposure and development of a tumor varies greatly, usually between 20 and 40 years. Asbestos exposure determines the age incidence and geographical distribution of mesothelioma but about 10% of cases appear unrelated [2] and tumors occasionally occur in childhood [3].

Gross Appearances [4, 5]

In its early stages mesothelioma appears as multiple tumor nodules on pleural surfaces. These coalesce to form a sheet of tumor covering the surface of the lung or, less commonly, a localized mass. A blood-stained effusion is frequently present but as the tumor advances the pleural space becomes obliterated, often with loculation of residual fluid. At a later stage the lung is encased by tumor, as a dense white sheet up to several centimeters thick. Infiltration of the chest wall makes the lung difficult to remove from the chest at autopsy and infiltration of diaphragm or pericardium may lead to compression of large veins. Direct infiltration of lung parenchyma is usually superficial but serosal spread occurs into fissures and lymphatic involvement results in spread along bronchovascular bundles toward the hilum. Involvement of the serosal surface and subserosal parenchyma of the liver and other viscera follows infiltration through the diaphragm, and lymph nodes are frequently involved. Multiple deposits may occur on the surface of the opposite lung. Distant metastasis is less common and sites include lung, brain, adrenal, kidney, and liver. Pleural mesothelioma is often accompanied by hyaline fibrous plaques on uninvolved pleural surfaces, a common manifestation of asbestos exposure.

Microscopic Appearances [4, 5]

The very varied microscopic appearances of mesothelioma are due to the ability of neoplastic mesothelial cells to assume the characteristics of epithelial cells, mesenchymal cells, and intermediate forms. This is reflected in the traditional classification into epithelial, mixed, and fibrous types. The recent concept of "mesodermoma" emphasizes the mesodermal nature of mesothelium and its potential for multidirectional differentiation [6].

Epithelial Mesothelioma. Cells are generally cuboidal or polygonal with moderate amounts of eosinophilic cytoplasm and rather uniform nuclei with a single nucleolus. They form cohesive groups with either a papillary pattern, with several layers of cells around a delicate fibrovascular core (Fig. 1), or a tubular pattern, with cords of cells surrounding a central glandular lumen (Fig. 2). Commonly the two patterns are mixed so that cell clusters contain complex, slit-like, branching intercellular clefts (Fig. 3). Cytoplasmic vacuolation is frequently present and if vacuoles are large and numerous a microcystic pattern may be produced (Fig. 4). The surrounding stroma frequently appears myxoid. Increasing cellular pleomorphism or anaplasia is accompanied by loss of recognizable pattern and areas of tumor may consist of sheets of large cells with few characteristic features (Fig. 5). Such areas may resemble squamous cell carcinoma and true squamous metaplasia is occasionally seen.

Mixed (Biphasic) Mesothelioma. Most mesotheliomas, if adequately sampled, contain areas where cells assume an oval or spindle-cell form and the resulting

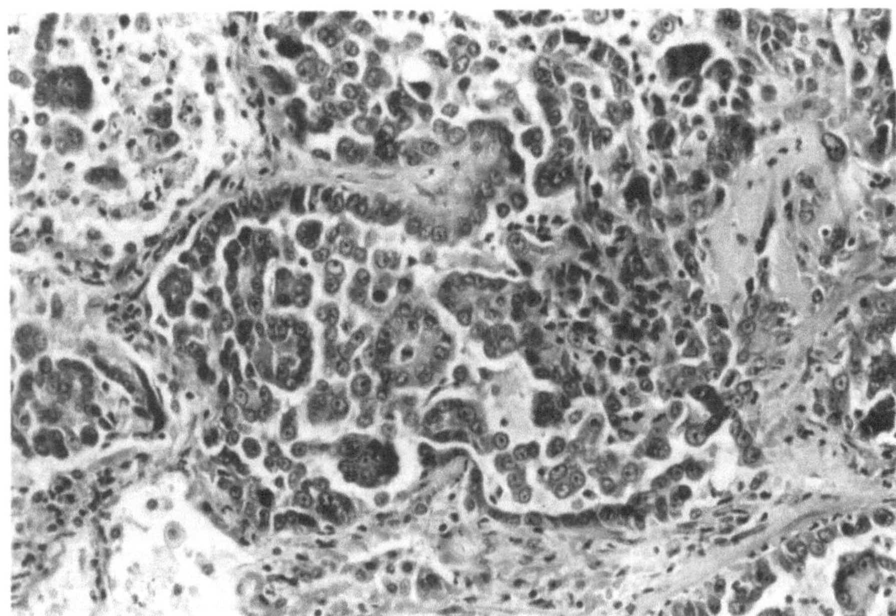

Fig. 1. Epithelial mesothelioma – groups of cells form papillary structures projecting into an irregular space

206

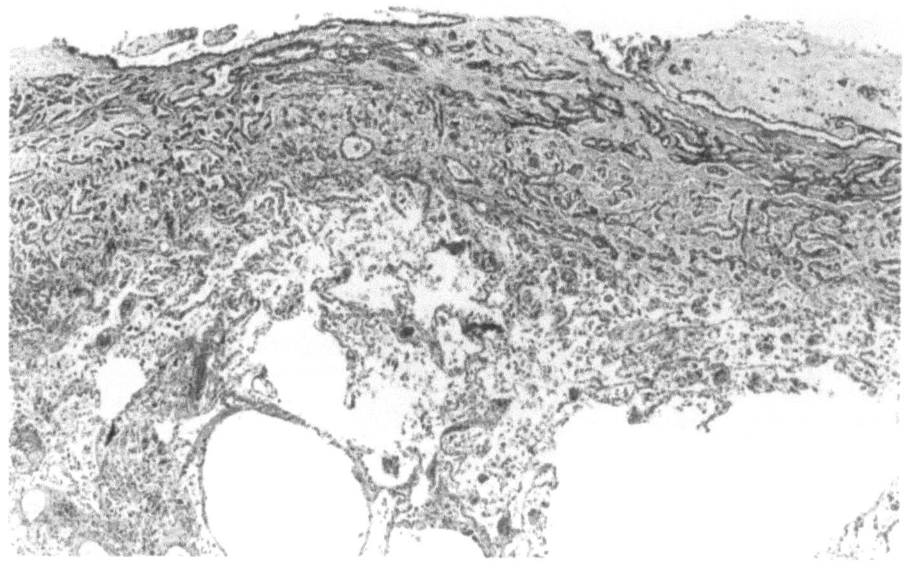

Fig. 2. Early mesothelioma – the thickened pleura is infiltrated by cells forming irregular gland-like spaces

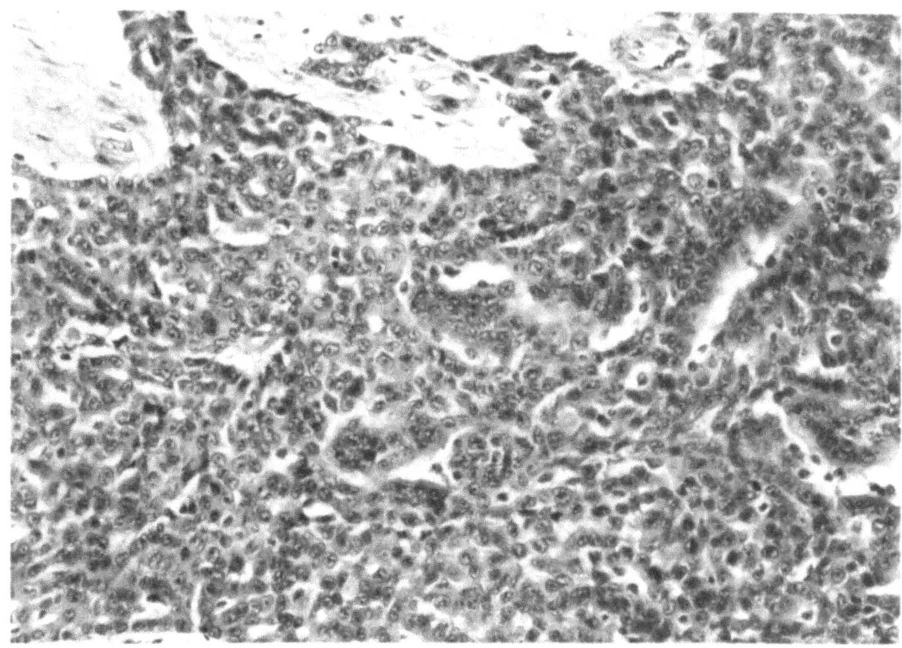

Fig. 3. Epithelial mesothelioma – frequently cells form a complex tubulopapillary pattern with slit-like spaces

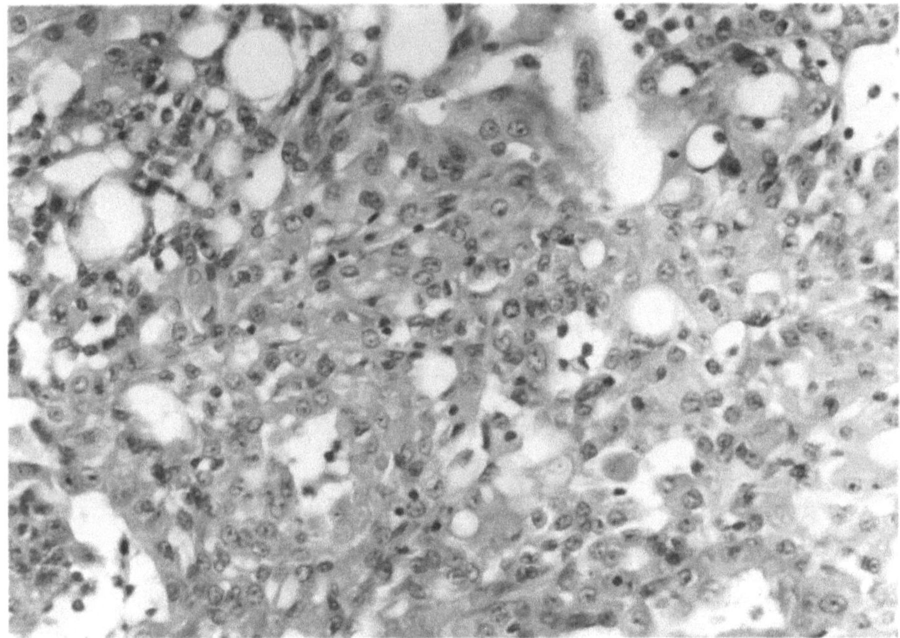

Fig. 4. Epithelial mesothelioma – prominent cytoplasmic vacuolation gives this tumor a microcystic appearance

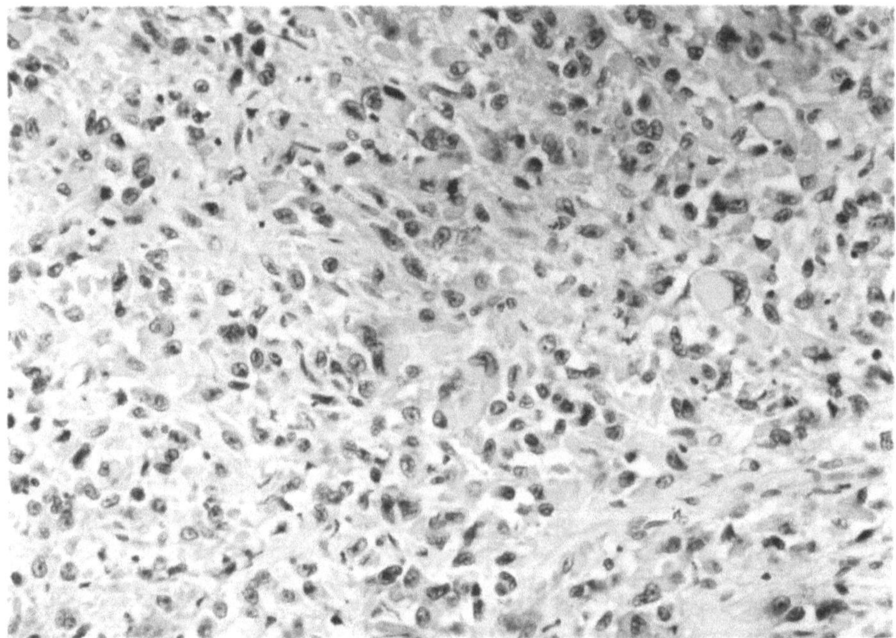

Fig. 5. Mesothelioma – tumor cells show an unusual degree of pleomorphism and cellularity with no discernible pattern

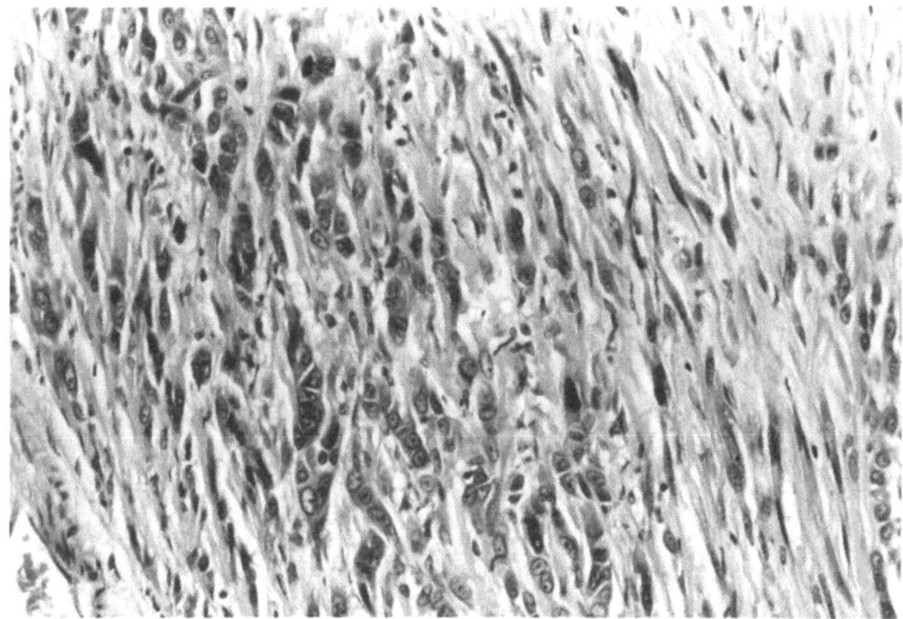

Fig. 6. Mixed mesothelioma – cords of cohesive polygonal cells *on the left* merge with spindle cell areas *on the right*

biphasic pattern is one of the most helpful diagnostic features. In transitional areas the two components of the tumor can be seen to merge (Fig. 6). The transition from epithelial to spindle-cell morphology is accompanied by dissociation of cells and an increase in stroma with collagen deposition. The cellularity of the spindle-cell areas varies greatly: from scattered, rather bland spindle cells resembling fibroblasts in a densely collagenized stroma, to cellular sarcomatous foci where cells show marked pleomorphism. Clear evidence of mesenchymal differentiation, with cartilage or bone formation, is rare.

Fibrous (Sarcomatous or Mesenchymal) Mesothelioma. When no clearly epithelial component can be identified the tumor is of the fibrous type. Frequently much of the tumor is densely fibrotic but further sampling usually reveals more cellular areas.

Differential Diagnosis

Mesotheliomas often present difficult diagnostic problems. The epithelial type must be distinguished from atypical reactive mesothelial hyperplasia and from carcinoma [8]. Reactive proliferation of mesothelial cells may produce cohesive cell clusters closely resembling mesothelioma. These tend to be confined to the surface with no tendency to infiltration but their site may be difficult to establish in a small biopsy. Surface papillary structures may also be nonneoplastic but their presence in a needle biopsy is very suggestive of malignancy [9]. A papillary or tubular configuration in mesothelioma may mimic adenocarcinoma, either peripheral adenocarcinoma of lung involving the pleura or pleural deposits from adenocarcinoma elsewhere.

Mixed mesothelioma may be confused with other biphasic tumors, particularly spindle-cell carcinoma of the lung, pulmonary carcinosarcoma, or metastatic renal carcinoma.

Fibrous mesotheliomas resemble spindle-cell sarcomas, such as fibrosarcoma, malignant fibrous histiocytoma, and leiomyosarcoma. If neoplastic bone or cartilage is formed the distinction from chondrosarcoma or osteogenic sarcoma is extremely difficult on histological grounds.

Cytology [10, 11]

Pleural fluid can be used for cytological diagnosis or, after centrifugation, as a source of cell blocks for light or electron microscopy. Epithelial mesotheliomas frequently shed papillary aggregates of cells. These morulae may contain a hundred or more cells and are typically rounded with a knobbly border. Their presence in large numbers is characteristic of mesothelioma but cannot be regarded as diagnostic. Both nuclear size and cytoplasmic area tend to be increased in mesothelioma but the nuclear-cytoplasmic ratio is often not significantly raised [12]. Binucleate or multinucleate cells are frequent and the presence of cells within cells or engulfed cells is a feature rarely seen in benign effusions. The zonal cytoplasmic staining characteristic of mesothelial cells is present together with multiple small lipid vacuoles. The large vacuoles and irregular nuclei of adenocarcinoma are not seen. Extracellular hyaluronic acid may produce a characteristic pink granular background in smears stained by a Romanovsky method.

Electron Microscopy [5, 13, 14, 15, 16]

In epithelial mesotheliomas cells are closely apposed on a well-defined narrow basement membrane. Desmosomes are numerous and abundant intermediate filaments (tonofilaments) form bundles that may converge on cell junctions. Long thin microvilli project into intercellular spaces, on both apical and lateral surfaces, and into intracellular lumena. Glycogen and lipid are present in the cytoplasm. The absence of other secretory granules, particularly mucin, and the length of the microvilli are among the features that help to distinguish between mesothelioma and adenocarcinoma. In spindle-cell areas, although cells appear more widely separated, points of contact are maintained and well-developed junctions may be seen. Bundles of filaments are present and surface microvilli remain but are more focal and comparatively sparse. The basement membrane becomes discontinuous and collagen fibrils are deposited between cells.

Histochemistry and Immunohistochemistry

Until recently the distinction between mesothelioma and adenocarcinoma depended heavily on mucin staining. Immunohistochemistry now provides additional evidence and frequently enables a firm diagnosis to be made. As yet there is no reliable marker of malignancy that helps make the distinction between benign and malignant mesothelial cells.

Mesothelial cells contain finely dispersed glycogen and lack epithelial mucin. Both of these features can be demonstrated by use of the periodic acid-Schiff (PAS) stain, with and without diastase digestion. Mesothelial cells may contain a few fine PAS-positive granules even after diastase digestion but large intracellular mucin vacuoles are not found. Stains for hyaluronic acid should also be interpreted with care. Hyaluronic acid is a glycosaminoglycan produced by mesodermal cells, including mesothelium. Although it is present in the stroma of mesotheliomas in large amounts it is also present in the stroma of carcinomas. The presence of intracytoplasmic hyaluronic acid is characteristic of mesothelioma but in practice its demonstration is difficult. Staining with colloidal iron or Alcian blue at pH 2.5 should be done with and without digestion by hyaluronidase [17]. The material may be seen in intracellular vacuoles but these frequently appear empty as hyaluronic acid washes out during fixation. The measurement of hyaluronic acid in effusions may provide additional useful evidence as very high levels are seen in mesothelioma [7].

The presence of carcinoembryonic antigen (CEA), detected by an immunohistochemical method, is valuable in making the distinction between mesothelial cells, which are either negative or weakly positive, or adenocarcinoma, which is usually strongly positive [18, 19, 20, 21, 22]. Staining for cytokeratins, the intermediate filaments characteristic of epithelial cells, is invariably positive in both types of cell as they share several cytokeratins characteristic of simple epithelium [19]. However, coexpression of cytokeratins and vimentin is found in the fusiform cells of biphasic and fibrous mesotheliomas [23]. Epithelial membrane antigen (EMA) may be of some value in distinguishing between benign and malignant mesothelial cells: in general reactive cells stain only weakly whereas mesothelioma and adenocarcinoma are strongly positive [7, 24].

Pleural Fibromas [25, 26, 27, 28]

The many synonyms for this tumor include benign localized mesothelioma and localized fibrous mesothelioma. It occurs over a wide age range, but is most frequent in the 5th and 6th decades with a mean age of 50. No association with asbestos exposure has been established and this tumor appears unrelated to malignant mesothelioma. Extrapulmonary symptoms include pyrexia, hypertrophic pulmonary osteoarthropathy, and hypoglycemia; and chest symptoms are often minimal until the tumor has reached a large size.

Gross Appearances

Smaller tumors may be intrapulmonary but larger tumors lie within the pleural cavity attached to the visceral pleura by a narrow pedicle. Those arising from the parietal pleura are less common and more sessile, being attached over a wider area. Pleural fibromas are usually well-circumscribed lobulated masses which may fill the pleural cavity, compressing the lung, and usually show no evidence of infiltration. The surface is smooth and the cut surface is firm with a uniform, white whorled appearance resembling a uterine fibroid. Larger lesions may show areas of hemorrhage and necrosis.

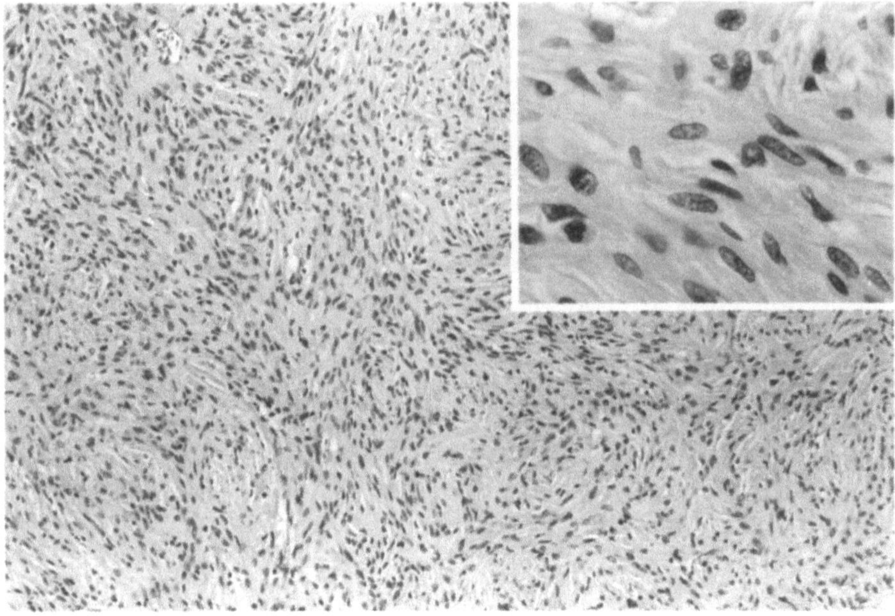

Fig. 7. Pleural fibroma – moderately cellular area with interlacing bundles of small uniform spindle cells. *Inset* shows cellular detail

Microscopic Appearances

Wide variations in cellularity are seen in the same tumors with areas of loose, sparsely cellular, edematous connective tissue alternating with more densely cellular areas. Cells are spindle shaped with regular fusiform nuclei (Fig. 7). Nuclear chromatin is uniformly dispersed and nucleoli are not prominent. In larger tumors cellular pleomorphism may be more marked. The mitotic rate is very variable: in smaller tumors mitoses are scarce but in larger tumors they may be more frequent. Nuclear palisading is occasionally seen. Cells form interlacing bundles and may reproduce the storiform pattern characteristic of fibrous histiocytomas. Irregular clefts or channels are lined by flattened cells and some tumors have prominent blood vessels, occasionally reminiscent of hemangiopericytoma. Mesothelial cells cover the surface and if there is significant infiltration of adjacent lung parenchyma, alveolar epithelial inclusions may be seen.

Ultrastructural Appearances

On electron microscopy most cells have the features of mesenchymal cells and resemble fibroblasts. The basement membrane, microvillous processes, and intermediate filaments characteristic of mesothelial cells are not seen, although cell junctions are described [25].

212

Histogenesis

The origin of pleural fibromas is uncertain. On the basis of ultrastructural and immunohistochemical studies a mesothelial derivation seems unlikely and an origin from subpleural connective tissue is currently favored.

Behavior

Most tumors, irrespective of their cellularity and mitotic rate, do not recur provided that removal is complete. This is more easily achieved with pedunculated lesions than with sessile ones, which are more likely to infiltrate locally and recur following resection. Therefore there is some justification for regarding these tumors as low-grade sarcomas.

Other Primary Tumors of the Pleura

Isolated case reports of primary mesenchymal tumors of the pleura, including liposarcoma [29, 30], malignant fibrous histiocytoma [31], and rhabdomyosarcoma [32], suggest that these are extremely rare. However, sarcomatous mesotheliomas may reproduce other types of connective tissue tumor, particularly if heterologous elements are present [6].

Secondary Involvement of the Pleura

Carcinoma of the Lung

Peripheral pulmonary adenocarcinoma, and occasionally squamous cell carcinoma, may mimic malignant mesothelioma clinically and macroscopically by spreading over serosal surfaces to obliterate the pleural cavity and encase the lung ("pseudomesotheliomatous carcinoma") [33, 34]. The origin of the tumor in the lung is rarely apparent and the distinction from mesothelioma is based on histology, electron microscopy, and (immuno)histochemistry.

More typical pulmonary adenocarcinomas may give rise to metastatic pleural deposits. This is less often seen with other types of lung carcinoma although infiltration of pleura overlying the tumor is common.

Metastatic Carcinoma from Other Sites [35, 36].

Metastatic carcinoma is a frequent cause of pleural effusion. Adenocarcinoma is by far the most common type and primary sites include lung, breast, thyroid, ovary, stomach, pancreas, kidney, and large bowel. In a significant percentage of cases the primary site is not apparent [37].

Malignant Lymphoma

Both Hodgkin's disease and non-Hodgkin's lymphoma may manifest themselves as solid pleural deposits, with or without evidence of disease at other sites. Nodules occur immediately beneath the visceral pleura and may spread to involve the soft tissues of the chest wall [38].

Tumors of the Chest Wall

Carcinoma and Mesothelioma

Mesotheliomas characteristically infiltrate the thoracic wall and occasionally extend along a biopsy track to the skin surface. Less commonly the chest wall is directly infiltrated by an underlying lung carcinoma.

Thoracic wall metastases may involve bone and soft tissue as well as pleura. Adenocarcinoma is the most frequent type (see above) [36, 37]. Prostatic and breast carcinoma, and occasionally carcinoid tumors, may give rise to osteosclerotic bone metastases.

Malignant Lymphoma

Up to 10% of patients with Hodgkin's disease and non-Hodgkin's lymphoma develop evidence of thoracic wall involvement, with soft tissue masses beneath the pectoral muscles or lesions related to ribs [39].

Soft Tissue Tumors [40]

Tumors of Nerve Sheath Origin [37, 41, 42, 43, 44, 45]

Benign and malignant tumors of nerve sheath origin, arising from intercostal nerves, form one of the largest groups of soft tissue tumors involving the chest wall. In patients with neurofibromatosis these may be multiple and malignancy may supervene at an earlier age. These tumors are more fully discussed in the section dealing with mediastinal tumors.

Tumors of Adipose Tissue [43, 44, 45].

Benign Lipomas. These are extremely common tumors which often involve the subcutaneous fat of the back, shoulder, and neck. Here they form well-circumscribed, thinly encapsulated tumors of mature adipose tissue. Spindle-cell and pleomorphic variants are often found on the shoulder region, and benign tumors of brown fat (hibernomas) most commonly occur on the chest wall and in the interscapular region. Intramuscular and intermuscular lipomas are more deeply located, infiltrative lesions that may be difficult to excise and are therefore likely to recur. Rarely a lipoma may extend through the chest wall with extra- and intrathoracic components [46].

Liposarcoma. This is the most common soft tissue sarcoma of adults but only a small percentage occur in the chest wall. They are usually well-circumscribed lobulated masses and most have a soft, fatty, or mucoid consistency. Excision may be incomplete because of separate satellite nodules. The well-differentiated and myxoid variants tend to recur repeatedly, often over long periods, without metastasizing. Myxoid liposarcomas may produce serosal metastases. The round cell and pleomorphic variants metastasize more readily and survival rates are correspondingly poor.

Tumors of Fibroblastic and Fibrohistiocytic Origin

Extraabdominal Desmoid Tumor (Extraabdominal Fibromatosis) [44, 45, 47]. The chest wall is a favored site for this lesion, which arises from deep fascia and the connective tissue of muscles. The shoulder girdle is most frequently involved and in over one-third of patients the tumors extend to involve the upper chest wall. They appear as hard, fixed, unencapsulated masses which invade and replace muscle. Subcutaneous fat may be involved but underlying bone is rarely included. The surface is dense and white. Microscopically they consist of uniform, spindle cells in a collagenized stroma (Fig. 8). Variation in cellularity is seen and the stroma may appear myxoid. Cartilage or bone formation is rare. At the infiltrating margins included muscle fibers may be atrophic or appear as rounded multinucleated cells. In common with the other fibromatoses desmoids are characterized by a tendency to recur.

Dermatofibrosarcoma Protruberans (DFSP). DFSPs are dermal tumors of low-grade malignancy, about half of which are situated on the chest wall. Nodules of tumor extend into subcutaneous tissue and may occasionally involve deeper structures. Microscopicaly they consist of spindle cells with a characteristic storiform pattern. Excision is frequently followed by recurrence and metastases are recorded.

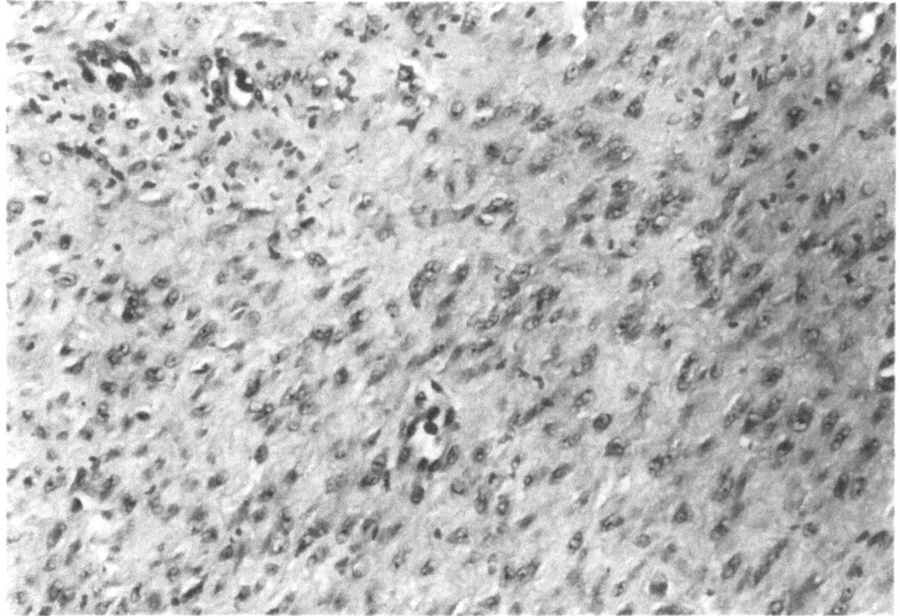

Fig. 8. Fibromatosis (desmoid) of chest wall - plump benign fibroblasts are separated by dense collagen

Fibrosarcoma and Malignant Fibrous Histiocytoma (MFH). In some series of chest wall tumors fibrosarcomas form the majority of malignant soft tissue tumors [43, 44, 45]. Nowadays, diagnostic criteria are more strict and some tumors previously called fibrosarcoma would be reclassified as MFH. Nevertheless, even by current criteria it seems that fibrosarcomas are more frequently seen on the trunk than MFHs.

Fibrosarcomas are characterized by a uniform histological pattern, consisting of closely packed spindle cells and a fine intercellular collagen network. A "herringbone" pattern is typical of better-differentiated tumors. Some examples have followed irradiation of the chest wall for breast carcinoma [48]. The distinction from a malignant tumor of nerve sheath origin may be difficult on purely histological grounds.

The five subtypes of MFH (storiform-pleomorphic, myxoid, giant cell, inflammatory, and angiomatoid) embrace a great variety of soft tissue sarcomas and a detailed description is beyond the scope of this manual.

Tumors of Vascular Origin

Benign Hemangiomas [43] *and Lymphangiomas of the Chest Wall.* These may involve cutaneous and subcutaneous tissues, muscle, rib, and pleura [49]. Tumors are poorly circumscribed and the distinction between hemangioma and angiosarcoma may occasionally be difficult. This is particularly true of a type of hemangioma of muscle that involves the trunk in 35% of cases and has alarming histological features [50].

Hemangiopericytomas. These occur rarely in the chest wall [51].

Angiosarcomas. These are rare tumors which occasionally involve the soft tissues of the chest wall with or without pleural involvement [42, 43, 52, 53, 54]. The vascular nature of the tumor is usually apparent, with irregular anastamosing vascular channels lined by atypical endothelial cells. In some variants the neoplastic cells may assume an epithelioid or spindle-cell morphology; the endothelial nature of the malignant cells may be demonstrated by immunochemistry with antibody to factor-VIII-related antigen. Angiosarcoma is recorded following mastectomy and irradiation of the chest wall [55] and angiosarcoma associated with postmastectomy lymphedema may spread from the affected arm to the chest wall.

Other Tumors

Other soft tissue sarcomas which occasionally occur on the chest wall include synovial sarcoma [56], leiomyosarcoma [57], and adult rhabdomyosarcoma [44].

Chest Wall Tumors in Childhood

Benign Mesenchymoma. A mesenchymoma is defined as a mixed tumor containing two or more cell types of mesenchymal origin and may be benign or malignant. In children tumors consisting of immature or mature mesenchyme with cartilaginous, bony and vascular elements may cause rib erosion [62, 63].

Malignant Small Tumors of Childhood. These tumors form the principal soft tissue tumors of childhood. They consist of small hyperchromatic cells and many lack features of differentiation. The chest wall may be primarily involved by three variants:

Malignant Small Cell Tumor of the Thoracopulmonary Region (Peripheral Neuroectodermal Tumor, Peripheral Neuroblastoma). This rare tumor occurs almost exclusively in the first 2 decades and 75% of the patients are female. It occurs as solitary or multiple nodules in the chest wall with rib erosion and subsequently spreads to involve pleura, pericardium, or diaphragm. Distant metastases are unusual. Microscopically there are few distinctive features. Tumor cells form sheets, nests, or irregular bands. Rosette formation, with fibrillary cytoplasmic extensions at the center of clusters of radially arranged cells (Homer Wright rosettes), may be present (Fig. 9). Some contain intracytoplasmic glycogen. Electron microscopy demonstrates blunt cytoplasmic processes and dense core neurosecretory granules. The cells are positive for S-100 protein and neuronspecific enolase, both immunohistochemical markers of a neuroectodermal origin [59, 60].

Ewing's Sarcoma. Ewing's sarcoma of bone may rarely arise in a rib but the chest wall and paravertebral region are favored sites for the soft tissue or extraosseous variant. This occurs in a somewhat older age group than conventional Ewing's sarcoma, with a median age of 20, and lacks the male predominance shown by the latter. Grossly the tumors are grayish-white with focal necrosis and may appear attached to rib periosteum. Two types of cells are described: primary cells with oval

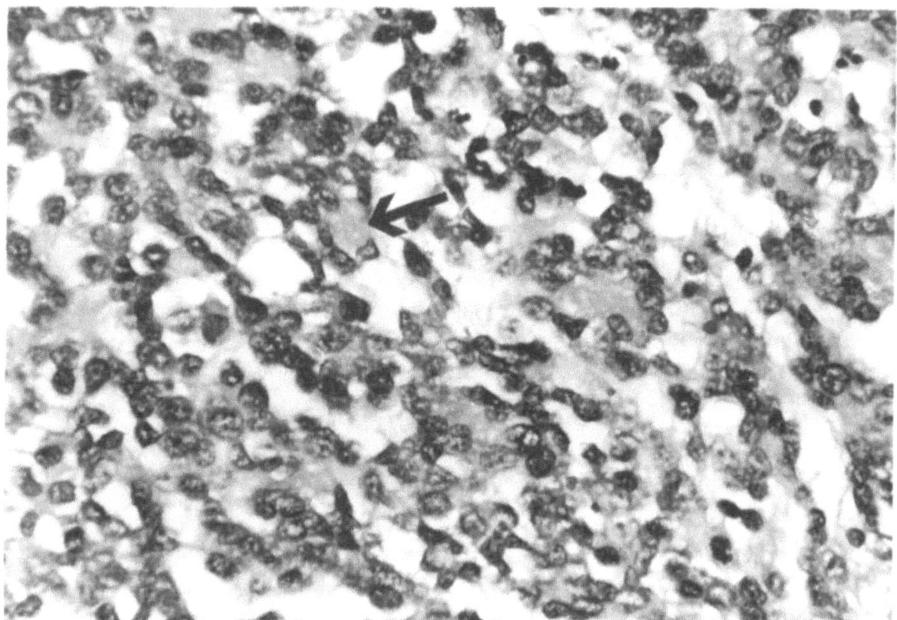

Fig. 9. Malignant thoracipulmonary tumor of childhood - small cells form occasional rosettes with central fibrillar material (arrow)

nuclei and moderate finely granular or clear cytoplasm and secondary (dark) cells with smaller, more hyperchromatic, irregular nuclei and minimal cytoplasm. The primary cells contain variable amounts of PAS-positive glycogen, either finely dispersed or en bloc but this is less conspicuous than in the bone variant. Electron microscopy confirms the presence of glycogen and shows occasional junctional complexes. The histogenesis of Ewing's sarcoma and the relationship between the conventional and soft tissue variants is uncertain [58].

Rhabdomyosarcoma. Although rhabdomyosarcoma is the commonest soft tissue tumor in children, primary chest wall or pleural involvement is uncommon [61]. Cells may have variably acidophilic cytoplasm, frequently with cytoplasmic glycogen, and electron microscopy may reveal bundles of alternating actin and myosin filaments. Immunochemical diagnosis depends on the demonstration of myosin, actin, desmin, or myoglobulin [58].

Bone Tumors

Virtually any type of bone tumor may occur in the thoracic skeleton. Those encountered most frequently are briefly described below. Detailed descriptions are given in standard texts [64, 65].

Tumors of Cartilage

These form the largest group of tumors of the thoracic skeleton [41, 42, 43, 55, 66, 67, 68]. About 80% arise in ribs and 20% in the sternum. In ribs they tend to arise near the costochondral junction and in the sternum more occur in the manubrium than the gladiolus.

Osteochondroma. Cartilage-capped exostoses comprise about one-fourth of all benign rib tumors. Hereditary multiple osteochondromatosis frequently affects the ribs. Lesions may be pedunculated or sessile and the bony component merges with cortical bone. The cap is of hyaline cartilage and endochondral ossification takes place at the junction.

Chondroma. Benign tumors of cartilage form the most common benign sternal tumors. They arise in the medulla and expand the cortex. Macroscopically they appear as bluish-gray, semitranslucent lobulated tissue and histologically they consist of mature cartilage with areas of calcification. Nuclei are uniform and lack mitotic activity.

Chondrosarcoma. This is the most common primary malignant tumor of the chest wall: 19% of chondrosarcomas in one large series were located in the ribs and sternum [68]. Some arise in preexisting benign lesions. Grossly most resemble benign chondromas and microscopically the distinction may be difficult. Nuclear atypia, with large or double nuclei and mitoses, is a better indication of malignancy than cellularity (Fig. 10).

Chondromyxoid Fibroma [44] *and Benign Chondroblastoma* [69]. These tumors rarely involve the chest wall but occasional cases are recorded.

218

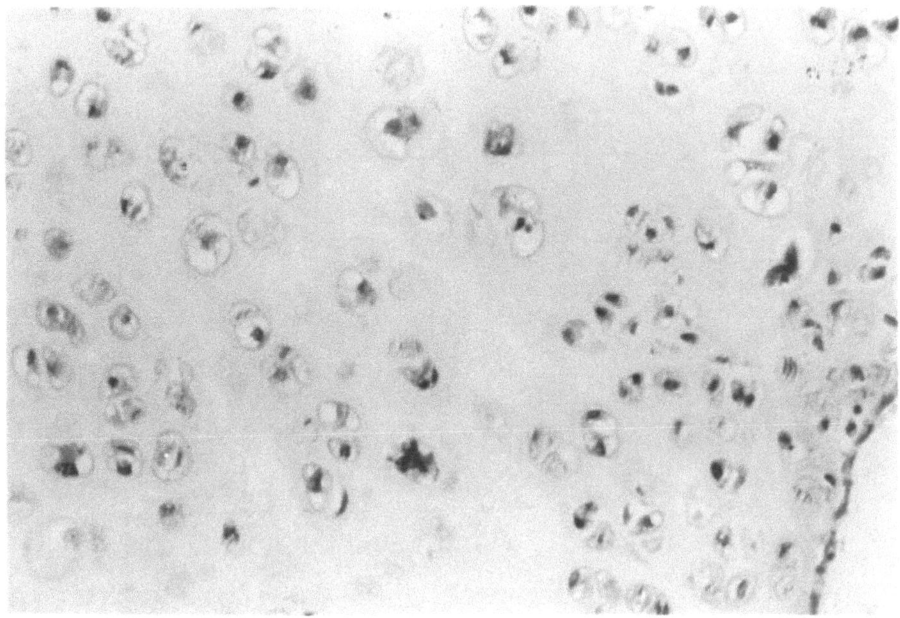

Fig. 10. Chondrosarcoma – although not particularly cellular, nuclei appear hyperchromatic and irregular with occasional mitoses

Tumors of Bone

Fibrous Dysplasia. Fibrous dysplasia, although not strictly speaking a neoplasm, accounts for one-third of all benign rib tumors, and 42% of all lesions occur in the ribs [44, 70]. The monostotic form has an equal sex incidence and usually presents before the age of 40. Multiple (polyostotic) unilateral fibrous dysplasia may be associated in females with increased pigmentation and precocious puberty (Albright's syndrome).

Typically lesions involve the posterior parts of the ribs as fusiform lytic swellings with erosion of the cortex. The cut surface is gray, soft, and gritty. Microscopically irregular spicules of woven bone, which lack osteoblastic rimming, are present in a spindle-cell, fibroblastic stroma (Fig. 11). The stroma may contain myxoid or cartilaginous areas and osteoclast-like giant cells may be present.

Benign Tumors and Tumors of Borderline Malignancy. Aneurysmal bone cyst [56, 57], osteoblastoma [43, 56, 67], osteoma [56], osteoid osteoma [56], chondroblastoma [56], nonossifying fibroma [64], and fibrous histiocytoma [65] rarely involve the thoracic wall. Giant cell tumors may occur in the ribs [42, 43] and histologically may closely resemble the bone lesions of hyperparathyroidism.

Osteogenic Sarcoma. Only about 3% of all osteosarcomas occur in the chest wall [69, 70], usually in the 2nd or 3rd decades. In older patients tumors may be associated with Paget's disease. The gross and microscopic appearances are very variable but the essential feature is the presence of neoplastic osteoblasts and the for-

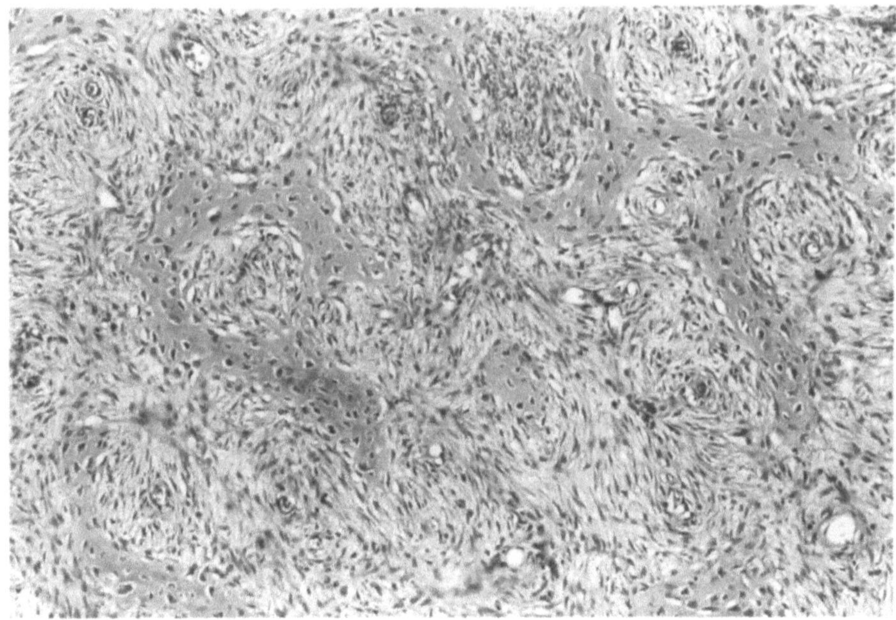

Fig. 11. Fibrous dysplasia – osteoid is formed in a background of cellular fibrous tissue

mation of osteoid. Cartilage may be present and spindle-cell areas may resemble fibrosarcoma or malignant fibrous histiocytoma. Vascular (angiomatoid) examples may be mistaken for aneurysmal bone cysts.

Ewing's Sarcoma [41, 42, 43, 56, 67]. In a recent large series 6.5% of Ewing's sarcomas were primary rib lesions [71]. Sternal involvement is rare. The appearances are described under soft tissue tumors. Metastatic neuroblastoma should always be excluded.

Tumors of Lymphoid and Histiocytic Origin

Myeloma and Plasmacytoma [41, 42, 43, 44, 56, 67]. Deposits of myeloma frequently produce multiple lytic lesions in ribs and sternum, making this the most common malignant tumor of the chest wall. Solitary plasmacytoma of bone is less frequent and in a high proportion of cases multifocal disease, with paraproteinemia and the other manifestations of multiple myeloma, eventually becomes evident [72]. The tissue appears soft and hemorrhagic and consists of closely packed plasma cells. The degree of cellular atypia varies greatly: in a well-differentiated tumor immunohistochemistry may be required to differentiate between a neoplastic and inflammatory origin by demonstrating the monotypic nature of the plasma cell population.

Histiocytosis-X (Eosinophilic Granuloma) [43, 44, 56, 66, 67, 73, 74]. Bone involvement is present in 80% of cases of histiocytosis-X. Ribs are more frequently involved in patients with multifocal disease whereas solitary eosinophilic granuloma

220

usually occurs in the skull and long bones. The lesions, which are more common in males, usually appear before the age of 20 and the prognosis is good. Eosinophilic granuloma originates in the medulla and erodes the cortex, occasionally extending into soft tissue. Macroscopically the tissue appears yellow or hemorrhagic and histologically the essential diagnostic feature is the presence of histiocytes with the characteristics of Langerhans cells. By electron microscopy they contain distinctive racquet-shaped pentalaminar inclusions (Birbeck granules) and by immunohistochemistry the presence of S-100 protein and the OKT6 antigen can be demonstrated. Variable numbers of eosinophils are present, often with eosinophil abscess formation, together with neutrophils, plasma cells, and lymphocytes. The presence of fibrous tissue may represent a healing stage.

Malignant Lymphoma [42, 44, 56]. The term "reticulum cell sarcoma" of bone is now regarded as obsolete and malignant lymphomas of bone should be classified according to the same criteria as lymphoma in other sites. Rib and sternal lesions account for only 3%-4% of recent series [75, 76]. About half are solitary bone lesions but in other patients lymphoma can be demonstrated elsewhere at the time of presentation. With immunohistochemical methods the distinction from Ewing's sarcoma and other small cell tumors should no longer present a problem.

Tumors of Vascular Origin

Benign Hemangioma: Although hemangiomas of bone are rare tumors, they feature in some series of chest wall tumors [56].

Angiosarcoma. Malignant vascular tumors are among the rarest of primary bone neoplasms. The term hemangioendothelioma is generally used to describe tumors with a more indolent course than angiosarcoma. Rare examples occurring in the ribs are recorded [77].

"Pseudotumors" of the Chest Wall

A number of nonneoplastic conditions may simulate chest wall neoplasms. These include hydatid disease [37], actinomycosis [78], osteomyelitis, and healing fracture with callus formation.

References

1. Wagner JC, Sleggs CA, Marchand P (1960) Diffuse pleural mesothelioma and asbestos exposure in the North Western Cape Province. Br J Ind Med 17: 260-271
2. Peterson JT, Greenberg SD, Buttler PA (1984) Non-asbestos related malignant mesothelioma. Cancer 54: 951-960
3. Brenner J, Sordillo PP, Magill GB (1981) Malignant mesothelioma in children - report of seven cases and review of the literature. Med Pediatr Oncol 9: 367-373
4. Jones JSP, Lund C, Planteydt HT (1985) Colour atlas of mesothelioma. MTP, Lancaster
5. Suzuki Y (1980) Pathology of human malignant mesothelioma. Semin Oncol 8: 268-282

6. Donna A, Betta PG (1981) Mesodermomas: a new embryological approach to primary tumors of coelomic surfaces. Histopathology 5: 31-44

7. Whitaker D, Shilkin KB (1984) Diagnosis of pleural malignant mesothelioma in life - a practical approach. J Pathol 143: 147-175

8. Kwee WS, Veldhuzan RW, Golding RP, Mullink H, Stam J, Donner R, Boon ME (1982) Histologic distinction between malignant mesothelioma, benign pleural lesion and carcinomae metastasis. Virchows Arch (Pathol Anat) 397: 287-299

9. Herbert A, Gallagher PJ (1982) Pleural biopsy in the diagnosis of malignant mesothelioma. Thorax 37: 816-821

10. Spriggs AI, Boddington MM (1968) The cytology of effusions. Heinemann, London

11. Tao L (1979) The cytopathology of mesothelioma. Acta Cytol 23: 209-213

12. Kwee WS, Veldhuzen RW, Alons CL, Morawetz F, Boon ME (1982) Quantitive and qualitative differences between benign and malignant mesothelial cells in pleural fluid. Acta Cytol 26: 401-406

13. Wang NS (1973) Electron microscopy in the diagnosis of pleural mesotheliomas. Cancer 31: 1046-1054

14. Suzuki Y, Churg J, Kannerstein M (1976) Ultrastructure of human malignant diffuse mesothelioma. Am J Pathol 85: 241-262

15. Warhol MJ, Hickey WF, Carson JM (1982) Malignant mesothelioma: ultrastructure distinction from adenocarcinoma. Am J Surg Pathol 6: 307-314

16. Dardick I, Srigley JR, McCaughey WTE, van Nostrand AWP, Ritchie AC (1984) Ultrastructure aspects of the histogenesis of diffuse and localized mesothelioma. Virchows Arch (Pathol Anat) 402: 373-388

17. Wagner JC, Munday DE, Harington JS (1962) Histochemical demonstration of hyaluronic acid in pleural mesotheliomas. J Pathol Bacteriol 84: 73-78

18. Wang N-S, Huang SN, Gold P (1979) Absence of carcinoembryonic antigen-like material in mesothelioma. Cancer 44: 937-943

19. Carson JM, Pinkus G (1982) Mesothelioma: profile of keratin proteins and carcinoembryonic antigen: an immunoperoxidase study of 20 cases of comparison with pulmonary adenocarcinomas. Am J Pathol 108: 80-87

20. Holden J, Churg A (1984) Immunohistochemical staining for keratin and carcinoembryonic antigen in the diagnosis of malignant mesothelioma. Am J Surg Pathol 8: 277-279

21. Loosli H, Hurlimann J (1984) Immunohistochemical study of malignant diffuse mesotheliomas of the pleura. Histopathology 8: 793-803

22. Gibbs AR, Harach R, Wagner JC, Jasani B (1985) Comparison of tumor markers in malignant mesothelioma and pulmonary adenocarcinoma. Thorax 40: 91-95

23. Blobel GA, Moll R, Franke WW, Kayser KW, Gould VE (1985) The intermediate filament cytoskeleton of malignant mesothelioma and its diagnostic significance. Am J Pathol 121: 235-247

24. To A, Dearnley DP, Ormerod MJ, Canti G, Coleman DV (1983) Indirect immunoalkaline phosphatase staining of cytologic smears of serous effusions for tumor marker studies. Acta Cytol 27: 109-113

25. Dalton WT, Zolliker AS, McCaughey WTE, Jacques J, Kannerstein M (1979) Localized primary tumors of the pleura. An analysis of 40 cases. Cancer 44: 1465-1475

26. Briselli M, Mark EJ, Dickersin R (1981) Solitary fibrous tumors of the pleura. Eight new cases and review of 360 cases in the literature. Cancer 47: 2678-2689

27. Said JW, Nasg G, Banks-Schlegal S, Sassoon AF, Shintaku IP (1984) Localized fibrous mesothelioma: an immunohistochemical and electron microscopic study. Hum Pathol 15: 440-443

28. Janssen JP, Wagenaar SJ Sc, van den Bosch JMM, Vanderschueren RGJRA, Planteydt HT (1985) Benign localized mesothelioma of the pleura. Histopathology 9: 309-313

29. Gupta RK, Paolini FA (1967) Liposarcoma of the pleura, report of a case with a review of the literature and views on histogenesis. Am Rev Respir Dis 95: 298-304

30. Evans AR, Wolstenholme RJ, Shettar SP, Yogish H (1985) Benign pleural liposarcoma. Thorax 40: 554-555

31. Yang H-Y, Weaver LL, Foti PR (1983) Primary malignant fibrous histiocytoma of the pleura. Acta Cytol 27: 683-687

32. Duhig JT (1969) Solitary rhabdomyosarcoma of the pleura. Report of a case with a note on the nomenclature of pleural tumors. J Thorac Surg 37: 236–241
33. Harwood TR, Gracey DR, Yokoo H (1976) Pseudomesotheliomatous carcinoma of the lung – a variant of peripheral lung cancer. Am J Clin Pathol 65: 159–167
34. Nishimoto Y, Tomohiko O, Saito K (1983) Pseudomesotheliomatous carcinoma of the lung with histochemical and immunohistochemical study. Acta Pathol Jpn 33: 415–423
35. Chernow B, Sahn SA (1977) Carcinomatous involvement of the pleura. An analysis of 96 patients. Am J Med 63: 695–702
36. Shepherd MP (1982) Thoracic metastases. Thorax 37: 366–370
37. Rami-Porta R, Bravo-Bravo JL, Aroca-Gonzolez MJ, Alix-Treuba A, Serrano-Munoz F (1985) Tumors and pseudotumors of the chest wall. Scand J Thorac Cardiovasc Surg 19: 97–103
38. Shuman LS, Libshutz HI (1984) Pictorial essay. Solid pleural manifestations of lymphoma. AJR 142: 269–273
39. Press GA, Glazer HS, Wasserman TH, Aronberg DJ, Lee JKT, Sagel SS (1985) Thoracic wall involvement by Hodgkin's disease and non-Hodgkin's lymphoma: CT evaluation. Radiology 157: 195–198
40. Enzinger FM, Weiss SW (1983) Soft tissue tumors. Mosby, St. Louis
41. Spear HC, Daughtry DC, Chesney JC (1960) Chest wall tumors: a review of clinical experiences with 30 cases. Dis Chest 37: 520–531
42. Watkins E, Gerard FP (1960) Malignant tumors involving chest wall. J Thorac Cardiovasc Surg 39: 117–129
43. Threlkel JB, Adkins RB (1971) Primary chest wall tumors. Ann Thorac Surg 11: 450–459
44. Teitelbaum SL (1969) Tumors of the chest wall. Surg Gynecol Obstet 129: 1059–1073
45. Teitelbaum SL (1972) Twenty years' experience with soft tissue sarcomas of the chest wall at a large institution. J Thorac Cardiovasc Surg 63: 585–586
46. Saini VK, Wahi PI (1964) Hourglass transmural type of intrathoracic lipoma. J Thorac Cardiovasc Surg 47: 600–604
47. Dalshiell TG, Payne WS, Hepper NGG, Soule EH (1978) Desmoid tumors of the chest wall. Chest 74: 157–162
48. Oberman HA, Oneal RM (1970) Fibrosarcoma of the chest wall following resection and irradiation of carcinoma of the breast. Am J Clin Pathol 53: 407–412
49. Bhatti MAK, Ferranti JW, Giekhinsky I, Norman JC (1985) Pleuropulmonary and skeletal lymphangiomatosis with chylothorax and chylopericardium. Ann Thorac Surg 40: 398–401
50. Allan PW, Enzinger FM (1972) Hemangioma of skeletal muscle. Cancer 29: 8–22
51. Ingianni G, Mack D, Harlacher A, Gullotta U (1981) Haemangiopericytoma of the chest wall – case report. Praxis Klin Pneumol 35: 234–236
52. Tandon RK, Stivastava VK, Pandey RP (1971) Haemangioendotheliosarcoma of the chest wall and pleural cavity. Indian J Canc 8: 205–207
53. Ximenes M, Miziara HL (1981) Haemangioendothelioma of the lung and pleura – report of 3 cases. Int Surg 66: 67–70
54. Vaughan R, Moussali H, Lodge KV (1982) Haemangiosarcoma of the chest wall. Thorax 37: 222–223
55. Lo TCM, Silverman ML, Edelstein A (1985) Postirradiation haemangiosarcoma of the chest wall. Acta Radiol (Oncol 24: 237–240
56. Ochsner A, Lucas GL, McFarland GD (1966) Tumors of the thoracic skeleton: review of 134 cases. J Thorac Cardiovasc Surg 52: 311–321
57. Marshall DG, Bains M (1980) Massive leiomyosarcoma of the chest wall in a young child. J Pediatr Surg 15: 666–669
58. Variend S (1985) Small cell tumors in childhood. J Pathol 145: 1–25
59. Askin FB, Rosai J, Sibley RK, Dehner LP, McAlister WH (1979) Malignant small cell tumor of the thoracopulmonary region in childhood. Cancer 43: 2435–2452
60. Gonzalez-Crussi F, Wolfson SL, Misingi K, Nakajima T (1984) Peripheral neuroectodermal tumors of the chest wall in childhood. Cancer 54: 2519–2527
61. Raney RB Jr, Ragab AH, Ruyman FB, Lindberg RD, Hays DM, Gehan EH, Soule EH (1982) Soft-tissue sarcoma of the trunk in childhood: results of the intergroup rhabdomyosarcoma study centre. Cancer 49: 2612–2616

62. McLeod RA, Dahlin DC (1979) Hamartoma (mesenchymoma) of the chest wall in infancy. Radiology 131: 657-661
63. Campbell AN, Waggert J, Mott MG (1982) Benign mesenchymoma of the chest wall in infancy. J Surg Oncol 21: 267-270
64. Spjut HJ, Dorfman HD, Fechner RE, Ackerman LV (1971) Tumors of bone and cartilage, (Atlas of tumor pathology, 2nd Ser., fasc. 5). Armed Forces Institute of Pathology, Washington DC
65. Spjut HJ, Dorfman HD, Fechner RE, Ackerman LV (1981) Tumors of bone and cartilage (Supplement), (Atlas of tumor pathology, 2nd Ser., fasc. 5). Armed Forces Institute of Pathology, Washington DC
66. Teitelbaum SL (1972) Twenty years' experience with intrinsic tumors of the bony thorax at a large institution. J Thorac Cardiovasc Surg 63: 776-782
67. Sabanathan S, Salama FD, Morgan WE, Harvey JA (1985) Primary chest wall tumors. Ann Thorac Surg 39: 4-15
68. O'Neal LW, Ackerman LV (1951) Cartilaginous tumors of ribs and sternum. J Thorac Surg 51: 71-108
69. Dahlin DC (1967) Bone Tumors: General aspects and data on 3,987 cases. 2nd edn. Thomas, Springfield
70. Pascuzzi CA, Dahlin DC, Clagett OT (1957) Primary tumors of the ribs and sternum. Surg Gynecol Obstet 104: 390-400
71. Thomas PRM, Foulkes MA, Gilula LA, Burgert EO, Evans RG, Kissane J, Nesbit ME, Pritchard DJ, Tefft M, Vietti TJ (1983) Primary Ewing's sarcoma of the ribs: a report from the intergroup Ewing's sarcoma study. Cancer 51: 1021-1027
72. Wiltshaw E (1976) The natural history of extramedullary plasmacytoma and its relation to solitary myeloma of bone and myelomatosis. Medicine 55: 217-238
73. Lichtenstein L (1953) Histocytosis X: integration of eosinophilic granuloma of bone, "Letterer-Siwe disease" and "Schüller-Christian disease" as related manifestations of a single nosologic entity. Arch Pathol 56: 84-102
74. Watanabe S, Shimosato Y, Nakajima T (1983) Proliferative disorders of histiocytes. In: Sommers SC, Rosen PP (eds) Malignant Lymphomas: a Pathology Annual Monograph. Appleton-Century-Crofts, Connecticut
75. Boston HC Jr, Dahlin DC, Ivins JC, Cupps RE (1974) Malignant lymphoma (so-called reticulum cell sarcoma) of bone. Cancer 34: 1131-1137
76. Dosoretz DE, Raymond AK, Murphy GF, Doppke KP, Schiller AZ, Wang CC, Suit HD (1982) Primary lymphoma of bone. Cancer 50: 1009-1014
77. Hartmann WH, Stewart FW (1962) Haemangioendothelioma of bone. Cancer 15: 846-854
78. Scully RE, Mark EJ, McNeely BU (1983) A young man with a mass involving the lung, pleura and chest wall. (Case 45-1983). N Engl J Med 309: 1171-1178

16. Primary Mediastinal Tumors

T. Treasure

Introduction

There are many tumors that can occur within the anatomical confines of the mediastinum, either primarily, or as a result of secondary spread. They include some pathological entities, perhaps typically found in, or even specific to, the mediastinum. Some of these are extremely rare. In addition, the multifocal malignant diseases, the common cancers, and many less common ones, can spread to, or present with the clinical features of, mediastinal involvement. The presenting features, symptoms, and signs are usually a result of the anatomical site and invasive behavior of the tumor rather than its exact pathological characteristics. In this section, most emphasis will therefore be placed on presentation, diagnosis, and the principles of management.

Anatomical Boundaries

The term "mediastinum" covers all the structures and tissues below the thoracic inlet and above the diaphragm, behind the sternum and in front of the vertebral column, and is bounded on either side by the mediastinal pleura. For descriptive purposes, the mediastinum is subdivided, arbitrarily, into the superior mediastinum, above the level of the manubriosternal joint; the anterior mediastinum, anterior to the pericardium; the middle mediastinum, within the pericardium; and the posterior mediastinum, lying posterior to it. Structures lying in the paravertebral gutters are usually included within the posterior mediastinum (Fig. 1).

The heart, great vessels, trachea, and esophagus are, of course, within this anatomical territory, but for pathological and surgical purposes it is convenient and much more useful to discuss the diseases of those structures in their own right. We are left with the thymus gland, lymphatics, sympathetic and other nerves, and the interstitial areolar and connective tissue which fills the interstices between the major structures that crowd this anatomical area.

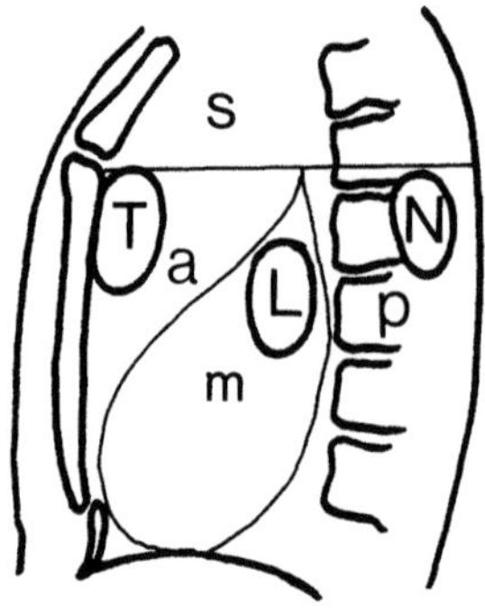

Fig. 1. A diagrammatic view of the left side of the mediastinum as if from a lateral chest X-ray. The lower case letters *(s, a, m, p)* identify the superior, anterior, middle, and posterior parts of the mediastinum respectively. The upper-case letters show the typical sites of thymoma and teratoma *(T)*, lymphoma involving the hilum *(L)*, and neurogenic tumors *(N)*

Classification

The major classifications of the primary tumors characteristic of this area are given in Table 1.

Thymoma

The commonest primary tumor of the mediastinum is thymoma, located in the superior-anterior compartment. Histological examination does not help in distinguishing benign from malignant lesions: malignancy is determined by invasive behavior of the tumor. Local invasion into the pericardium, sternum, pleura, lung, and blood vessels is common, but metastases are rare. Resection is therefore always advisable when a thymoma is detected because biopsy gives no reassurance about subsequent behavior of the tumor. Resection may, however, be impossible if the tumor is already invading major structures, or it may be undesirable for other reasons. Thymoma may respond to radiotherapy.

Neurogenic Tumors

These are typically in the posterior mediastinum, arising from intercostal nerves or the sympathetic chain, in the paravertebral gutter. Pressure on adjacent structures

Table 1. Classification of primary mediastinal tumors (from [1])

Thymoma	25%
Neurogenic tumors	25%
Lymphoma	16%
Germ-cell neoplasm	13%
Mesenchymal tumor	9%
Endocrine tumor	8%
Primary carcinoma	4%

226

may cause pain, but most of these tumors are detected on roentgenography while they are still asymptomatic. They include neuroblastoma, a highly invasive childhood tumor; neurofibroma and neurilemoma (schwannoma), which arise from nerve sheaths and fibers and have a wide range of behavior; pheochromocytoma, which arises from the sympathetic chain and is associated with the characteristic endocrine syndrome; and ganglioneuroma, which usually occurs in childhood and is said to not grow further after puberty. If the tumor originates near an intervertebral foramen, there may be a substantial proportion within the canal, a "dumbbell" tumor. Evidence of erosion of a pedicle and enlargement of the foramen should always be sought with tumors in the paravertebral gutter.

Lymphoma

Lymphomata of all types may originate in or involve the mediastinal lymphatics. Surgical resection is not indicated but adequate tissues for thorough histological assessment should be obtained and treatment should then be with whatever combination of radiotherapy and chemotherapy is judged best for the particular histological type.

Germ-cell Neoplasm

These tumors are usually found anteriorly and include the most differentiated form of dermoid cyst, which differentiates along ectodermal lines and characteristically contains teeth and hair. A careful search usually reveals muscle or cartilage, indicating that they are part of the spectrum of teratomata which contain a mixture of tissues, of all three germ layers. About 80% are benign but may cause trouble by compression. Elevated serum levels of α-fetoprotein, β-human chorionic gonadotrophin, and carcinoembryonic antigen are typical of malignant teratodermoid tumors. A blood sample for these markers should always be taken in young males (<40 years) with an anterior mediastinal mass. If the serum levels are elevated, this is diagnostic of a germ-cell tumor.

Mesenchymal Tumors

About 5% of the mediastinal tumors are mesenchymal in origin, and of these, half are malignant. Lipomas are usually located in the anterior mediastinum, while liposarcomas tend to occur in the posterior compartment. Fibrosarcoma, liposarcoma, and mesothelioma are other examples of malignant tumors.

Endocrine Tumor

The most common example is intrathoracic extension of a thyroid tumor; true mediastinal thyroid tumors are rare. About 10% of all parathyroid adenomata are in the mediastinum, usually anteriorly, amongst thymic tissue.

Symptoms and Signs

In countries with either widely available health screening programs, or a readiness to perform chest roentgenograms as a preoperative routine and for minor ailments, an increasing number of mediastinal masses are detected in asymptomatic patients. It is interesting to note, however, that as many as 95% of these coincidentally discovered lesions are benign. The tumors that present with symptoms, in particular with pain, are much more likely to be malignant.

In many instances there are relatively nonspecific symptoms such as cough or pain. There are also several characteristic modes of presentation.

Superior Vena Cava Compression

Tumors of the mediastinum which grow in the restricted space behind the sternum cause compression. The superior vena cava is the vessel with the lowest pressure, and therefore is the first to produce symptoms of obstruction. The typical features are secondary to venous engorgement of the upper extremities, and include edema of the head and neck, particularly the eyelids, which is at its worst in the morning and improves after a while in the upright position. The venous distension, however, persists even when the patient is upright. There is often cyanosis due to the poor flow in the superficial capillaries and dilated collaterals may be seen over the chest wall. At its worst, it may cause engorgement of the brain with resulting neurological impairment. This symptom, when due to malignant disease, is rapidly alleviated by radiotherapy, so tissue diagnosis is important. The commonest cause of the syndrome is bronchial carcinoma, either with direct extension from the right upper lobe, or with generalized lymphatic spread. In benign disease, surgery may be attempted to relieve localized obstruction, but collateral channels will often open with time, relieving the symptoms. Attempts at surgical bypass from the jugular or innominate veins above the obstruction to the right atrium below it are rarely successful, and not justified other than in a few carefully selected cases.

Tracheo-esophageal Compression

Extrinsic compression or, less commonly, invasion of the trachea or esophagus, may cause presentation with dyspnea, stridor, or dysphagia. As with superior vena cava obstruction, radiotherapy can provide useful palliation, while surgical relief of compression from malignant causes is not of great benefit. Insertion of stents into either hollow viscus may relieve obstruction, but must be carefully considered, because results are not predictably good.

Invasion of Nerves

Invasion of the vagus or recurrent laryngeal nerve on the left may cause a hoarse voice due to cord paralysis; invasion of the phrenic nerve may cause paralysis of a hemidiaphragm; and sympathetic nerve involvement causes Horner's syndrome. All are features of malignancy, are irreversible, and are usually contraindications to any attempt at surgical relief.

Pericardial Involvement

Direct invasion of the pericardium, most characteristically with malignant thymoma, may cause pain and the features of pericarditis, including ECG changes. Bleeding into the pericardium results in cardiac compression and the clinical signs of tamponade. Cardiac dysrhythmias, typically atrial fibrillation, may also result.

Chylothorax

The uncommon finding of an opaque, fatty, or milky fluid on tapping a pleural effusion, i.e., the discovery of chylothorax, suggests a mediastinal tumor obstructing the thoracic duct and its major collaterals. This is usually due to extensive, malignant tumor, possibly of lymphatic origin.

Paraplegia

Neurogenic tumors, originating in the paravertebral gutter, may have intraspinal as well as thoracic components, the so-called dumbbell tumors. The intrathoracic component has plenty of room and may cause no symptoms at a stage when the intraspinal growth is causing severe compression, and results in paraplegia.

Myasthenia Gravis

The association between myasthenia and thymoma is a curious one. In patients with myasthenia, screened for thymic tumors, a lesion is found in less than 20%. Patients with a thymoma have an incidence of myasthenia of about 30%. Of course, series collected by neurologists and those collected by thoracic surgeons are very difficult to compare, and both of these estimates may be unrepresentative.

Endocrine Syndromes

Pheochromocytoma may occur in the chest, usually in the paravertebral gutter, and may present with paroxysmal hypertension. Other neurogenic tumors, such as ganglioneuroma and neuroblastoma, may also have systemic effects, such as sweating, flushing, hypertension, and diarrhea.

Other Systemic Effects

Thymoma has been associated with red-cell aplasia and hypogammaglobulinemia. Fever is a feature of mediastinal lymphoma.

Investigation

Routine Radiology

Standard posteroanterior and lateral chest roentgenograms provide a large amount of information about some of these tumors, particularly if they lie well anteriorly of posteriorly. Tumors overlying the hilum are much more difficult to evaluate. The addition of swallowed barium will help in the evaluation of superior and posterior lesions, especially if dysphagia has been one of the clinical features.

Tomography

Conventional tomography is of value in some cases where the lesion cannot be separated from related structures on routine films.

Nuclear Imaging

If a method is available to mark a particular tissue with a radiopharmaceutical, this will help in confirming the nature of the mass and identifying its position. Thyroid tissue, which will take up radioactive iodine, is the best example, and more recently, pheochromocytomata have been reliably imaged with ^{131}I-labeled meta-iodobenzylguanidine (MIBG).

Computed Tomography

There is no doubt that this technique is very valuable in imaging mediastinal masses, and with the aid of intravascular contrast medium and skilled interpretation of attenuation densities, a large amount of information can be gleaned. It does not, however, replace a histological diagnosis, and there are many examples where, although the lesion has been skilfully imaged, the diagnosis and, therefore, the prognosis and management have not been greatly advanced.

Angiography

If there is real doubt about the nature of a lesion, arterial or pulmonary angiography may save an unnecessary, inappropriate, or hazardous surgical exploration of a vascular mass in the belief that it is a solid tumor. Venous angiography is also valuable in defining the site and nature of superior vena caval obstruction.

Bronchoscopy

In any patient with respiratory symptoms, or in the investigation of a mass in the upper part of the mediastinum or near the hila, bronchoscopy is essential for diagnosis and assessment of the lesion. If evidence of extrinsic compression is found, this helps in localization of the mass, but may still leave the operator without a tissue diagnosis.

Percutaneous Biopsy

Possible approaches include fine needle aspiration or cutting needle biopsy, under the guidance of an image intensifier or ultrasonography. Many radiologists are reluctant to use these techniques in the mediastinum or hila for fear of striking a large blood vessel. Tissue diagnosis is more often in the hands of the surgical team.

Mediastinoscopy

Through a small, transverse, cervical incision, a plane can be developed immediately on the trachea, and a specially designed speculum passed down into the mediastinum and as far as the hilum, on the right. Lymph nodes may be removed for histology and solid masses of tumor biopsied. Our own policy is to always aspirate through a long needle before taking tissue from the depths of the mediastinum, because of the number of large vessels close to the mediastinoscope.

Anterior Mediastinotomy

This technique supplements mediastinoscopy and is more usually performed on the left, where the hilum is less accessible due to its relationship with the aortic arch. We approach the mediastinum through the second interspace, cutting the intercostal muscles, much preferring this approach to the alternative method which involves resecting costal cartilage. The internal mammary artery may be divided if access is required more medially. Through this incision the nodes under the aortic arch may be biopsied and disease in the hilum or anterior mediastinum may be assessed.

Surgical Exploration

If other attempts at biopsy fail, or reveal a lesion best dealt with by surgery, operating may be planned. Advanced malignancy in the mediastinum is usually not helped by surgery, but localized malignancy or tumors with malignant potential should be considered for resection. The best approach to the anterior or superior mediastinum is through a median sternotomy. The posterior mediastinum should be approached through a posterolateral thoracotomy at an appropriate level. It is wise to plan the operation carefully, because the range of problems that can be encountered is considerable.

Reference

1. Sabiston DC, Oldham HN (1983) The Mediastinum. In: Sabiston DC, Spencer FC (eds) Gibbon's Surgery of the Chest. 4th edn. Saunders, Philadelphia London, p 407

17. Chest Wall Tumors

T. Treasure

Introduction

The skin and each of the connective tissues of the chest wall may develop malignant disease, each appropriate to the particular tissue. Treatment is as for any other area, and it is only when surgical management results in a defect or impairment of the mechanics of the chest wall that this becomes a specialist chest problem. The tumors that particularly involve the thoracic surgeon are, therefore, primary growths of the ribs and sternum.

The majority of primary tumors of the chest wall fall into the classification of chondroma or chondrosarcoma. Tumors involving the sternum are almost without exception malignant. Those of the ribs often recur if locally excised and many, in time, behave as malignant tumors with invasion and pleural seeding. Histological diagnosis may be very difficult, and even among experts there may be differences of opinion. Osteogenic sarcoma of the chest wall is extraordinarily rare, and there are a number of other primary tumors, similarly uncommon, that have been reported.

Presenting Symptoms and Signs

The usual presentation is of a palpable lump, hard and painless or slightly tender. If it is hot, the possibility of an infected lesion should be considered. A hot, pulsatile swelling over the sternum may be due to a mycotic or luetic aneurysm, and this possibility should be remembered before ill-considered attempts at biopsy. Alternatively, thyroid or renal secondary tumors can present in this way.

Lytic lesions are usually secondaries, those in breast and bronchus being two of the commonest types. They are usually recognized on roentgenography but may present as pathological fractures. Solitary plasmacytoma of the sternum or rib has been reported.

Investigation

Routine chest roentgenograms may not be particularly helpful in the assessment of chest wall tumors. Tomograms and oblique views of the ribs are usually necessary, and should be planned in discussion with the radiologist. CT scanning is helpful, but not necessary for management.

Surgical Management

Chondrosarcoma of the chest wall should be surgically removed whenever feasible because the response to radiotherapy and chemotherapy is poor, and the tumors have a relentless pattern of locally invasive growth. The practical points apply, in general, to the management of other chest wall tumors.

The first issue is whether preoperative tissue diagnosis will help in the management. As stated above, histological classification may be difficult, and the separation of benign from malignant lesions is not always easy. If resection is practicable and seen as the best way of dealing with the tumor, then it is best to resort to excision biopsy in the first instance, knowing that local removal of apparently benign chondromata is associated with a high incidence of recurrence. This avoids the anxiety about seeding into a biopsy incision or needle track and the surgical problem of knowing how to deal with a less than ideally sited biopsy incision, when the definitive operation is being performed.

Nevertheless, chest wall resection for tumor may be very extensive, and under many circumstances the patient and surgeon would prefer to have histological confirmation of some sort before proceeding.

In planning surgical resection, local recurrence is the problem which has to be anticipated. It appears that the tumor may spread in the bone marrow, periosteum, or tissue planes, and the principle is that the whole of the rib (or ribs) involved and the healthy ribs above and/or below should be resected for a length well clear of the width of the tumor.

The Incision

It is best to place the incision so that it does not overlie the defect in the chest wall. Thought must also be given to the possible need to extend the incision for added access, how muscles may be spared, and finally, how the wound is to be closed. Use of flaps for closure is worth considering and planning for.

234

Resection

Through an intercostal incision, away from the tumor, the tumor's inner content may be palpated. Uninvolved overlying muscles may be spared and mobilized as necessary. A full-thickness panel of chest wall is removed, following the rules outlined above.

Closure

Surprisingly large defects are tolerated, especially deep to the scapula, near the costal margin, or deep to thick musculature, where respiratory paradox is minimized. Closure is helped by prosthetic material such as Marlex (C.R.Bard, Billerica) and home-made plates of acrylic or metal can be devised. The use of wires, such as are employed to close chest incisions, is tempting, but with regular movement they fatigue, leaving sharp ends with potentially damaging consequences. Finally, for an elective procedure such as this, collaboration with a surgeon familiar with plastic surgial techniques and the use of myocutaneous flaps may help. The wound should be closed with underwater seal drainage as a general principle, and it is wisest to leave the patient intubated until fully recovered from the anesthetic, so that the functional effect of any chest wall paradox can be assessed.

18. Malignant Mesothelioma

M. E. Hodson

Introduction

Primary tumors of the pleura are rare compared with carcinoma of the bronchus. The most common pleural tumor is a metastatic deposit from carcinoma of the lung or from carcinomas elsewhere in the body. Benign connective tissue tumors, such as fibromas and hemangiomas, occur, as does another benign tumor which is composed of fibrous tissue and mesothelial cells and is often called a "benign mesothelioma". It is the malignant counterpart of this tumor, the "malignant mesothelioma", which will be considered here. It has often been suggested that the term "mesothelioma" should be restricted to the malignant tumor, and that is how the term is used here.

Epidemiology

In most cases mesothelioma is related to asbestos exposure [1]. The term asbestos comes from the Greek *asbesta,* meaning unconsumable. Asbestos has been used for thousands of years, particularly for its fibrous and heat-resistant properties. By the mid-1970s, 5 million tons were mined per year. Asbestos consists of a number of naturally occurring fibrous silicates. There are two varieties:

1. The serpentine group, e.g., chrysotile, or white asbestos. This is mainly hydrated magnesium silicate and comprises over 90% of the asbestos mined.
2. The amphibole group.
   a) Crocidolite, or blue asbestos, which is generally thought to be the most dangerous.
   b) Amosite, or brown asbestos.
   c) Anthophyllite, found only in Finland.
   d) Tremolite.
   e) Actinolite.

The amphiboles are mainly composed of ferrous-ferric silicates. Crocidolite has a straight fiber which readily penetrates to the pleura, whereas chrysotile is a thicker and more curled fiber. Asbestos is widely used because of its fire-resistant properties, and for the preparation of paints, textiles, cements, plastics, and brake and clutch linings. The majority of asbestos mined is from South Africa, the USSR, and Canada. Workers most at risk are those in the asbestos mining and processing industry, and those involved in transporting the fibers. Also at risk are some of those who work in the building and textile industries and demolition workers. Almost all urban dwellers have some asbestos bodies in their lungs at autopsy.

Patients with mesothelioma have a higher count of asbestos fibers in their lungs than do controls [2]. There may only be a history of trivial asbestos exposure and often this has occurred 20-40 years before the mesothelioma develops. People living near asbestos mines and members of the family of asbestos workers who handle dusty clothes are also at risk. Some sources of asbestos exposure go unrecognized for many years, such as gas mask assemblies [3].

Other fibers may cause mesothelioma. In the villages of Karain, in Turkey, the dangerous material appears to be zeolite [4], and probably other dangerous fibers, possibly some of them man-made, have still to be identified [5]. There are also definitely a number of cases of mesothelioma without a history of asbestos exposure [6].

Mesothelioma is not the only disease associated with asbestos exposure. Pulmonary fibrosis, carcinoma of the bronchus, pleural plaques, and gastrointestinal tumors also have a higher incidence among people exposed to asbestos dust.

Some workers have suggested that patients who develop a mesothelioma may have some underlying immunological abnormality. However, recent work [7] suggests that the abnormalities of immune function detected are due to advanced malignant disease, rather than a causal factor.

Pathology

The tumor grows in diffuse sheets of thick tissue, encasing the lung (Fig. 1). The tumor infiltrates between the fissures and spreads into the mediastinum and the diaphragm, and it can invade the pericardium and the heart. The tumor may invade the lung and can become bilateral. Areas of collapse and pneumonia occur in the affected lung. Large pleural effusions are common. Metastases occur in mediastinal and hilar lymph nodes in about 50% of cases [7]. Blood-borne spread to other organs used to be considered rare, but it is now well recognized that metastases may occur in liver, adrenal, kidney, brain, bone, meninges, and other organs [8–10]. Histologically, the tumor may be of several types [11] (see Chap. on "Pathology of Tumors of Pleura and Chest Wall").

Clinical Features

The clinical behavior of this tumor is now well recognized, and varies with the different histological types of mesothelioma. Epithelial mesotheliomas are associated with clinical features more characteristic of carcinomas than sarcomas including

238

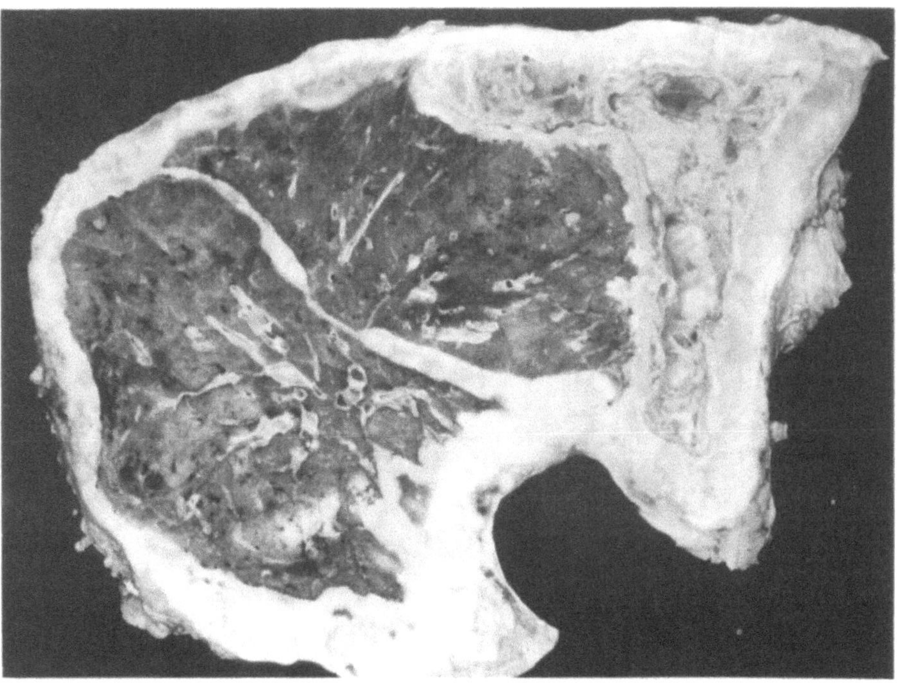

Fig. 1. Mesothelioma: a specimen showing the tumor encasing the lung

spread of tumor by direct extension, large pleural effusions, contralateral pleural effusions, ascites, metastases to regional lymph nodes, and occasional responses to radiotherapy. By contrast, sarcomatous mesotheliomas are associated with clinical features more like sarcomas, namely, there are more distant metastases, little or no pleural effusions, and a shorter survival [12]. It also appears that the epithelial type of tumor has a better prognosis than the sarcomatous type [12, 13] (Fig. 2).

In the series reported by Law et al. [10], 78 patients (61%) presented with large pleural effusions, whereas the remaining 49 cases had no or little effusion. They noted that the patients who presented with a large effusion presented early, when they were not very ill, and experienced dyspnea, whereas the patients without a pleural effusion tended to present later, complaining of chest pain, with or without dyspnea, and by that time they were sicker with weight loss, fever, and evidence of tumor extension. The erythrocyte sedimentation rate (ESR) was significantly higher in this second group of patients. Patients can also present with weight loss, hemoptysis, intermittent episodes of chest pain, fever, or a spontaneous pneumothorax.

At the time of presentation, the disease is nearly always extensive. CT scans performed by Law et al. [10] showed the majority of patients had disease not only in the chest wall, but also extending to the mediastinum, diaphragm, and lung. Physical signs at the time of presentation are usually those of a pleural effusion.

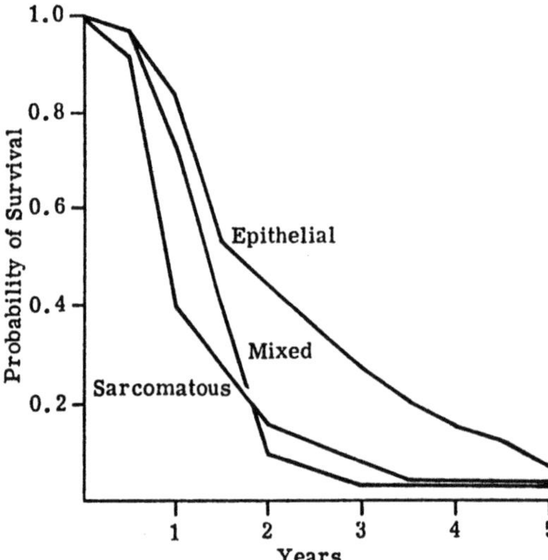

Fig. 2. Mesothelioma: the effect of histology on prognosis

However, patients who present later may also have signs of paraplegia, superior vena caval obstruction, Horner's syndrome, or bronchial obstruction. A few patients have finger clubbing.

Diagnosis

Radiology

The chest radiograph commonly shows a massive pleural effusion, which may initially hide the mesothelioma until after chest aspiration has been performed. Scalloped masses may then be discernable along the costal margin and on the mediastinal surface of the pleura (Fig. 3a, b). If exposure to asbestos has been heavy, pleural plaques may be found on the opposite pleura. There may be some contraction of the affected hemithorax, and the diaphragm may be raised. CT scans (Fig. 4) performed on patients with mesothelioma show a good correlation with thoracotomy and autopsy findings, but may not be superior over plain chest radiographs in delineation of the tumor. The greater sensitivity of CT is of limited value when the tumor is extensive, and the CT is not particularly helpful in detecting diaphragmatic involvement [15].

Tissue Diagnosis

Examination of cytological fluid and small samples of tissue obtained by needle biopsy are not usually very helpful in the diagnosis [10, 16] and can easily be con-

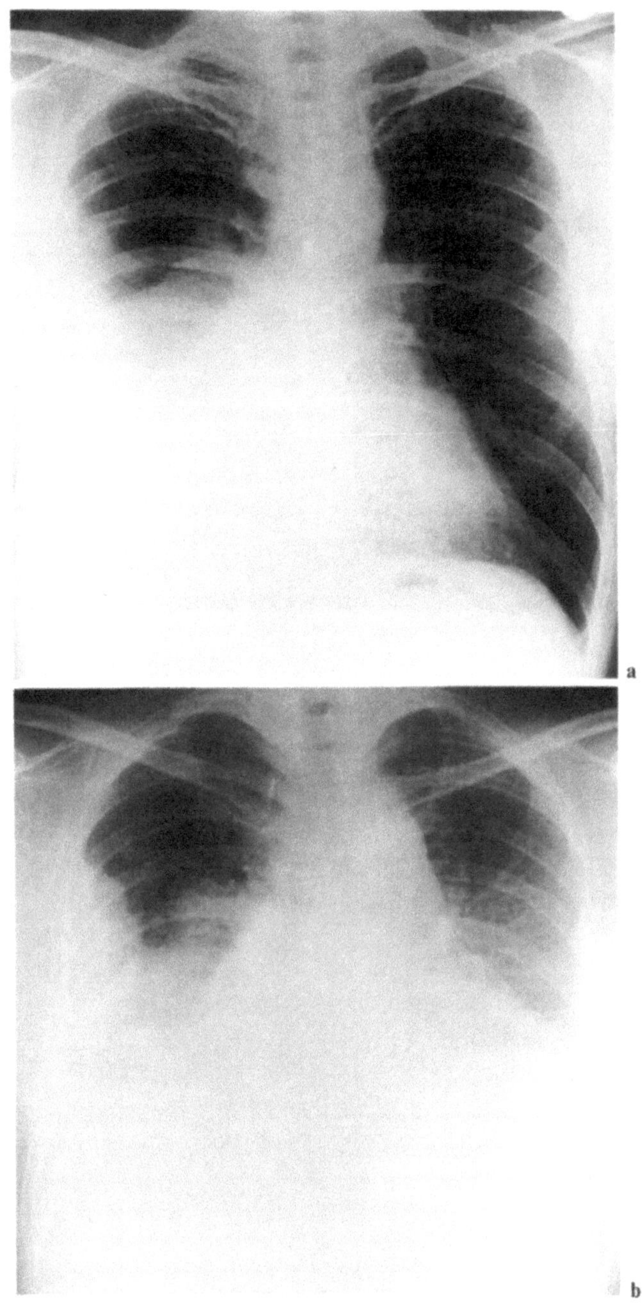

Fig.3a, b. Mesothelioma – chest radiographs: **a** There is an effusion *on the right* which overlies the extensive nodular tumor involving the pleura, both laterally and against the mediastinal surface. The *left side* is normal. **b** There is now an effusion at the left base, although the pleura is thickened. The typical nodularity is not yet apparent. Following aspiration, the extent of the right-sided mesothelioma is now visible on the lateral chest wall and diaphragm, and on the mediastinal pleura

241

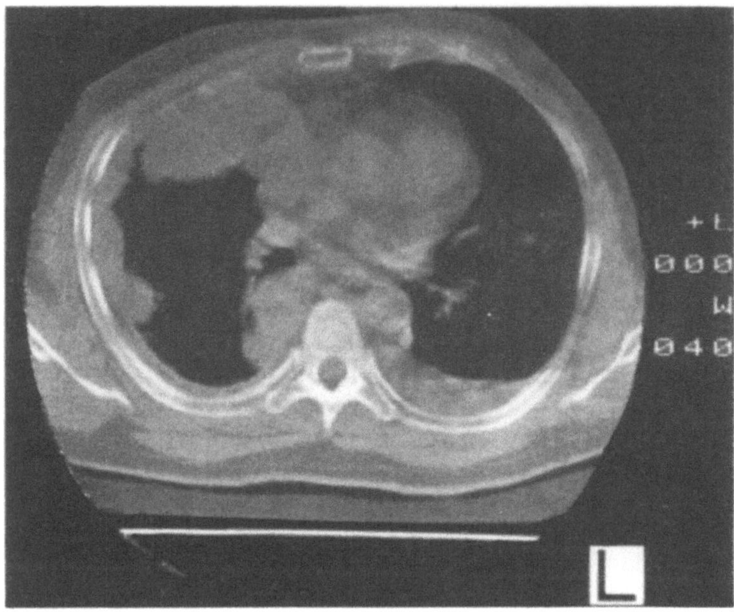

Fig. 4. Mesothelioma: CT scan below the carina shows massive involvement of the pleura, circumferentially constricting the lung. There is also an effusion posteriorly *on the left*

fused with adenocarcinoma. It is essential to distinguish mesothelioma from metastases of primaries in the lymphatic system, ovary, or thyroid. The most reliable way to obtain a definite histological diagnosis is by thoracoscopy, open biopsy, or decortication, done at the time of thoracotomy. The success rate of diagnostic procedures are quoted by Law et al. [10] as follows:

Closed pleural biopsy	21%
Needle biopsy	50%
Thoracoscopy	57%
Open pleural biopsy	88%
Decortication	98%

It has been persistently stated that following surgical intervention the tumor will grow through the site of the incision causing painful nodules [17]. However, that has not been our experience [10]. In our series of 140 patients, 94 of whom had thoracotomy, we did not find infiltration of tumor through aspiration sites and thoracotomy scars.

As the histological appearance of a mesothelioma can resemble that of an adenocarcinoma, special histological tests have to be performed. In an alcohol-fixed preparation of tissue it is found that a metachromatic acid mucopolysaccharide is secreted by mesotheliomas, which can be removed by prior digestion with hyaluronidase. Secretions are also positive in adenocarcinoma when stained by the PAS method, and with alcian blue, but this cannot be altered by prior hyaluronidase digestion [18].

242

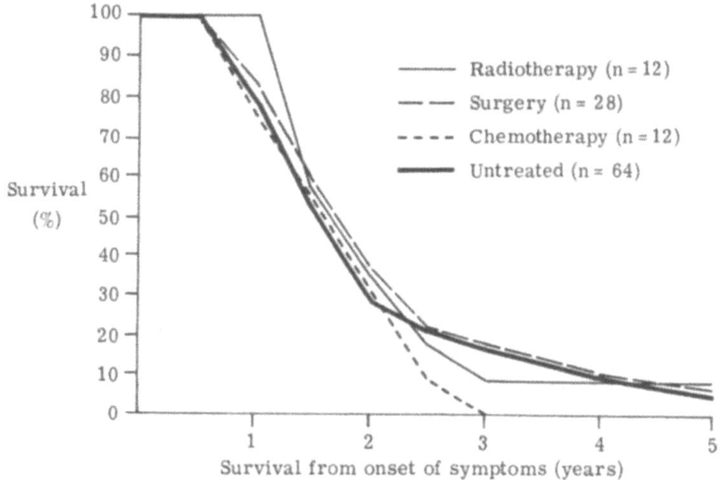

Fig. 5. Mesothelioma: the effect of treatment

Staging

Mesothelioma is conventionally stages as follows: Stage 1 is confined to the parietal pleura of one hemothorax. In stage II, there is invasion of chest wall, mediastinum, or intrathoracic lymph nodes. In stage III, there is spread to peritoneum, the other hemithorax, or extrathoracic lymph nodes. In stage IV, there is hematogenous spread.

Treatment

Curative

De Larie et al. [19] have reported a 27%, 2-year survival following pleuropneumonectomy for mesothelioma. However, most other authors report high mortality following this operation, and no improvement in survival. Indeed, Law et al. [20] studied 116 patients and compared the effect of treatment by pleurectomy, chemotherapy, multivoltage radiotherapy, and symptomatic treatment only, and found survival not to be improved by any of the treatments used (Fig. 5). The median survival for all groups was about 19 months. There was a suggestion by Brenner et al. [13] that very occasionally, in a localized lesion, local surgical treatment may be useful, but in the vast majority of patients it does not prolong survival. Radiotherapy may occasionally relieve chest wall pain, and chemotherapy is of minimal value [21]. Lerner et al. [22] reported the experience of the Eastern Cooperative Oncology Group, that in 96 patients the response to chemotherapy in most cases was nonexistent, and in those patients who did respond the response was very limited.

Brenner et al. [13] reported that only three patients responded to chemotherapy out of 111 treated. We currently have no treatment that will cure this disease, and research must be continued to find effective treatments; meanwhile, our efforts must be toward palliation [10].

Symptomatic Treatment

Recurrent pleural effusions – these reaccumulate rapidly after aspiration, and it is very unpleasant for a patient to keep needing recurrent aspirations. The success rate for treating recurrent pleural effusions as reported by Law et al. [10] was: intrapleural cytoxic or radioactive gold 0%, radiotherapy 50%, decortication 88%, and in five patients treated with aspiration and intrapleural bleomycin, followed by suction, there were no recurrences. It would seem sensible, therefore, that if a patient needs surgery for diagnosis, a decortication should be performed at the same time to prevent recurrent pleural effusions. If a patient is reaching the terminal stage, then intrapleural bleomycin (80–100 mg), preceded by aspiration to dryness and followed by suction, appears to be a successful form of treatment.

Pneumothorax – this is a rare complication and when present it can often be treated by intercostal drainage, but in some cases decortication is necessary.

Skin deposits – when they occur they are not always painful. If they are painful in some patients, this can be relieved by radiotherapy; in others, analgesics are necessary.

Fever and sweating – this is a problem in a number of patients even in the absence of infection. Indomethacin, or prednisolone, may be of some benefit, and prednisolone also improves the appetite and sense of well-being.

Pain – chest pain is probably the most difficult symptom to control in patients with mesothelioma. It can often be constant and severe long before the terminal stage. Occasionally, radiotherapy is helpful. Initially, simple analgesics should be used, but later these will not control the symptoms. Various procedures, such as intercostal nerve blocks, paravertebral blocks, and cervical anterior spinothalamic tractotomies have been used, but in the experience of the author, these are rarely successful. The best way to control severe pain is to use opiates. Patients can be maintained on oral morphine at home for many months. This is the most effective way to control their pain, and to give them a reasonable quality of life for the time remaining to them.

Prognosis

Most reported series report the median survival from time of first symptoms as being between 1 and 2 years [6, 14]. Treatment, as yet, does not influence these distressing figures. Malignant mesothelioma is a rapidly lethal disease, nonresponsive to treatment, for which we require new therapies. Most patients die of respiratory failure, arrhythmias, or cachexia [23]. It is established, however, that patients with

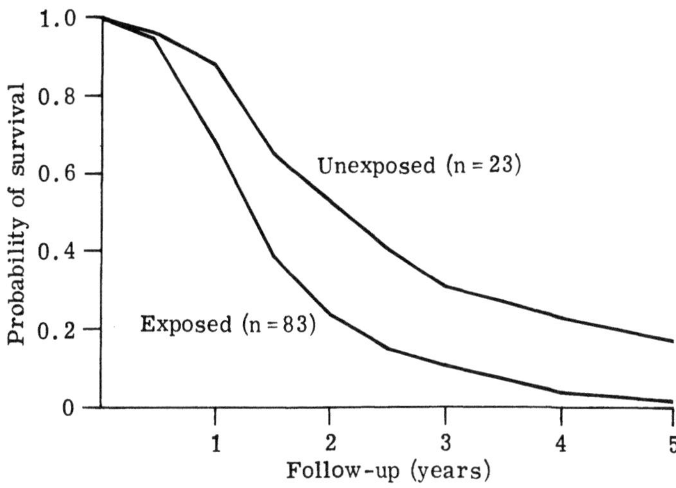

Fig. 6. Mesothelioma: survival in relation to exposure or non-exposure to asbestos

an epithelial type of histology have a better survival [12] than those with a sarcomatous histology.

Patients without a history of asbestos exposure [6] (Fig. 6) have better survival than those with such a history, median survival from time of first symptoms being 25 months in those without a history of exposure, compared with 15 months in those who had a history of definite asbestos exposure. Patients with limited disease have a better survival than those with extensive disease [13].

Conclusions

Patients with mesothelioma present commonly with the symptoms of a large pleural effusion, and less often with localized chest pain. Diagnosis by needle biopsy is often unsuccessful, and many patients require surgical procedures, such as open biopsy or thoracotomy. No treatment has yet been shown convincingly to prolong life, and efforts should be concentrated on relieving symptoms. The management of recurrent pleural effusions by intrapleural bleomycin, preceded by aspiration, and followed by suction, is a useful alternative to surgery. If surgery is being undertaken for diagnostic purposes, then a pleurectomy should be performed at the same time to reduce the incidence of troublesome, recurrent pleural effusions. Pain relief is difficult, and opiates should be used early and in adequate doses to control this symptom.

Acknowledgments. I would like to thank Professor B. Corrin for providing Figure 1; Dr. B. Strickland for the radiographs; the Editor of *Thorax* for permission to reproduce Fig. 4, 7, and 8; and Miss Sally Hockley for typing this manuscript.

References

1. Wagner JC, Slegg CA, Marchand P (1960) Diffuse pleural mesothelioma and asbestos exposure in the North West Cape Province. Br J Ind Med 17: 260-271
2. Whitewell F, Scott J, Grimshaw M (1977) Relationship between occupations and asbestos-fibre content of the lungs in patients with pleural mesothelioma, lung cancer, and other diseases. Thorax 32: 377-386
3. Jeffreys DB, Vale JA (1978) Malignant mesothelioma and gas mask assemblers. Br Med J 2: 607
4. Baris I, Elmes PC, Pooley FD, Sahim A (1978) Mesotheliomas in Turkey. Thorax 33: 538
5. Editorial (1983) Mesotheliomas, minerals and man-made fibres. Thorax 35: 561-563
6. Law MR, Ward FG, Hodson ME, Heard BE (1983) Evidence for longer survival of patients with pleural mesothelioma without asbestos exposure. Thorax 38: 744-746
7. Law MR, Smith MJ, Millband C, Haslam PL, Hodson ME (1985) Immune function and survival in pleural mesothelioma. Clin Exp Immunol 61: 214-215
8. Harrison RN (1984) Sarcomatous pleural mesothelioma and cerebral metastases; case report and a review of eight cases. Eur J Respir Dis 65: 185-188
9. Manfredi F, Rosenbaum D, Childress RH (1986) Diffuse malignant mesothelioma of the pleura. Am Rev Respir Dis 92: 269-279
10. Law MR, Hodson ME, Turner-Warwick M (1984) Malignant mesothelioma of the pleura: clinical aspects and symptomatic treatment. Eur J Respir Dis 65: 162-168
11. Dunnill MS (1982) In: Pulmonary pathology. Churchill Livingstone, London Chap 21, p 422
12. Law MR, Hodson ME, Heard BE (1982) Malignant mesothelioma of the pleura: relation between histological type and clinical behaviour. Thorax 37: 810-815
13. Brenner J, Sordillo PP, Magill GB, Golbey RR (1982) Malignant mesothelioma of the pleura. Cancer 49: 2431-2435
14. Elmes PC, Simpson MJC (1976) The clinical aspects of mesothelioma. Q J Med 45: 427-449
15. Law MR, Gregor A, Husband JE, Kerr IH (1982) Computed tomography in the assessment of malignant mesothelioma of the pleura. Clin Radiol 33: 67-70
16. Herbert A, Gallagher PJ (1982) Pleural biopsy in the diagnosis of malignant mesothelioma. Thorax 37: 816-821
17. Emerson P (1981) In: Thoracic medicine. Emerson P (ed) Buttersworth, Chap 48, p 602
18. Wagner JC, Munday DE, Harington JS (1962) Histochemical demonstration of hyaluronic acid in pleural mesotheliomas. J Path Bact 84: 73-78
19. de Larie GA, Hensik R, Faber LP, Kittle CF (1978) Surgical management of malignant mesothelioma. Ann Thorac Surg 26: 375-382
20. Law MR, Gregor A, Hodson ME, Bloom HJG, Turner-Warwick M (1984) Malignant mesothelioma of the pleura: a study of 52 treated and 64 untreated patients. Thorax 39: 255-259
21. Aisner J, Wiernik PH (1981) Chemotherapy in the treatment of malignant mesothelioma. Semin Oncol 8: 335-341
22. Lerner HJ, Schoenfeld DA, Martin A, Falkson G, Bordon E (1983) Malignant mesothelioma. Cancer 52: 1981-1985
23. Antman KH (1981) Benign and malignant mesothelioma. Semin Oncol 8: 313-320

19. Radiotherapy of Mediastinal and Chest Wall Tumors

J. S. Tobias

Tumors of the Mediastinum

To the radiotherapist, a simple anatomical classification of mediastinal tumors is of great value since different tumors occur predominantly at different sites, and the role of radiotherapy varies considerably with both tumor type and location.

In the *anterosuperior mediastinum,* the commonest malignant tumors are thymoma and germ cell tumors, including both teratomas and seminomas. Carcinoma of the thyroid may occasionally arise from the retrosternal portion of the gland. Radiotherapy is employed for tumors of the anterosuperior mediastinum in three situations:

1. As definitive therapy of highly radiosensitive conditions, for example in mediastinal seminoma.
2. As an adjunct to surgery, for example in thymoma, in which surgical resection is undertaken where possible, but postoperative radiotherapy is employed in order to reduce the chance of local recurrence. It is important to remember that in this condition the histological appearance is a rather poor guide to clinical behavior, and postoperative irradiation is valuable wherever there is doubt about the adequacy of surgical resection.
3. In combination with chemotherapy. This situation arises in the management of germ cell tumors in which chemotherapy may have been used to shrink the tumor mass, but in which there is residual disease still present. This is a highly individualized and uncommon clinical problem in which special expertise is required. In general, tumors which are chiefly, or completely, seminomatous are more radioresponsive than teratomatous tumors. However, even in the latter, radiotherapy may have a role particularly where surgical resection of residual tumor is felt to be inadvisable.

It is usually appropriate to employ an anteroposterior parallel pair of treatment fields, though for deep-seated tumors of small volume, a multifield arrangement, using three or four fields, may give a better distribution (Fig. 1), with less unwanted irradiation of normal lung. For thymoma, a postoperative dose of 3500-4500 rad (35-45 Gy) in 3-5 weeks, is commonly employed. Higher doses are sometimes used, particularly where the thymoma is unresectable or poorly encapsulated. For medistinal seminoma, a total dose of 4000 rad (40 Gy) in 20 daily fractions over 4 weeks is generally considered adequate even for fairly bulky tumors. If treatment with both radiotherapy and chemotherapy is to be used together as definitive therapy, it is wise to avoid irradiation until the

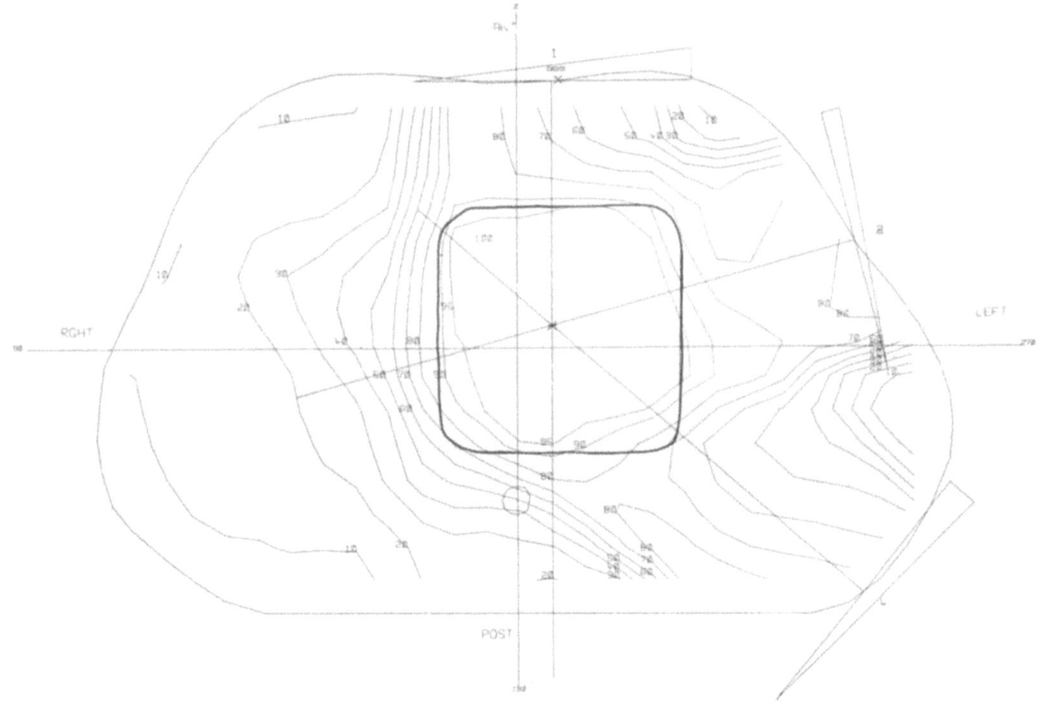

Fig. 1. Multifield irradiation of a mediastinal tumor. For deeply situated tumors, a three- or four-field arrangement usually gives better distribution without overirradiation of normal structures, particularly lung and spinal cord

chemotherapy has been completed. There is evidence that this sequence produces a lower rate of toxicity. This problem arises not only in treatment of germ cell tumors of the mediastinum, but also in mediastinal lymphoma (see below).

In the *middle mediastinum,* lymphomas are the most frequent malignant tumors, and both Hodgkin's disease and non-Hodgkin's lymphomas occur commonly. Indeed, about one-fourth of patients with Hodgkin's disease have evidence of mediastinal involvement. Tissue diagnosis is essential, though a superficial lymph node biopsy is usually diagnostic and mediastinoscopic biopsy is not generally necessary.

Radiotherapy plays an important part in the management of these conditions. In patients with Hodgkin's disease, localized to the upper half of the body ("supradiaphragmatic disease") and without constitutional symptoms of weight loss, fever, or sweating, radiotherapy is the most important method of treatment, curative in the majority of cases. There are two main approaches to the treatment by radiotherapy:

"Involved Field" Radiotherapy. In this technique, the affected lymph node group is treated without any attempt to irradiate more widely. The technique is suitable for very localized disease, particularly where histology is favorable (lymphocyte predominant or nodular sclerosis subtypes). Although suitable for asymptomatic

248

highly localized disease, it is not usually appropriate for treatment of mediastinal Hodgkin's disease, since it is unusual for mediastinal nodes to be affected in the absence of disease in the neck or axilla. For this reason, although involved field irradiation is often appropriate for localized Hodgkin's disease at superficial sites, it is not generally employed for mediastinal disease.

"Mantle" Radiotherapy. For patients with mediastinal Hodgkin's disease and evidence of involvement in the neck and/or axilla (it is usually superficial lymphadenopathy which is the presenting complaint, rather than the mediastinal involvement), radiotherapy using the classical "mantle" technique is still regarded as the most appropriate form of treatment. In this technique (Fig. 2), the mediastinum is irradiated in continuity with other lymph node groups. An important feature of this treatment is the careful lung shielding which is achieved by the use of tailor-made lung blocks. Treatment is administered via large anteroposterior fields, and most centers insist on daily dosage in order to reduce long-term toxicity. A total dose of 3500 rad (35 Gy) in 3½ weeks is used to the clinically uninvolved areas, with boosting to 4000 rad (40 Gy) total dose to clinically involved areas, treated over a period of 4–4½ weeks. Doses higher than this give significant risk of pericarditis. Other long-term complications include hypothyroidism (usually asymptomatic but detectable biochemically) and spinal cord damage (easily avoidable if the cord is shielded by introducing a narrow strip of lead into the posterior treatment beam after the cord has received a total dose of 2000 rad (20 Gy). In general, the bulkiness of the mediastinal disease should influence management. Where the total mediastinal contour is less than one-third of the transverse diameter of the chest at that level, treatment with radiotherapy alone is appropriate, assuming that the patient does not have constitutional symptoms. If the mediastinal disease is more bulky, then chemotherapy should be employed to reduce the amount of disease. Once chemotherapy has been completed, then mantle irradiation is generally given, though there are certainly documented cases in which the chemotherapy alone has proved to be curative. It is therefore uncertain whether, in cases treated by chemotherapy, radiation should be given as a routine: in this department, he policy is to use both methods of treatment, with the chemotherapy preceding the treatment by irradiation. Even very large tumors can sometimes be cured by this approach (Fig. 3).

For non-Hodgkin's lymphoma of the mediastinum, the treatment approach is different. Unlike Hodgkin's disease, there is little to be gained by a wide field ("mantle") approach, since the disease characteristically spreads by noncontiguous routes. Treatment is therefore more individualized, and chemotherapy plays a larger role since a larger proportion of cases are disseminated at diagnosis. Nonetheless, local irradiation can be valuable, particularly where there are compression syndromes, such as dysphagia, resulting from paratracheal lymphadenopathy. A dose of 3500 rad (35 Gy) in 3½ weeks is generally adequate and normally achieved using an interoposterior parallel opposed pair of treatment fields.

Tumors of the *posterior mediastinum* are chiefly neurogenic in origin, usually arising from the thoracic sympathetic chain or intercostal nerves. The commonest of these tumors – neurofibromas, ganglioneuromas, and Schwannomas – should

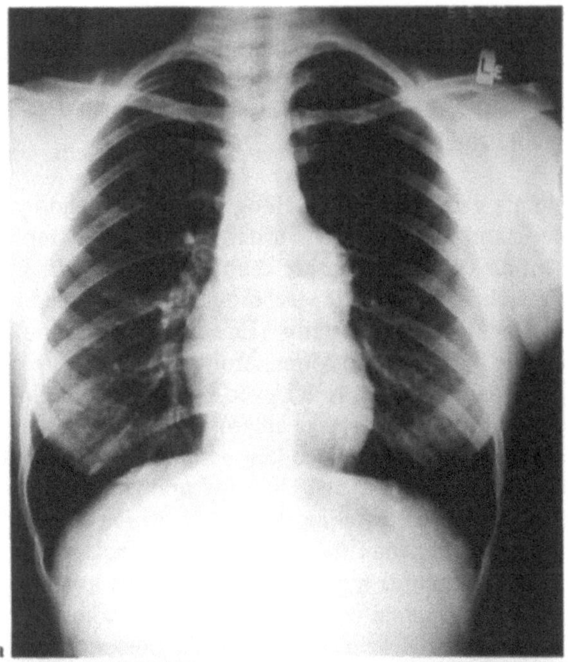

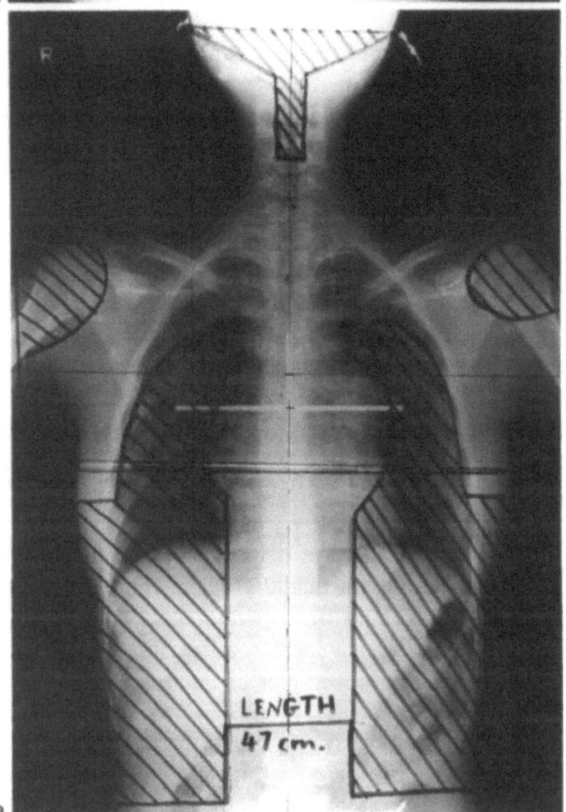

Fig. 2. a Typical X-ray findings in supradiaphragmatic Hodgkin's disease with mediastinal involvement. In this case, the mediastinal bulk was small and radiotherapy was the sole treatment. **b** Treatment technique using "mantle" irradiation. Tailor-made lung shielding, together with shielding of the floor of the mouth, larynx, and humeral heads, ensures that sensitive structures are shielded while treating supradiaphragmatic lymph node groups in contiguity. Four years later the patient, a young nurse, is alive and well

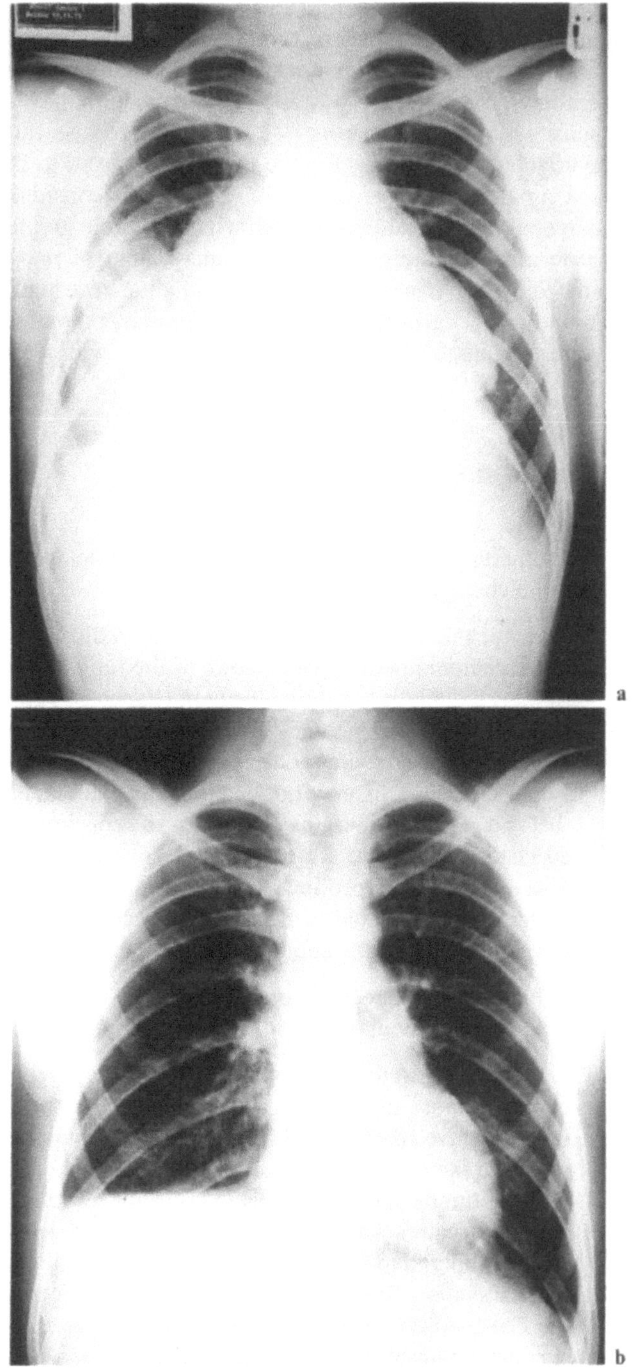

Fig. 3a, b. Huge mediastinal involvement from Hodgkin's disease. Treatment was by combination chemotherapy followed by "mantle" irradiation. **a** Before treatment. **b** After treatment. This patient is alive and well 10 years after treatment

be surgically removed, and radiotherapy plays little if any part in their management. However, malignant tumors, including neurofibrosarcoma, neuroblastoma, and (rarely) malignant pheochromocytoma or chordoma, may be difficult to resect entirely. In these cases, postoperative irradiation may be valuable though the radiosensitivity of these tumors is low, so a high dose must be contemplated. This is particularly difficult where the tumor is adjacent to the spinal cord. Neuroblastoma, a partly chemosensitive tumor, should be considered separately from the adult sarcomatous neural tumors and, where possible, treated in centers of special pediatric interest. Radiotherapeutic management of chordoma is unsatisfactory, but may be worth considering where residual or recurrent tumor in the upper mediastinum or neck has resulted in severe pain or pressure symptoms (Fig. 4). Unfortunately, palliation is difficult to achieve, even with a high dose.

Tumors of the Chest Wall and Pleura

Radiotherapy has an important role in the management of tumors of the pleura and the chest wall, for three main reasons:

1. Many of these tumors are at least partly radiosensitive; for example, squamous cell carcinoma arising at the apex of the lung and involving the chest wall with rib and brachial plexus involvement (Pancoast's tumor).
2. Surgical resection may be difficult or impossible, particularly with extensive tumors. Even where surgery has been performed, there may still be evidence of residual disease. This may not be clinically evident, and it is important to confirm that the resection margins of the excised specimen have been carefully inspected histologically and are free of disease.
3. These tumors may produce severe symptoms, particularly pain (a characteristic feature of the Pancoast syndrome). In such cases, radiotherapy may be especially valuable for symptomatic relief.

There are no specific contraindications to radiotherapy for chest wall and pleural tumors, though the following guidelines should always be considered.

1. Is the tumor surgically resectable? If so, then surgery should be the treatment of choice in most clinical situations. If, however, the tumor is known to be highly radiosensitive (for example non-Hodgkin's lymphoma or seminoma), surgical resection is usually unnecessary.
2. Has the tumor been completely surgically resected? In most cases, where complete surgical excision has confidently been achieved, there is no role for routine postoperative radiotherapy. Opinions are divided as to whether postoperative irradiation should routinely be given following surgery for a melanoma of the chest wall: in general, unless there has been wide excision of the primary site, postoperative treatment of the surrounding area might be helpful, since tumor satellite deposits may be present, but clinically undetectable. Where possible, surgical excision of these tumors should clear a wide area, and in most cases grafting will have been necessary. For soft tissue sarcomas arising on the

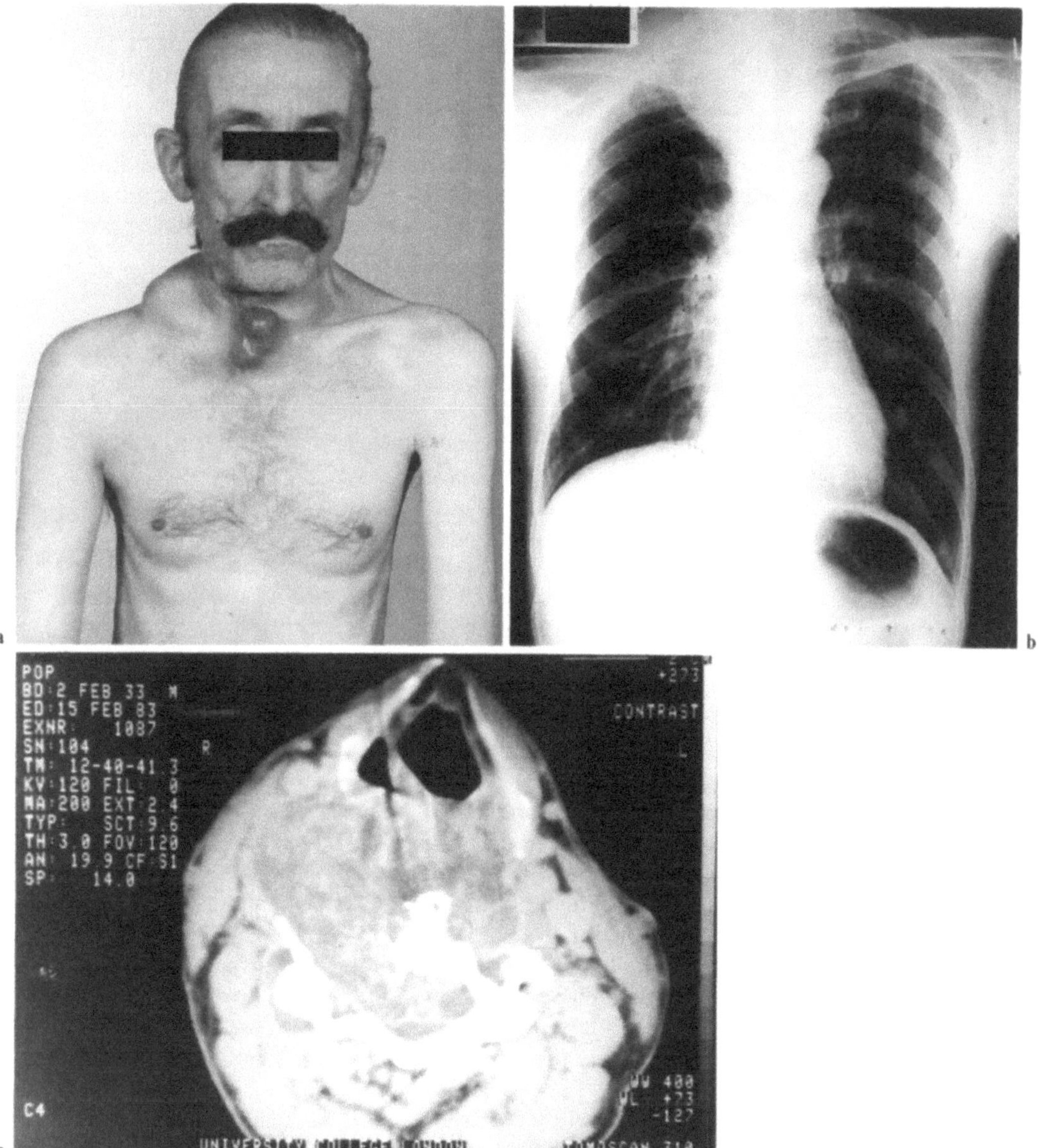

Fig. 4 a–c. Chordoma. **a** The primary tumor, initially present in the region of the lower cervical spine, erupted through the supraclavicular fossa and upper part of the anterior mediastinum. **b** Chest X-ray showing involvement of the posterior mediastinum. **c** CT scan at the level of the lower cervical spine, showing the tumor erupting forwards and across the midline as well as into the spinal canal

chest wall, wide local excision should ideally be followed by local irradiation of the tumor bed. Although there are no firm data to support this approach, the analogy is with compartmental resection of soft tissue sarcoma of the extremity, a technique which has largely replaced amputation, but must be followed by postoperative irradiation in all cases, in order to give equivalent results. Postoperative radiotherapy is also indicated in postoperative treatment of sarcomas of bone, such as osteosarcoma or Ewing's tumor of a rib. Ewing's tumor is in fact highly radiosensitive, and if this diagnosis has been established by biopsy, it is probably unnecessary to undertake further surgery at all.

3. Most patients are fit for radiotherapy, even where there is evidence of distant disease. However, in patients with widespread metastases the role of radiotherapy is limited to palliation. If there is severe pain from the primary tumor, the radiotherapist should not hesitate to treat such a patient, even where widespread metastases are present. Where pleural effusion is the only evidence of disease, palliative treatment should again be considered if necessary, though most would agree that such patients are surgically and radiotherapeutically incurable.

4. Is the tumor likely to be radiosensitive? This question is an important one. Some tumors (for example Ewing's tumor, seminoma, lymphoma), are highly responsive to radiotherapy and, therefore, a low or modest dose may be sufficient to ensure local control. On the other hand, tumors such as melanoma and soft tissue sarcoma are much more resistant, and higher doses are necessary, with risk of damage to local normal tissues. Mesothelioma is a good example in the latter category, and radiotherapy has very little role in this disease. Most of the common tumors are in an intermediate category: partly radiosensitive and well worth treating, though requiring considerable skill to avoid unnecessary damage. Small cell carcinoma of the bronchus is the most radiosensitive type of lung cancer, and squamous cell carcinoma is generally agreed to be rather more radiosensitive than adenocarcinoma or large cell carcinoma. These points will also influence the judgment of the radiotherapist regarding treatment of any individual tumor. In addition, tumor bulk is an important consideration; the smaller the tumor, the more likely is control by radiotherapy.

5. Are there alternatives to radiotherapy? Patients with small cell lung cancer, seminoma, lymphoma, and neuroblastoma should be considered for treatment by chemotherapy, particularly where the tumor is bulky and radiotherapy alone is unlikely to cure. However, in many (probably most) of these situations, local treatment with radiotherapy should be offered as well, in order to ensure local control wherever possible.

6. What are the disadvantages of radiotherapy? Radiotherapy-induced side effects vary sharply with the dose administered. At low dose, it is unusual to encounter side effects at all, particularly if the treatment is fractionated carefully over several days or weeks. At higher doses (or if the treatment is given more briskly over a shorter period), skin reactions of varying intensity will occur, ranging from mild erythema to dry and then moist desquamation, sometimes with permanent pigmentation. Later skin changes include subcutaneous fibrosis, loss of elasticity, and telangiectasia. All of these changes are particularly common where a superficial chest wall tumor has been treated, with deliberate intent to

raise the skin surface itself to a high dose. Rib fracture will also occur in a proportion of patients treated for chest wall or pleural disease, particularly where orthovoltage equipment has been used, in which bone absorption of radiation energy is preferentially high. For this reason, supervoltage equipment should always be preferred, where available, for treatment of chest wall tumors. If large portions of the heart are unavoidably included in the field of treatment, a dose-dependent pericarditis (with or without effusion) may occur, especially where the dose received by the heart exceeds 4500 rad (45 Gy), given over 4–5 weeks, and particularly if a large volume of the pericardium is included. Brachial plexus damage is also important as a radiation side effect following treatment of apical chest wall or pleural tumors, particularly where retreatment with radiotherapy has occurred. Treatment of apical or axillary tumors may also lead to local lymphatic obstruction and lymphedema, particularly where axillary lymph node dissection has taken place (for example as part of the surgical treatment of a melanoma of the chest wall). In children, local growth failure should be anticipated. There may be loss of height, often with scoliosis, if a portion of the spine has been included in the radiation beam. For more laterally placed tumors, reduction in rib growth may result in local and permanent loss of pulmonary volume and distortion of the chest wall. In girls, such treatment may also lead in later life to failure of breast development on the affected side.

Radiation Techniques

As tumors of the pleura and chest wall are in superficial sites, it is unnecessary to employ sophisticated multifield treatment approaches. As with radiotherapy treatment at any site, technique will be governed by the size, site, and depth of the tumor. Total dose, dose rate, and fractionation technique also vary, depending on the histological type of tumor, as well as its size and location. Unnecessary treatment of underlying lung must be avoided since the lung is sensitive to irradiation, and lung damage can be permanent, causing persistent and disabling symptoms. Although this is a greater problem with radical irradiation for carcinoma of the lung, it is important to remember that the exit beam will usually pass through lung when irradiation of the chest wall or pleura is undertaken. Fortunately, this is usually unilateral.

Although the simplest method of treatment is to use a single radiation field, placed perpendicularly against the chest wall (Fig. 5), unwanted irradiation of underlying lung may be considerable. This varies with the treatment energy used and will obviously be greater with supervoltage irradiation (telecobalt or linear accelerator) than with orthovoltage treatment (for example 250 kV). This and other radiation-induced damage will be greater with a large volume and with nondaily fractionation. In general, it is unwise to employ this technique to treatment fields greater than 10×10 cm, though there are always exceptions – for example, the treatment of multiple rib metastases, a common clinical situation in which speed and simplicity of treatment are important.

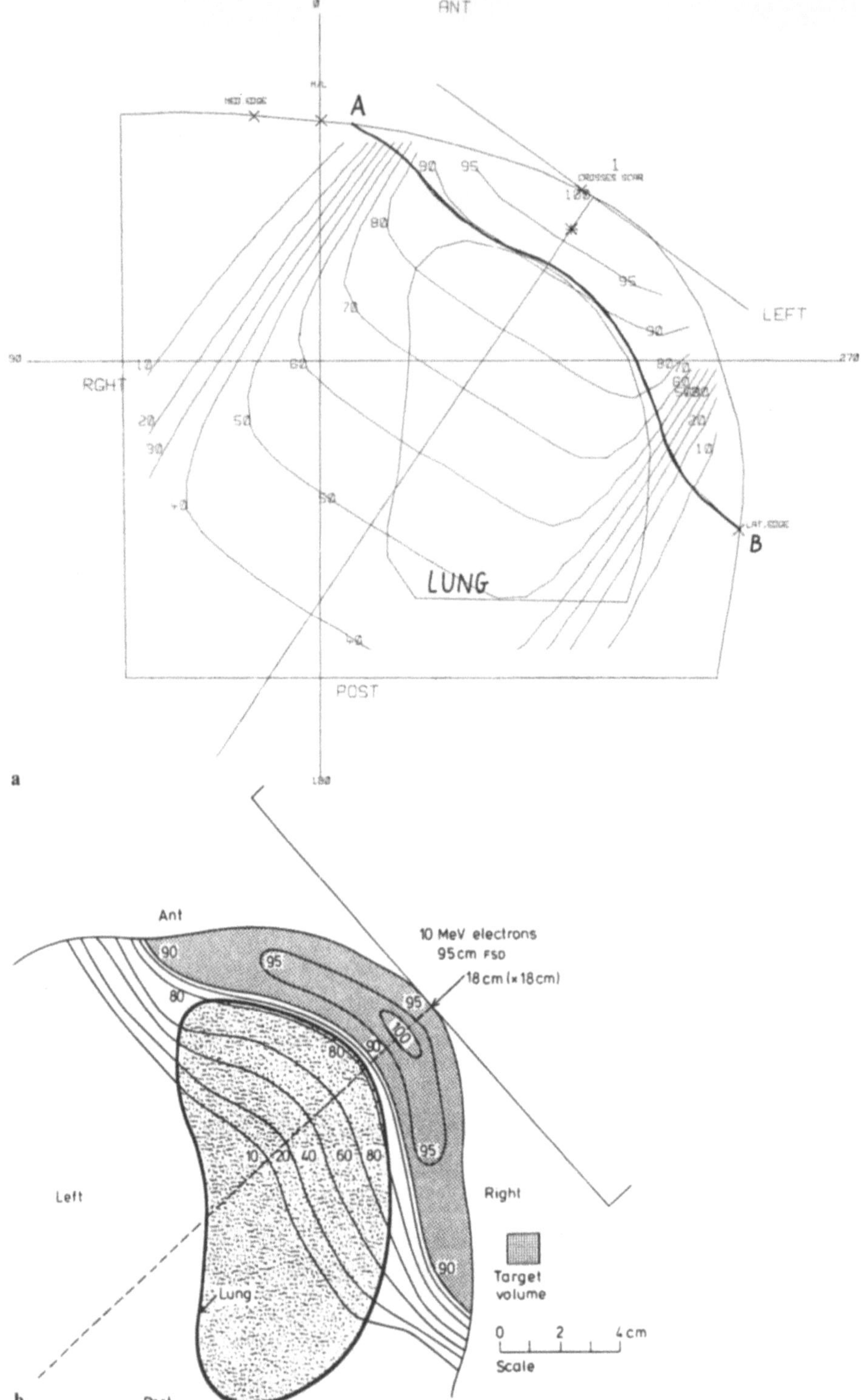

Fig. 5a, b. Treatment of superficial chest wall tumor using a single direct field. **a** Treatment with X-ray (photon) irradiation, using cobalt-60. Note the substantial but unwanted irradiation of the underlying lung by the exit beam, in addition to inadequate coverage of the marked volume *A B*. **b** Direct electron beam irradiation. Note that the underlying lung is relatively spared because of the different radiation characteristics of the electron beam

Even with very superficial chest wall tumors, orthovoltage irradiation should be avoided if a radical dose (above 5000 Rad (50 Gy) in 5½–6 weeks) is contemplated because of the probability of radionecrosis. However, for palliative treatment (e.g., treatment of rib metastases), orthovoltage irradiation is often appropriate as the dose is very much lower and the expected survival time shorter.

A more satisfactory treatment can usually be achieved by the use of a two-field arrangement, often a "wedged pair" using supervoltage treatment such as telecobalt or a 4–10 MeV linear accelerator (Fig. 6). A radical dose can generally be achieved, though once again it is important to obtain a field arrangement which offers minimal unwanted irradiation to underlying lung. If the tumor (or even part of it) is superficially placed, the obliquity of the radiation beams gives a useful increase in skin dose, though in many cases tissue bolus will also be necessary in order to bring up this dose to the desired 100%. Nonetheless, this is usually still preferable to direct field treatment, especially where the treatment area is greater than 10×10 cm, since the risk of bone necrosis is much lower than with orthovoltage.

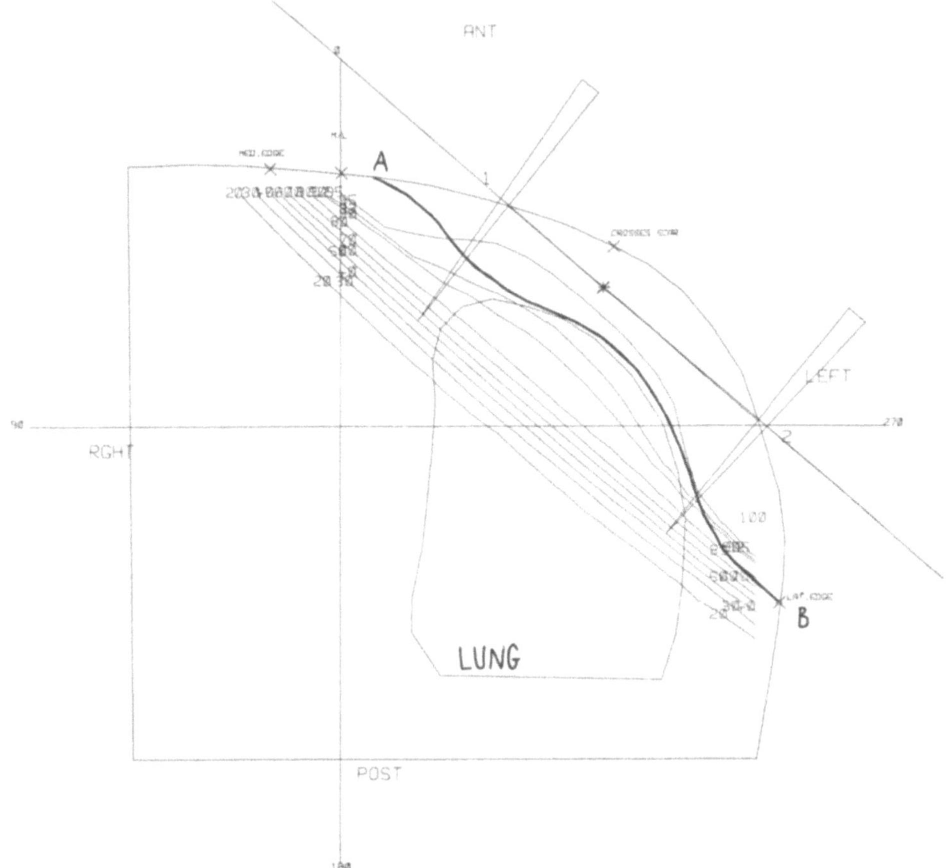

Fig. 6. Irradiation of chest wall tumor using a wedged tangential pair of X-ray beams. This give a better distribution than in Fig. 5, with less irradiation to the lung

257

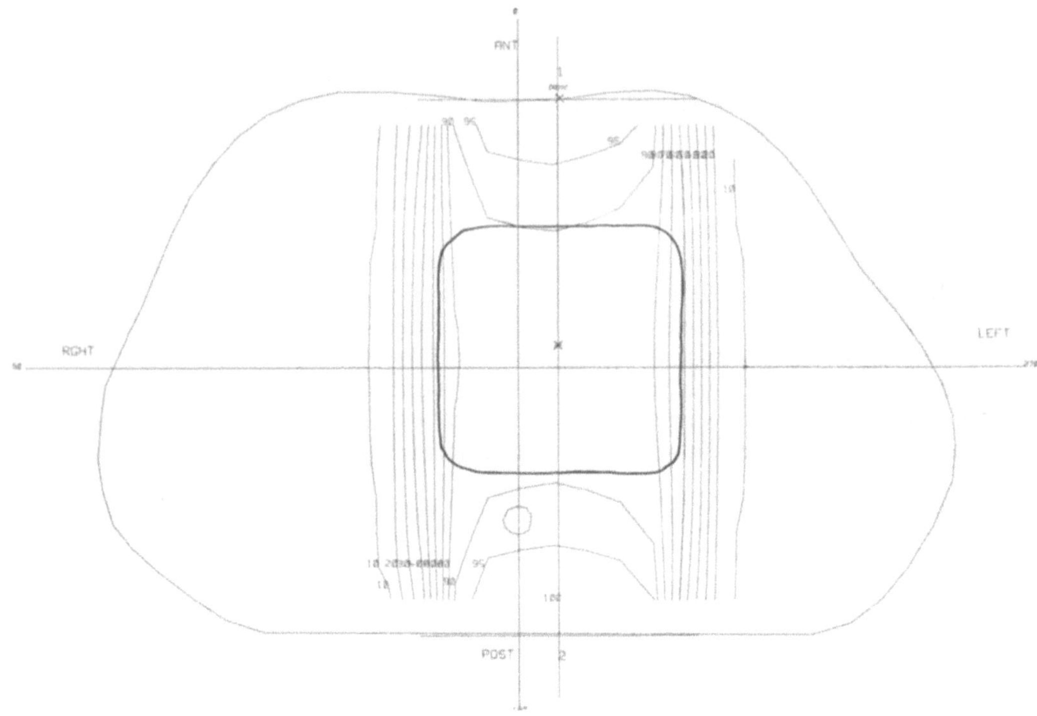

Fig. 7. Irradiation of a medistinal or chest wall tumor using a "parallel-pair" of radiation beams. In this case, the primary tumor was in the mediastinum and the radiation beams were applied anteroposteriorly

Furthermore, tumors which are both superficial but deeply extensive (up to 6–8 cm in depth) can generally be encompassed by this approach.

In other circumstances, particularly with apical tumors, a "parallel pair" of fields (usually placed anteriorly and posteriorly) may give the best distribution (Fig. 7). Although the beams will pass directly through the lungs, this is less of a problem at the apex than elsewhere, since less lung will be included in the treatment volume. Treatment by an anteroposterior parallel pair of fields also has the advantage that lead shielding can easily be introduced so that lung or spinal cord sparing can often be achieved.

Radiation Dosage

For radical treatment, a dose of 6000 rad (60 Gy), given in daily fractions over 6 weeks, is often recommended, particularly for relatively insensitive tumors such as a soft tissue sarcoma or melanoma of the chest wall. This may be difficult to achieve where the volume is large. In many departments, where throughput is

258

high, nondaily treatment schedules may be preferred in order to treat the maximum number of patients. In this situation, a total of 4000 rad (40 Gy) given in 10 fractions over 4 weeks, on a 5×2 weeks basis (Mon, Weds, Fri, Tues, Thurs, then repeat), is a suitable alternative. Many departments feel it unnecessary to subject their patients to treatment for 6 weeks, and prefer a treatment schedule of 4500 rad (45 Gy) in 15 fractions over 3 weeks. Although both acute and long-term reactions are possibly slightly greater with this approach, this technique is widely employed and gives good results. Particular care should be taken with dose and fractionation in patients where a portion of spinal cord is included in the treatment volume. In general, a dose of 4000 rad (40 Gy) in 20 fractions over 4 weeks to 10 cm cord is regarded as a safe dose, and radiation myelopathy increases in incidence above this dose. The risk of this side effect seems particularly high when nondaily fractionation is employed. Similar guidelines should also be borne in mind when a substantial portion of the brachial plexus is to be included in the treatment volume.

A special problem arises in the treatment of mesothelioma. This is a highly radioresistant tumor, often diffuse in nature and frequently associated with malignant pleural effusion. There is little evidence to suggest that radiotherapy plays an important part in its management, even for palliation of severe pain caused by this tumor. However, where there is local disease and other treatment is felt to be inappropriate, radiotherapy can occasionally produce a short-term benefit. Attempts to irradiate the whole of the pleural surface, using sophisticated rotational or other planning techniques, have so far been unsuccessful.

Further Reading

Dobbs HJ, Barrett A (1985) Practical radiotherapy planning: Royal Marsden Hospital Practice. Arnold, London
Kaplan HS (1972) Hodgkin's disease, 1st edn. Cambridge, Mass: Harvard University Press
Meredith WJ, Massey JB (1977) Fundamental physics of radiology, 3rd edn. Wright, Bristol
Moss WT, Brand WN, Battifora H (1979) Radiation oncology: rationale, technique, results, 5th edn. Mosby, St. Louis
Souhami RL, Tobias JS (1986) Cancer and its management. Blackwell Scientific, London

20. Chemotherapy of Mediastinal Tumors

R. L. Souhami

Many tumors of the mediastinum are benign; others are of low-grade malignancy. Complete surgical excision is frequently curative. There are some tumors which are either locally invasive or have a tendency to metastasize, and which are sensitive to treatment with cytoxic drugs. Indeed, with some tumors, chemotherapy is a principal component of treatment, surgery being necessary only for diagnosis. Malignant mediastinal tumors which respond to cytoxic drugs are listed below:

1. Tumors that are highly sensitive to chemotherapy
   a) Hodgkin's disease
   b) Non-Hodgkin's lymphoma
   c) Germ cell tumors
2. Tumors that are partially sensitive to chemotherapy
   a) Thymoma
   b) Some sarcomas

The decision on whether to treat a patient with a malignant mediastinal tumor with chemotherapy, therefore, depends on (a) accurate histological diagnosis and (b) staging of the neoplasm, in particular the demonstration of metastatic disease.

Hodgkin's Disease

A mediastinal mass may be the only clinically apparent site of Hodgkin's disease. The mass may be due to involvement of lymph nodes or to thymic Hodgkin's disease. Presentation with mediastinal Hodgkin's disease is particularly common in young women with the nodular sclerosing form of the disease. Even if there are no clinically apparent lymph nodes at other sites, it is essential to determine the degree of spread of the tumor before making a treatment decision. Such staging investigations will typically include bipedal lymphography, or CT scanning of the abdomen, and possibly bone marrow and liver biopsy, depending on the clinical circumstances. Staging laparotomy and splenectomy are sometimes employed if the treatment decision depends greatly on knowledge of whether there is splenic disease.

Hodgkin's disease confined to the mediastinum can be successfully treated with radiotherapy alone, but very large masses are usually treated by a combination of chemotherapy and radiation. There is an increasing tendency to use chemotherapy in the first instance, with radiotherapy in the middle or at the end of the chemotherapy program. Initial chemotherapy controls possible systemic

Table 1. Chemotherapy for Hodgkin's disease

---

1. MOPP
    Mustine 6 mg/m^2 day 1 and 8
    Vincristine 1.4 mg/m^2 day 1 and 8
    Procarbazine 100 mg/m^2 day 1–14
    Prednisolone 40 mg/m^2 day 1–14

The cycle is repeated every 4 weeks for 6 cycles or is alternated with the ABVD regimen shown below.

2. ABVD
    Doxorubicin (Adriamycin) 25 mg/m^2 day 1 and 15
    Bleomycin 10 mg/m^2 day 1 and 15
    Vinblastine 6 mg/m^2 day 1 and 15
    Dacarbazine 375 mg/m^2 day 1 and 15

---

disease and causes the mediastinal mass to shrink, allowing smaller radiation fields to be employed.

Typical chemotherapy protocols employ drug combinations such as mustine, vincristine, procarbazine, and prednisone (MOPP), or with chlorambucil substituted for mustine. Often these are alternated with "non-cross-resistant" drugs such as doxorubicin, bleomycin, vinblastine, and dacarbazine (ABVD) (see Table 1).

Non-Hodgkin's Lymphomas

When mediastinal masses occur in non-Hodgkin's lymphoma, there is usually disease elsewhere, necessitating drug treatment. Chemotherapy of these disorders varies with the histological type.

There is a form of non-Hodgkin's lymphoma which arises in the thymus, and which presents with a mediastinal swelling, sometimes without clinically apparent involvement of the peripheral nodes. This is a T-cell lymphoma, which characteristically occurs in young males (Sternberg sarcoma). The disease usually disseminates rapidly to bone marrow and central nervous system, and is then indistinguishable from T-cell acute lymphoblastic leukemia. The principles of treatment are the same as for that disorder. Some T-cell lymphomas of the mediastinum are clearly less aggressive, but at present, pending better definition of subtypes of T-cell disease, the mainstay of treatment is intensive combination chemotherapy.

B-cell lymphomas may rarely be confined to the mediastinum at presentation, but spread to the bone marrow and liver is commonly found on investigation. These are almost always high-grade immunoblastic lymphomas and are treated with intensive combination chemotherapy.

262

Germ Cell Tumors

Each of the different types of germ cell tumors which arise in the testis or ovary may arise in the mediastinum. They constitute an extremely important group of mediastinal tumors because they may be mistaken for other histological types and because there is a high likelihood of cure with correct treatment. Germ cell tumors which may present with a mediastinal mass include:

1. Seminoma (germinoma)
2. Non-seminomatous germ cell tumors
   a) Teratoma (differentiated, intermediate, undifferentiated)
   b) Embryonal carcinoma
   c) Choriocarcinoma

The tumors probably arise from residual germ cells in the thymus and most of the tumors appear to be of thymic origin. In most cases, there is no evidence of an associated testicular or ovarian tumor. The tumors usually arise in the anterior mediastinum and spread to the mediastinal lymph nodes.

Seminoma

This tumor occurs in men between the ages 20–40, and the female equivalent (germinoma) is very rare. The majority of patients have an invasive tumor which cannot be surgically removed. The tumor is extremely sensitive to irradiation, which produces long-term control of the disease in 50%–80% of patients. It is not clear whether chemotherapy will improve these results, but it seems likely that it will. Chemotherapy is clearly indicated if there is evidence of spread of the disease outside the thorax into supraclavicular or other nodes or metastatic to the lung or brain.

Most chemotherapy regimens include *cis*platin as the most active drug. This is usually used in combination with bleomycin, vinblastine, and etoposide, as in other germ cell tumors (Table 2).

Non-Seminomatous Germ Cell Tumors

These tumors are more common in men (M:F = 3:1). The histological appearances are similar to those found in the testis. The presentation is the same as for any mediastinal tumor with cough, central chest discomfort, and dyspnea. The serum HCG and AFP may be elevated, and these markers are used as a guide to treatment as in testicular tumors.

Table 2. Chemotherapy of malignant teratoma

PVB
*Cis*platin 20 mg/m² for 5 days every 3 weeks × 4
Bleomycin 30 mg i.v. weekly × 12
Vinblastine 0.3 mg/kg every 3 weeks × 4

Chemotherapy is the mainstay of treatment using combination chemotherapy regimens based on *cis*platin, bleomycin, etoposide, vinblastine, and actinomycin. Using these regimens, the prognosis has been markedly improved, compared with the results obtained in the early 1970s. Over 65% of patients will now be free of disease at 5 years and probably cured.

Thymomas

Thymomas are usually slowgrowing tumors and spread outside the mediastinum is uncommon, and occurs late. Chemotherapy is usually considered when there has been a local recurrence which has not responded to radiation. There have been few systematic studies of chemotherapy in this tumor, but responses have been reported to alkylating agents such as cyclophosphamide, and more recently, to ifosfamide. *Cis*platin and doxorubicin may also produce responses. Combinations of these drugs may improve the response rate, but it is not clear if survival is improved.

Sarcomas

Sarcomas may arise in mesenchymal and neurogenic tumors in the mediastinum, but are rare. The mainstay of treatment is surgical excision, followed by radiotherapy. Chemotherapy may be indicated for local recurrence, or if there is evidence of distant spread at the time when the patient first presents. The drugs commonly used are the same as for sarcomas at other sites. Doxorubicin, vincristine, cyclophosphamide, and actinomycin are the most useful agents.

Chemotherapy of Primary Malignant Chest Wall Tumors

Sarcomas may develop in the muscle and connective tissue of the chest wall as at other sites. A classification is shown below:

1. Bones
    a) Osteosarcoma
    b) Chondrosarcoma
    c) Ewing's tumor
2. Muscle and connective tissue
    a) Fibrosarcoma
    b) Malignant fibrous histiocytoma
    c) Rhabdomyosarcoma
    d) Dermatofibrosarcoma protruberans

Management

The mainstay of management for tumors which have not metastasized is surgical excision, which should be as radical as possible, since the risk of local recurrence is high both for bone and soft tissue sarcomas. With bone sarcomas arising in the ribs, this will necessitate resection of part of the chest wall. Following surgical excision, radiotherapy is usually recommended for soft tissue sarcomas to decrease the likelihood of local recurrence. Radiotherapy is of little value following complete excision of an osteosarcoma or chondrosarcoma, but may be considered when there has been incomplete resection.

Chemotherapy is indicated in the following circumstances: (1) as an adjunct to surgery in operable osteosarcoma and Ewing's tumor (2) as an adjunct to surgery in soft tissue sarcoma, (3) in metastatic soft tissue sarcoma and osteosarcoma, and (4) in inoperable osteosarcoma and soft tissue sarcoma as an adjunct to radiotherapy.

Chemotherapy for Operable Osteosarcoma and Ewing's tumor

If the diagnosis has been established by biopsy before excision, there is much to be gained by preoperative chemotherapy to attempt to shrink the tumor, followed by continued treatment postoperatively. If the tumor has been resected, treatment should be given as an adjuvant. The most useful agents are *cis*platin, doxorubicin, very high dose methotrexate (HDMTX), actinomycin and ifosfamide. Treatment regimens using these agents must be intensive, and there is much to be said for such treatment to be concentrated in specialist centers with the necessary resources.

Chemotherapy for Operable Soft Tissue Sarcoma

In children and young adults, preoperative chemotherapy is often given in an attempt to reduce the tumor mass and to assess the sensitivity of the tumor to cytotoxic agents. As with osteosarcoma, chemotherapy is continued postoperatively. If the tumor is large and has been completely excised, many oncologists would nevertheless use postoperative chemotherapy, especially in a child or young adult, since the risk of metastasis is considerable, and many of these tumors are sensitive to cytotoxic agents. The drugs employed are those used for metastatic disease.

Chemotherapy for Metastatic Osteosarcoma and Soft Tissue Sarcoma

Metastatic osteosarcoma can be treated by chemotherapy, but cures are seldom obtained even with intensive treatments. Nevertheless, intensive treatment should be given and progress assessed by repeated chest X-rays or CT scans. In pretreated patients, second-line chemotherapy is of little value. If a solitary metastasis develops after chemotherapy has been completed, surgical removal should be considered.

Many regimens have been developed for soft tissue sarcomas. The most useful agents are doxorubicin, ifosfamide, actinomycin, vincristine, and cyclophosphamide. These regimens should be given intensively in children, especially if the diagnosis is embryonal rhabdomyosarcoma, which is a relatively chemosensitive tumor. In adults, the question of whether to treat will be a matter of clinical judgment, depending on the age of the patient, the diagnosis, and the fitness of the patient.

Chemotherapy for Inoperable Osteosarcoma and Soft Tissue Sarcoma

Some chest wall tumors are far advanced or arise from unresectable structures. In these circumstances radiotherapy and chemotherapy are frequently used together. The dose of radiation will usually need to be very high. There is much to be said for initial treatment with chemotherapy, both to assess response and to increase the likelihood of control of the tumor by subsequent irradiation if the tumor regresses. The drugs used are the same as those employed in the adjuvant situation. In adults, many of these tumors are highly resistant to both chemotherapy and radiation, and drug treatment should not be continued unless there is clear evidence of response.

Subject Index

272

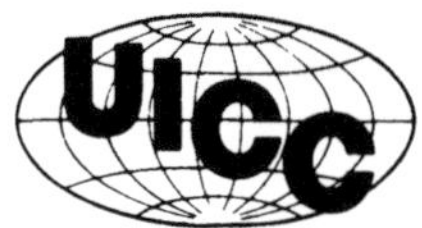

TNM Classification of Malignant Tumours

Editors: UICC, P. Hermanek, L. H. Sobin

4th fully revised edition. 1987. XVIII, 197 pages. ISBN 3-540-17366-8

After four years of international collaborative activity, a revised, unified fourth edition of the TNM Classification is published as the result of a joint venture by the American, British, Canadian, French, German, Italian and Japanese National TNM Committees. Specific changes in the fourth edition include:

- elimination of all differences between the AJCC (American Joint Committee on Cancer) and the UICC TNM classifications of head and neck tumours and lung tumours,
- revision of the T classifications of esophageal and gastric carcinomas based on Japanese studies,
- modification of the classification of colorectal tumours to provide direct congruence with the Duke's classification and allow for a finer degree of subdivision,
- redrafting in collaboration with FIGO of the FIGO classification of gynecological tumours in the format of TNM,
- addition of TNM classification for sites not previously covered in earlier UICC editions.

Prices are subject to change without notice

Springer-Verlag
Berlin Heidelberg New York
London Paris Tokyo

Manual of Adult and Paediatric Medical Oncology

Editors: S. Monfardini, K. Brunner, D. Crowther, S. Eckhardt, D. Olive, S. Tanneberger, A. Veronesi, J. M. A. Whitehouse, R. Wittes

1987. 25 figures. 184 tables, XVIII, 401 pages. ISBN 3-540-15347-0

This volume provides a rapid reference not only for specialists in medical oncology, but also for nonspecialists in oncology, such as the haematologist, radiologist, paediatrician, and general surgeon, who also care for the cancer patient. It is divided into four sections which deal respectively with general aspects (including antitumor drugs, endocrine therapy, and immunotherapy, patient evaluation and response to treatment); therapeutic strategy for adult tumors by site, with emphasis on clinical chemotherapy; the management of paediatric malignancies by site; and tumors of specific importance in Africa and Asia.

Manual of Clinical Oncology

Editor: C. D. Sherman, K. C. Calman, S. Eckhardt, I. Elsebai, D. Firat, D. K. Hossfeld, I.-P. Paunier, B. Salvadori

4th fully revised edition. 1987. 33 figures, XVII, 372 pages. ISBN 3-540-17367-6

The strength of this manual lies in the outstanding cooperation of international committees and institutions to produce the revised fourth edition. Part I covers basic aspects felt to be of clinical importance and has been compiled in close collaboration with the International Agency for Research in Cancer. Part II considers the clinical aspects of all the important tumor sites and has been concisely written with the general physician in mind. Part III outlines research of imminent impact on clinical oncology and has been developed by the Cancer Information and Dissemination Analysis Center of the U.S. National Cancer Institute.

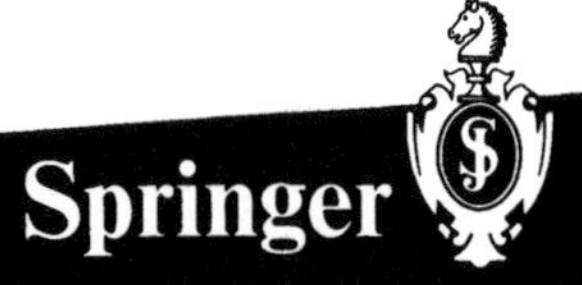

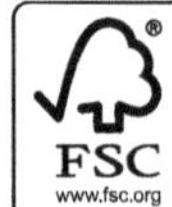